Immune Modulation and Anti-Inflammatory Therapy in Ocular Disorders

AF290248

Uwe Pleyer · Jorge L. Alió
Talin Barisani-Asenbauer
Phuc Le Hoang · Narsing A. Rao
Editors

Immune Modulation and Anti-Inflammatory Therapy in Ocular Disorders

IOIS Guidelines

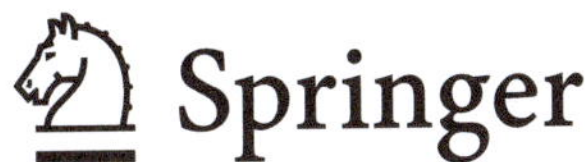

Editors
Uwe Pleyer
Department of Ophthalmology
Charité Campus Virchow-Klinikum
Berlin
Germany

Jorge L. Alió
Division of Ophthalmology
Miguel Hernandez University
Vissum-Instituto Oftalmologico de
Alicante
Spain

Talin Barisani-Asenbauer
Centre of Ocular Inflammation
and Infection OCUVAC
Medical University of Vienna Laura
Bassi Centre of Expertise
Vienna
Austria

Phuc Le Hoang
Department of Ophthalmology
Pitié-Salpêtrière's University Hospital
Paris
France

Narsing A. Rao
Doheny Eye Institute
University of Southern California Keck
School of Medicine
Los Angeles, CA
USA

ISBN 978-3-662-50738-4   ISBN 978-3-642-54350-0   (eBook)
DOI 10.1007/978-3-642-54350-0
Springer Heidelberg New York Dordrecht London

© Springer-Verlag Berlin Heidelberg 2014
Softcover reprint of the hardcover 1st edition 2014
This work is subject to copyright. All rights are reserved by the Publisher, whether the whole or part of the material is concerned, specifically the rights of translation, reprinting, reuse of illustrations, recitation, broadcasting, reproduction on microfilms or in any other physical way, and transmission or information storage and retrieval, electronic adaptation, computer software, or by similar or dissimilar methodology now known or hereafter developed. Exempted from this legal reservation are brief excerpts in connection with reviews or scholarly analysis or material supplied specifically for the purpose of being entered and executed on a computer system, for exclusive use by the purchaser of the work. Duplication of this publication or parts thereof is permitted only under the provisions of the Copyright Law of the Publisher's location, in its current version, and permission for use must always be obtained from Springer. Permissions for use may be obtained through RightsLink at the Copyright Clearance Center. Violations are liable to prosecution under the respective Copyright Law.
The use of general descriptive names, registered names, trademarks, service marks, etc. in this publication does not imply, even in the absence of a specific statement, that such names are exempt from the relevant protective laws and regulations and therefore free for general use.
While the advice and information in this book are believed to be true and accurate at the date of publication, neither the authors nor the editors nor the publisher can accept any legal responsibility for any errors or omissions that may be made. The publisher makes no warranty, express or implied, with respect to the material contained herein.

Printed on acid-free paper

Springer is part of Springer Science+Business Media (www.springer.com)

We dedicate this book to our teachers: patients and colleagues. In particular to the members of IOIS in their efforts to care, fight, and teach on the many aspects of ocular inflammation.

Preface

This IOIS guideline on "immune modulation and anti-inflammatory therapy in ocular disorders" is a continuation of our efforts to provide relevant details on ocular inflammations to the practicing clinician. All segments of the eye can be affected by often destructive and sight-threatening inflammatory diseases. Frequently the management of such disorders provides a challenge to physicians to handle them and for patients to follow instructions in avoiding complications of therapy. The rapid advance of our knowledge base and development of new immunomodulatory agents have culminated in a new era of medical care. Such advances allow us proper management of ocular inflammatory conditions.

This IOIS guideline on treatment of ocular inflammation is intended to provide the practitioner evidence-based practical information on therapeutic interventions based on recent advances in immunomodulatory agents. Therapeutic interventions in the broad area of ocular surface disorders, post-surgical noninfectious inflammations, uveitis related to systemic autoimmune disorders, and organ-specific inflammatory and immune diseases are covered by international experts. In addition, these experts provided relevant discussions on mechanisms underlying these conditions by incorporating results of most recent research literature.

We are grateful to all authors who have contributed to this edition of the IOIS guidelines and invested their valuable time with primary goal of providing succinctly proper and cutting-edge management of ocular inflammations. We believe that this book by providing proper guidelines for the management of the ocular inflammatory disorders will help both clinicians and patients suffering from potentially preventable blindness globally.

Berlin, Germany Uwe Pleyer, MD, FEBO
Los Angeles, CA, USA Narsing Rao

Contents

Contributors

Jorge L. Alió, MD, PhD Division of Ophthalmology,
Miguel Hernandez University, Vissum-Instituto Oftalmologico de
Alicante, Spain

Ilir Arapi, MSc, MD Department of Neuroscience,
Ospedali Riuniti di Ancona, Università Politecnica delle Marche,
Ancona, Italy

Björn Bachmann, MD, FEBO Department of Ophthalmology,
University of Cologne, Cologne, Germany

Neal P. Barney, MD Department of Ophthalmology and Visual Sciences,
University of Wisconsin School of Medicine and Science – Ophthalmology,
Madison, WI, USA

Soumyava Basu, MS Retina-vitreous and Uvea Service,
L V Prasad Eye Institute, Bhubaneswar, Odisha, India

Claus Cursiefen, MD Department of Ophthalmology,
University of Cologne, Cologne, Germany

John Kenneth George Dart, MA, DM, FRCS, FRCOphth
Corneal and External Disease, The National Institute of Health Research
Biomedical Research Centre (NIHR-BRC) at Moorfi elds Eye Hospital NHS
Foundation Trust and the UCL Institute of Ophthalmology, London, UK

Umberto De Benedetto, MD Ophthalmology – Ocular Immunology
and Uveitis Service, San Raffaele Scientific Institute, Milan, Italy

Marc D. de Smet, MDCM, PhD, FRCSC MIOS sa, Lavsanne,
Switzerland

Alfredo Vega Estrada, MD Department of Cornea, Cataract and
Refractive Surgery, VISSUM Corporation, Alicante, Spain

Marta S. Figueroa, MD, PhD Retina Section, Vissum Madrid, Spain

Stanley R. Fuller, MD John A. Moran Eye Center, University of Utah,
Salt Lake City, UT, USA

Alfonso Giovannini, MD Ospedali Riuniti "Umberto I-GM Lancisi-G Salesi", The Eye Clinic-Polytechnic University of Marche, Ancona, Italy

The Eye Clinic-Polytechnic University of Marche, Ancona, Italy

Claire Hooper, MBBS Department of Ophthalmology, Liverpool Hospital, Liverpool, NSW, Australia

Dana M. Hornbeak, MD, MPH Department of Ophthalmology, The Scheie Eye Institute, The University of Pennsylvania, Philadelphia, PA, USA

Jaime Javaloy, MD, PhD Department of Anterior Segment and Refractive Surgery, VISSUM Alicante (Spain), Alicante, Spain

Department of Ophthalmology, Miguel Hernández University of Elche, Alicante, Spain

John H. Kempen, MD, MPH, MHS, PhD Department of Ophthalmology, Biostatistics and Epidemiology, The Scheie Eye Institute, The University of Pennsylvania Perelman School of Medicine, Philadelphia, PA, USA

Moncef Khairallah, MD Department of Ophthalmology, Fattouma Bourguiba University Hospital, Monastir, Tunisia

Andrea Leonardi, MD Ophthalmology Unit, Department of Neuroscience, University of Padua, Padua, Italy

Anna-Karina Brigitte Maier, MD Department of Ophthalmology, Charité – Universitätsmedizin Berlin, Berlin, Germany

Nick Mamalis, MD Department of Ophthalmology, John A. Moran Eye Center, University of Utah, Salt Lake City, UT, USA

Cesare Mariotti, MD Ospedali Riuniti "Umberto I-GM Lancisi-G Salesi", Ancona, Italy

The Eye Clinic-Polytechnic University of Marche, Ancona, Italy

Peter McCluskey, MD, FRANZCO, FRACS Department of Ophthalmology, Save Sight Institute, South Block Sydney Hospital and Sydney Eye Hospital, Sydney, NSW, Australia

Elisabetta Miserocchi, MD Ophthalmology – Ocular Immunology and Uveitis Service, San Raffaele Scientific Institute, Milan, Italy

Giulio Modorati, MD Ophthalmology – Ocular Immunology and Uveitis Service, San Raffaele Scientific Institute, Milan, Italy

Piergiorgio Neri, BMedSc, MD, PhD Ospedali Riuniti "Umberto I-GM Lancisi-G Salesi", Ancona, Italy

The Eye Clinic-Polytechnic University of Marche, Ancona, Italy

Michele Nicolai, MSc, MD Department of Neuroscience, Ospedali Riuniti di Ancona, Università Politecnica delle Marche, Ancona, Italy

Vittorio Pirani, MSc, MD Department of Neuroscience, Ospedali Riuniti di Ancona, Università Politecnica delle Marche, Ancona, Italy

Uwe Pleyer, MD, FEBO Department of Ophthalmology, Charité, Berlin, Germany

Carolina Arruabarrena Sánchez, MD Retina Section, Hospital Príncipe de Asturias, Alcalá de Henares, Madrid, Spain

Valerie P. J. Saw, MBBS (Hons), FRANZCO, PhD Corneal and External Disease, The National Institute of Health Research Biomedical Research Centre (NIHR-BRC) at Moorfi elds Eye Hospital NHS Foundation Trust and the UCL Institute of Ophthalmology, London, UK

Ocular Allergy

1

Andrea Leonardi and Neal P. Barney

Contents

A. Leonardi, MD (✉)
Department of Neuroscience,
Ophthalmology Unit,
University of Padua,
Via Giustiniani 2, Padua 35128, Italy
e-mail: andrea.leonardi@unipd.it

1.1   Definition

Allergy is a pathologic condition that can occur in genetically predisposed individuals who generate an aberrant immune response against environmental antigens, defined allergens. This immune response is characterized by the differentiation of T-helper (Th) cells in the Th type 2 (Th2) cell and by the production of allergen-specific IgE.

Ocular allergy can involve all the components of the ocular surface including the lid and the lid margin, the conjunctiva, and the lacrimal system. Corneal involvement is typically restricted to the two most severe forms of ocular allergy, vernal keratoconjunctivitis (VKC) and atopic keratoconjunctivitis (AKC). In fact, anatomical, physiological, and immunological properties of the cornea render it relatively protected from allergic inflammation. The cornea is more frequently involved in autoimmune diseases, at times as the initial presenting sign of a new autoimmune disease or as a new sign in patients with a long-standing history of autoimmune systemic disease.

Approximately one-third of the world population is affected by some form of allergic disease and ocular involvement is estimated to be present in 40–60 % of this population. Allergic

N.P. Barney, MD
Department of Ophthalmology and Visual Sciences,
University of Wisconsin School of Medicine and
Science – Ophthalmology, 2880 University Avenue,
Madison, WI 53705, USA
e-mail: npbarney@wisc.edu

U. Pleyer et al. (eds.), *Immune Modulation and Anti-Inflammatory Therapy in Ocular Disorders*,
DOI 10.1007/978-3-642-54350-0_1, © Springer-Verlag Berlin Heidelberg 2014

1

conjunctivitis is a localized allergic condition frequently associated with rhinitis but often observed as the only or prevalent allergic sensitization. This disease ranges in severity from mild forms, which can still interfere significantly with quality of life, to severe cases characterized by potential impairment of visual function.

The term "allergic conjunctivitis" refers to a collection of hypersensitivity disorders that affects the lid and conjunctiva. Various clinical forms are included in the classification of ocular allergy (Table 1.1): seasonal (SAC) and perennial allergic conjunctivitis (PAC), vernal keratoconjunctivitis (VKC), atopic keratoconjunctivitis

Table 1.1 Ocular allergic diseases

Condition	Prevalence	Severity	Causes	Sign/symptoms
SAC/PAC	Most frequent ocular allergic disease 10–15 % of population	Mild/ moderate	Genetic predisposition Associated with rhinitis Seasonal allergens (pollens, molds, chemicals) Perennial allergens (dust, animal dander, foods, chemicals	Itching Redness Tearing Watery discharge Chemosis Lid swelling
VKC	Rare Ages 3–20 Under 14 M > F In adults M = F	Severe	Genetic predisposition? Associated with atopic disorders (50 %) Th2 upregulation Nonspecific eosinophil activation	Extreme itching Mucous discharge Giant papillae Trantas' dots SPK/ulcer Conjunctival eosinophilia
AKC	Rare 2nd to 5th decade of life M > F	Severe Sight threatening	Genetic predisposition Associated with atopic dermatitis Environmental allergens: food, dust, pollens, animal dander, chemicals	Itching Burning Tearing Photophobia Chronic redness Blepharitis Periocular eczema Mucous discharge SPK/ulcer Conjunctival and corneal scarring Cataract
GPC	Iatrogenic 2nd to 5th decade	Mild	Trauma induced by contact lens edge, ocular prosthesis, and exposed sutures and aggravated by concomitant allergy	Lens intolerance Blurred vision Foreign body sensation Giant papillae
Contact dermatitis of the eyelid	Not known	Moderate	Contact delayed-type hypersensitivity Exogenous haptens (cosmetics, metals, chemicals) Topical preparation (drugs, preservatives)	Eyelid eczema Eyelid itching Redness Follicles SPK
Drug-induced conjunctivitis	Any age/adults	Moderate	Epithelial toxicity Hyperosmolarity Indirect toxicity	Redness Lid eczema Follicles SPK

(AKC), giant papillary conjunctivitis (GPC), and contact or drug-induced dermatoconjunctivitis.

In 2001, the European Academy of Allergy and Clinical Immunology suggested a classification for allergic conjunctivitis, dividing them into IgE-mediated and non-IgE-mediated conjunctivitis, thus trying to provide a more schematic immunopathological approach to classification [23]. IgE-mediated conjunctivitis can be divided into intermittent and persistent conjunctivitis, the latter of which is classified into vernal and atopic keratoconjunctivitis. However, this classification has limitations and may create more confusion [6]. For example, contact blepharitis or dermatoconjunctivitis (CDC) is a non-IgE-mediated form of localized contact dermatitis that is immunologically different from VKC or AKC. Contact lens-related GPC should be considered a non-IgE-mediated disease, mechanically related to lens microtrauma, which shares some immunopathological aspects with VKC.

In the previous IOIS Guidelines on Blepharitis and Conjunctivitis [6], ocular allergy has been included in the classification of conjunctivitis under the chapter of "Non-Infectious Immune Mediated" and divided as seasonal and perennial allergic conjunctivitis, AKC, and VKC, while GPC has been included in the subchapter of "Specific ocular clinical entities."

In this chapter, we will use the traditional nomenclature for ocular allergy.

1.2 Etiology

1.2.1 Innate Immunity and Ocular Allergy

Innate immunity is the primary defense line for the ocular surface. It is essentially mechanical due to the anatomical characteristics and the position of the eye. These mechanical barriers are supported by nonspecific phagocytic and humoral responses produced by monocytes and macrophages and by ocular surface structural cells.

Induced immunity is the second specific defense line, involving the processing and recognition of antigen by antigen-presenting cells and lymphocytes and the development of a specific immune response through humoral- or cell-mediated mechanisms.

How innate immunity of the ocular surface might interact with the mechanisms that drive toward an allergic reaction remains unclear. Some of the players of innate immunity are modified in ocular allergy. Toll-like receptors (TLRs) play a crucial role in the activation of several immune cells, as well as possibly modulating the Th1/Th2 lymphocyte equilibrium. Recently, TLRs studied in normal subjects and VKC [11] and AKC patients showed different patterns when expressed in chronic allergic conjunctivitis. In VKC, TLR-4 was upregulated, TLR-9 was downregulated, and TLR-2 was slightly decreased relative to normal tissues. Whether this is a predisposing phenotype or a consequence of chronic inflammation remains a challenge for further studies. Activation of TLR-2 and TLR-4 induces mast cell degranulation and release of Th2 cytokines [58], suggesting a possible link between mechanisms that activate the adaptive immune response after microbial ocular infections and allergic inflammation.

There is also strong evidence supporting a role for a *Staphylococcus aureus* infection in the pathogenesis of AKC. In fact, in one study, most affected individuals had this pathogen identifiable on lid swabs [37]. It is believed that staphylococcal-derived superantigen is a potent adjuvant for allergen-specific Th2 responses and it may generically apply to other hypersensitivities, particularly when microorganisms have been implicated. In the ocular setting, these concepts are still unclear.

Recently, it was proposed that NK cells play a crucial role in the pathogenesis of allergic diseases by altering the balance between Th1/Th2 lymphocytes. NK cells might be triggered to secrete cytokines (IL-4, IL-5, and IL-13) that promote Th2 rather than Th1 responses. The recent finding of decreased circulating NK in VKC patients and significantly increased NK cells infiltrating the conjunctiva in inflamed VKC tissues [27] indicates that NK cells may be involved in the pathophysiology of chronic ocular allergy. By modulating allergic inflammation through the release of cytokines that influence the balance between Th1 and Th2 responses, and the resulting conjunctival eosinophil infiltration, these cells may provide a link between innate and specific immunity in allergic diseases.

1.2.2 The Allergic Process

The conjunctiva is normally exposed to picogram quantities of environmental allergens such as pollens, dust mite fecal particles, animal dander, and other proteins. When deposited on the mucosa, these antigens are processed by Langerhans cells or other antigen-presenting cells (APC) in the mucosal epithelium, bind to the antigen recognition site of major histocompatibility complex (MHC) class II molecules, and present to naive CD4+ lymphocytes at some unknown location that could be the local draining lymph nodes. Complex and multiple simultaneous contacts and cytokine exchanges between APC and T cells expressing antigen-specific T-cell receptors are necessary to trigger the antigen-specific T cells to differentiate into Th2 lymphocytes [34, 35]. Recently, more attention has been given to the role of dendritic cells in ocular allergic diseases. B7-1 and B7-2, co-stimulatory molecules on APC, interact with CD28 located on Th2 cells [2], activating them during the induction and effector phases. In contrast, CTLA-4 is expressed on activated T cells and transmits a negative signal that downregulates the ongoing T-cell responses upon engagement by B7-1 or B7-2 [51]. Other ligand interactions may also be crucial in the production of IgE; for example, conjunctival B cells expressing the ligands CD23, CD21, and CD40 are activated in individuals with vernal keratoconjunctivitis (VKC). These B cells may be responsible for the IgE production associated with VKC [2]. A direct activation of allergen-specific T cells by T-cell peptides or direct activation of dendritic cells bearing high-affinity receptors for IgE may be alternate pathways for initiating an allergic reaction in patients with or without evidence of specific IgE sensitization. In fact, specific IgE sensitization is identified in only 50 % of patients suggesting that non-IgE-mediated pathways may be present in

VKC. It is still unclear why disease incidence changes with age and in different geographical regions. The risk of disease may be influenced by genetic susceptibility factors, some of which affect the immune response, for example, polymorphisms of the FcεR1 and IL-4R genes [53]. We have shown recently that the number of DCs expressing the FcεRIg chain is increased and predominant in the substantia propria of the conjunctiva of VKC patients [34, 35]. This increased expression of the receptor is likely to increase the ability of DCs to capture and subsequently process antigens for presentation to CD4+ T cells, thereby initiating the immune cascade.

It is still unknown why one subject becomes allergic and one is tolerant to the same allergen. Nonatopic subjects usually develop a low-grade immunological response to aeroallergens with the production of allergen-specific IgG1 antibodies and, in vitro, a modest T-cell proliferative response to allergens with the production of IFN-γ, typical of Th1 cells. Nonatopics also appear to have a normal T-regulatory cell response [32]. In contrast, allergic subjects mount an exaggerated allergen-specific IgE response with elevated serum levels of IgE antibodies and positive skin tests to extracts of common aeroallergens. In fact, T cells derived from allergic subjects and grown in vitro proliferate in the presence of specific allergens, responding with the production of typical Th2-type cytokines, IL-4, IL-5, and IL-13. This may be the result of an inappropriate balance between allergen activations of regulatory T cells and effector Th2 cells.

The major driving force that polarizes CD4+ T cells to the Th2 phenotype is IL-4, whereas IL-12 favors a Th1 response. However, many other cytokines, chemokines, and mediators with potential relevance to allergy and allergic conjunctivitis, including histamine and histamine receptors, have been described since this initial definition of the Th1/Th2 paradigm. This may explain the disappointing results of single cytokine-directed therapy that have been recently proposed in allergy.

It has become evident that regulatory T cells (Treg) play a suppressive role in the development of allergy and that modulation of Treg function may be a possible therapy for allergic patients.

However, the role of Treg and regulatory cytokines such as IL-10 and TGFβ in ocular allergy is still unclear [18]. It has been shown that IL-10 and TGFβ do not have immunosuppressive roles in the development of experimentally induced allergic conjunctivitis. Moreover, these two cytokines increase the infiltration of eosinophils into the conjunctiva during the effector phase of experimentally induced allergic conjunctivitis.

1.2.3 Allergic Inflammation

Inflammatory mediators and inhibitors in the tear fluid have been extensively used in ocular allergy either to find a "disease marker," to better understand the immune mechanisms involved in the ocular surface inflammation, or to identify potential targets for therapeutic interventions. The presence of Th2 cells and Th2-type cytokines has been proven and confirmed in several studies. However, during the active inflammatory phase of the disease, multiple cytokines are overexpressed and produced including the typical Th1-type cytokine, INFγ, which probably contributes to increasing the ocular inflammation similar to what has been shown in animal models. The presence and distribution of multiple mediators, proteases, and angiogenic and growth factors in normal tears and in those of active VKC patients have been demonstrated using a modified microwell plate antibody array [30].

Massive infiltration of inflammatory cells is typical of chronic ocular allergy such as VKC and differentiates this disease from SAC and PAC. Chemokines such as IL-8, MCP-1, RANTES, and eotaxin are actively secreted in VKC and produced by mast cells, macrophages, epithelial cells, and fibroblasts [26].

Several enzymatic systems may be activated in chronic disease, contributing to cell migration, tissue damage, and remodeling.

Multiple mediators, cytokines, chemokines, receptors, proteases, growth factors, intracellular signals, regulatory and inhibitory pathways, and other unknown factors and pathways are differently expressed, ultimately resulting in the many clinical manifestations of ocular allergic disease. A better understanding of the mechanisms involved in ocular surface immunity is necessary for identifying new classification criteria and new therapeutic strategies.

1.2.4 Allergic Inflammation and Corneal Damage

During the ocular inflammatory process, allergic mediators are released onto the ocular surface and into the tear film, causing a wide range of corneal clinical manifestations.

Inflammatory cells, cytokines, and chemokines liberated from eosinophils, T-helper type 2 (Th2) cells, and tear film instability may act concomitantly in the pathogenesis of shield ulcer. Eosinophils and eosinophil-derived major basic (MBP) and cationic protein (ECP), neurotoxins, and collagenases, in particular MMP-9, have been shown to damage the corneal epithelium and basement membrane [29].

The fact that human corneal keratocytes and conjunctival fibroblasts, but not epithelial cells, are capable of producing eotaxin by stimulation with IL-4 and TNF-α suggests that eotaxin production in keratocytes may play an important role in eosinophil recruitment to corneal ulcers in allergic ocular disease [26]. Thus, eotaxin production by keratocytes, the increased production of cytokines on the ocular surface in the course of severe ocular allergies, and the increased expression of adhesion molecules by corneal epithelial cells stimulated by IL-4 and TNF-α are all responsible for the corneal involvement observed in the most severe allergic ocular diseases.

1.3 Clinical Symptoms and Signs of the Underlying Condition/Disorder

1.3.1 Seasonal and Perennial Allergic Conjunctivitis

Seasonal allergic conjunctivitis (SAC) is the most common form of ocular allergy. It is associated with sensitization and exposure to environmental allergens, particularly pollen (Table 1.1). The perennial form, *perennial allergic conjunctivitis*

(PAC), usually involves sensitization to mites or to multiple antigens. More than 95 % of patients with seasonal or perennial allergic conjunctivitis have allergic rhinitis, justifying the use of "allergic rhinoconjunctivitis" as a synonym for this disease. Allergic rhinoconjunctivitis may be associated with other airway disorders.

SAC and PAC are characterized by onset in childhood or early adulthood. They are typical IgE-mediated diseases, characterized by spikes of histamine and other mediators released from conjunctival activated mast cells that clinically correspond to episodes of ocular itching, redness, and lid swelling frequently associated with rhinitis. Other ocular signs of allergic conjunctivitis include mild serous or serous-mucous secretions and/or slight papillary or follicular hypertrophy of the conjunctiva. Symptoms may be occasional, seasonal, or persistent. Apart from the presence of itching, no sign or symptom related to SAC or PAC is specific or pathognomonic [39]. The most important diagnostic tool for SAC and PAC is a thorough medical history. While these conditions are not serious, they are very disturbing to patients and can significantly affect their quality of life. Correlations between allergic symptoms and psychological disturbances have been reported. Allergic rhinoconjunctivitis significantly reduces the patient's overall energy and negatively affects behavior, leading to increased school absenteeism and decreased work productivity (Table 1.1).

Acute or hyperacute episodes of ocular allergy, also called anaphylactoid reactions, are characterized by acute itching and eyelid swelling as either urticaria (hives and wheals) in the superficial layers of the skin or angioedema in the deeper, subcutaneous tissues or both. These reactions can be unilateral or bilateral and the conjunctiva may or may not be affected. Insect bites, food allergy, or contact hypersensitivity can be involved in the etiology of these reactions.

1.3.2 Vernal Keratoconjunctivitis

Vernal keratoconjunctivitis (VKC) is a severe ocular allergic disease that occurs predominately in children [28]. Most VKC patients complain of symptoms from early spring to fall, with differences among climate zones. Exacerbations of the disease and acute episodes arise, triggered by allergen exposure or, more frequently, by nonspecific stimuli such as wind, light, and dust. VKC is an IgE- and Th2-mediated disease; however, only 50 % of patients present a clearly defined allergic sensitization [10].

Intense itching, tearing, and photophobia are the classic symptoms of these patients. The presence of pain associated with photophobia is indicative of corneal involvement. Foreign body sensation may be caused by mucous hypersecretion, papillae hypertrophy, and superficial keratopathy. Various grades of conjunctival hyperemia and chemosis are always present in both forms of the disease. The tarsal form is characterized by irregularly sized hypertrophic papillae, leading to a cobblestone appearance on the upper tarsal plate and abundant mucus that may be incarcerated between them. A variation of the tarsal form of VKC may appear as diffuse upper tarsal conjunctival thickening with fine and diffuse subepithelial fibrosis without papillae formation. The limbal form of the disease is characterized by multiple gelatinous, yellow-gray limbal infiltrates and papillae, whose size and location may change over time. The limbus may appear thickened and opacified for 360°, accompanied by a peripheral, superficial neovascularization. The apices of infiltrates may appear as punctiform calcified concretions called Trantas' dots. In the mixed form of the disease, both tarsal and limbal signs are observed to varying degrees. Blepharospasm, tearing, and mucus hypersecretion may be present in all VKC forms, while pseudoptosis is usually secondary to the presence of heavy tarsal giant papillae (Table 1.1).

Corneal involvement is common in VKC and is more frequent in tarsal than limbal patients, taking the form of a superficial punctate keratitis, epithelial macroerosion or ulcers, plaque, neovascularization, subepithelial scarring, or pseudogerontoxon. Ulcer formation is preceded by a progressive deterioration of the corneal epithelium, which appears irregularly stained and covered with fine filaments. The ocular complications that lead to visual loss include steroid-induced cataract, steroid-induced glaucoma, central corneal scars, irregular astigmatism, keratoconus, limbal tissue hyperplasia, and dry eye syndrome.

1.3.3 Atopic Keratoconjunctivitis

Atopic keratoconjunctivitis (AKC) is a rare disease that comprises less than 1 % of all ocular allergies (Table 1.1). Generally, it emerges in children with active atopic dermatitis or in young adults and continues through the fifth decade of life, reaching its peak incidence between the ages of 30 and 50 [16]. A family history of allergic conditions is common, while 95 % of patients have a history of eczema and 87 % have a history of asthma. AKC presents as a chronic bilateral conjunctivitis with seasonal exacerbations corresponding to the offending allergen/s or food exposure. The common presenting symptoms are bilateral ocular itching, burning, tearing, and mucous discharge. The hallmark sign of AKC is erythematous, exudative lesions of the lids. Eyelids tend to be thickened, indurated, erythematous, and fissurated, due to eczema, which are often associated with chronic blepharitis, meibomian gland dysfunction, and staphylococcal infection. The lids of about 90 % of atopic patients are colonized with *Staphylococcus aureus* rather than the usual staphylococcal flora; however, their presence does not correlate with the incidence or severity of keratopathy [37]. The limbus may present Trantas' dots and the tarsal conjunctiva may present giant papillae similar to those observed in VKC patients. Cicatrizing conjunctivitis, subepithelial fibrosis, and symblepharon have also been reported, with the lower fornix possibly shrinking subsequent to scarring. Reduced tear function and tear volume may also be observed. Punctate keratitis, persistent epithelial defects, and ulcer with plaque formation are possible complications. Keratoconus is also often associated with AKC. Herpes keratitis, molluscum contagiosum, and microbial infections may complicate the disease, particularly if chronic topical steroid therapy is required. Severe keratopathy with corneal neovascularization, pannus formation, and stromal keratitis may develop as a consequence of repeated corneal inflammation. This can result in marked astigmatic changes and permanent visual impairment. Anterior "atopic" or posterior subcapsular cataract, more likely from steroid use, contributes to the visual deterioration associated with AKC.

1.3.4 Giant Papillary Conjunctivitis

Giant papillary conjunctivitis (GPC) is a non-IgE-mediated inflammation induced most frequently by the use of all types of contact lenses and ocular prostheses or the presence of corneoconjunctival sutures or protruding scleral buckling. The upper tarsal conjunctiva is subjected to repetitive or constant microtrauma generated by a conjunctival "foreign body"; this phenomenon is then complicated by an immune reaction against a protein or residue deposited on the lens. Suspension of contact lens wear initiates the immediate regression of the disease. Previously considered an allergic condition, GPC has similarities with VKC for the morphology of giant papillae and some immunopathological findings such as increased mast cell number, eosinophil and T-cell infiltration, and expression of Th2-type cytokines, such as IL-4 and chemokines [22]. GPC is mostly seen in young patients and is not related to gender but a history of atopy may be a predisposing factor. The early stages of GPC may be asymptomatic. In contact lens GPC, mild lens intolerance progresses to foreign body sensation, itching, blurred vision, and increased mucus production. Intolerance progresses until patients are no longer able to wear their lenses. In other forms of GPC, mild to severe irritation, discomfort, itching, and burning continue until removal of the external device or suture. The defining characteristic of GPC is the presence of giant papillae greater than 0.3 mm in diameter. There can be a single papilla or the entire tarsal plate may be covered. Conjunctival hyperemia, limbal infiltrates, Trantas' dots, and conjunctival thickening are common findings. Mucous discharge and lens deposits are typical.

1.3.5 Contact Blepharoconjunctivitis

Contact blepharitis or dermatoconjunctivitis involves the skin of the eyelid and/or conjunctiva [61]. It is related to contact T-cell-mediated delayed hypersensitivity reaction to haptens (incomplete antigens), which become immunogenic only after they bind to tissue protein. Various haptens and antigens that might come in contact with the eyelid and/or the conjunctiva have been implicated, including drugs, topical eyedrops, preservatives, metals, nail polish, and cosmetics. An "allergic" reaction may occur following instillation of topical antiglaucoma agents, such as beta-blockers, prostaglandins, and prostanoids, or mydriatics used for diagnostic purposes, usually phenylephrine. Other alpha-agonists are commonly used as decongestants in over-the-counter anti-allergy eyedrops. Topical antibiotics such as neomycin, as well as ocular solutions based on herbal extracts, can also provoke contact allergic reactions. Among preservatives, benzalkonium chloride, thimerosal, parabens, and ethylenediaminetetraacetic acid (EDTA) may cause either a toxic reaction or a cell-mediated (delayed) hypersensitivity (DH) response. The most prominent symptoms are itching and burning of the eyelid and eczematoid dermatitis. Other signs and symptoms are redness, eyelid swelling, tearing, and mucous discharge. The ocular surface may also be involved as conjunctival hyperemia; punctate staining of the cornea and conjunctiva, especially on the inferonasal bulbar conjunctiva; and a follicular reaction. Similar signs and symptoms and conjunctival staining patterns occur with drug or preservative toxicity. Marginal corneal infiltrates may rarely occur in reactions to neomycin, phenylephrine, dorzolamide, gentamicin, and atropine; however, the exact nature of these hypersensitivity reactions is not clear. Eczema on the eyelid skin in the absence of conjunctival hyperemia indicates that the cause of the reaction is due to something that has come in contact only with the eyelid. Diagnosis is based on accurate clinical history of agent/drug exposure and the results of patch tests on the dorsal skin (Table 1.1).

1.3.6 Drug-Induced Conjunctivitis or Keratoconjunctivitis

Drug-induced ocular surface toxicity is more frequent than ocular allergy and is only second in frequency to keratoconjunctivitis sicca (Table 1.1). Ocular discomfort may be the only manifestation after drug instillation. However, severe ocular surface reactions may develop. Often, these reactions develop slowly and exhibit subacute or chronic symptoms. Clinical manifestations of a drug's toxic effects may be mild with exacerbation occurring only several years later. Moreover, during the chronic use of topical medications, burning, itching, and other signs of intolerance may be attributed to the initial disease manifestations and the potential side effects of the drug remain underestimated.

Conjunctival irritations may result from a direct cytotoxicity of drugs, a low or high pH of the formulation, and/or a hyper- or hyposmolarity of the solution. Some substances can be allergenic at low concentrations and irritating at higher doses. Toxic compounds may cause corneal and conjunctival cell necrosis or induce cell death by apoptosis. Thus, initial impairment of ocular surface integrity stimulates a cycle of inflammatory reactions, with persistent inflammation leading to subepithelial fibrosis, symblepharon, corneal neovascularization, and scarring.

Unlike immunological reactions, which require prior sensitization, toxic effects can be observed after the first contact and can be dose dependent. Toxic adverse events may also be observed several months or even years after initiation of treatment when a cumulated concentration of the drug has been reached.

The toxicity of various topical medications can also be indirect as with the extensive use of antibiotics, antiviral agents, or corticosteroids due to toxicity on goblet cells, decreased lacrimal gland secretion or the detergent effect of preservatives on the lipid layer of the tear film, increased meibomian gland secretions, and seborrheic blepharitis.

Occlusion of the nasolacrimal system caused by inflammatory and fibrogenic mechanisms can induce alterations of tear film and bacterial flora that lead to secondary toxic effects on the ocular surface. Some types of drug may cause delayed wound healing (corticosteroids), deposits on the ocular surface (adrenaline), or pigment changes and growth of cilia (prostanoids).

1.4 Differential Diagnosis

Each of these clinical entities requires a differential diagnosis that is usually clinical, yet can be substantiated by objective laboratory parameters. Clinical characteristics allow a relatively convincing diagnosis of SAC, PAC, VKC, AKC, GPC, and contact blepharoconjunctivitis in the milder or initial stages of these diseases, but there can be some confusion as to which form of allergy is present. At times, pseudoallergic forms, with clinical manifestations similar to allergy but with a nonallergic equivocal pathogenesis, are difficult to distinguish from allergic forms that, in contrast, have precisely defined pathogenic mechanisms. Several clinical forms may mimic the clinical pictures of ocular allergy, including tear film dysfunction, subacute and chronic infections, and toxic and mechanical conjunctivitis (Table 1.2).

Bacterial, viral, or chlamydial infections should always be considered in the differential diagnosis of both acute and chronic conditions. In bacterial conjunctivitis, the discharge is usually purulent with morning crusting around the eyelids. It may be a unilateral condition, while allergy is usually bilateral. Viral conjunctivitis is often seen in conjunction with a recent upper respiratory infection. Conjunctival hyperemia, chemosis, serous discharge, and corneal subepithelial opacities indicate a viral infection. A chlamydial infection is caused by transfer of the organism from the genital tract to the eye. It is characterized by a follicular persistent or chronic conjunctivitis.

In most cases, allergy is confused with the different forms of dry eye that result from decreased tear production or disruption of tear stability. Even though dry eye is most common in adults or older people, and allergy in younger subjects, tear film dysfunction can occur at any age. Signs and symptoms include irritation, grittiness, burning, and foreign body sensation, but also itching. Dry eye may be worsened by certain medications including oral antihistamines, yet it can occur concomitantly to allergy.

Blepharitis is another common condition that can cause significant ocular irritation, itching, and discomfort. It is caused by an inflammation of the eyelid margin caused by staphylococcal infection with or without seborrhea. It is frequently associated with dry eye and skin diseases such as seborrhea, psoriasis, atopic dermatitis, and acne rosacea.

Table 1.2 Differential diagnosis of allergic from nonallergic conjunctivitis

	Allergy	Dry eye	Blepharitis	Toxic	Mechanical	Infections
History	Typical	Significant	–	±	–	–
Symptoms	Itching Tearing	Burning Foreign body sensation Discomfort Pain	Burning Itching Discomfort	Discomfort Burning	Discomfort Pain	Burning Discomfort Stickiness
Signs	Redness Lid swelling Papillae Eczema	SPK	Abnormal lid margin	Redness Follicles	Redness SPK	Intense redness Secretion Tearing Swelling
Discharge	Serous/mucus	Mucus	Serous/mucus	Serous	Mucus	Mucopurulent/purulent
Cytology	Eosinophils/neutrophils/lymphocytes	Altered epithelial cells/lymphocytes	Neutrophils	Neutrophils/altered epithelial cells/lymphocytes	Neutrophils	Neutrophils

Table 1.3 Diagnostic tests for ocular allergy

Test	Indication	Advantages	Disadvantages
Skin prick test	Suspected sensitization to environmental (pollens, molds, mites, animal dander) and food allergens	Simple, rapid inexpensive	Not always correlated with eye symptoms
Patch test	Eczematous blepharitis Contact sensitivity Drug-induced conjunctivitis		Time consuming Eyelid skin is quite different from that of the back Increasing number of haptens
Serum-specific IgE	In eczema, skin hyperreactivity, prolonged use of drugs	Quantify sensitization Diverse allergens simultaneously	Expensive Not always correlated with eye symptoms
Conjunctival provocation with allergens	Positive clinical history of allergic and prick test/IgE negative Define the most important allergen in patients with several positive skin tests	Confirm conjunctival responsiveness	Few allergens available Expensive Time consuming Rare systemic side effects
Cytology	To evaluate the quality and quantity of inflammation	Presence of eosinophils indicative of allergy	Absence of eosinophils does not exclude allergy
Tear IgE	Suspected sensitization and negative allergy tests	Local IgE production	Low-volume samples Not practical Not standardized

Toxic and mechanical conjunctivitis are frequently confused with allergy. In these cases, careful medical history and examination can exclude an allergic pathogenesis. An intense and persistent follicular reaction is the typical feature, associated with mild to intense hyperemia. Toxicity to single or repeated exposure to a particular chemical substance, eyedrop, or preservative does not produce a change in normal lysozyme or IgE levels but may result in low goblet cell levels, destruction of junctures between epithelial cells, and epithelial cell toxicity. The lacrimal puncta may be swollen or occluded by a cellular infiltrate with a consequent epiphora. The cornea is often involved as a diffuse punctate keratitis typically on the entire corneal surface. Dermal involvement of the eyelids includes injection, swelling, and excoriation. Medicamentosa is essentially a toxic response with no underlying immune dysfunction; however, contact sensitivity to drugs, preservatives, or cosmetics may be present.

1.5 Diagnostic Tests in Ocular Allergy

The first step in diagnosing allergy is to determine definitively that the inflammation is not nonspecific but is allergic in origin, caused by an IgE-mediated sensitization to antigen. The second phase of diagnosis consists in identifying which of the various forms of ocular allergy are present based on the clinical characteristics observed. Diagnostic tests are shown in Table 1.3.

1.6 Treatment of Ocular Allergy

The most common diseases, SAC and PAC, are classic IgE-mediated disorders, in which the therapeutic focus is mostly confined to the local suppression of mast cells, their degranulation, and the effects of histamine and other mast cell-derived mediators using topical drugs. Conversely, severe chronic disorders such as VKC and AKC are both IgE- and T-cell-mediated, leading to a chronic inflammation in which eosinophil, lymphocyte, and structural cell activations characterize the conjunctival allergic reaction. In these cases, stabilization of mast cells and histamine or other mediator receptor antagonists is frequently insufficient for control of conjunctival inflammation and the frequent corneal involvement.

Currently available topical drugs for allergic conjunctivitis belong to different pharmacological classes (Table 1.4): vasoconstrictors,

Table 1.4 Topical ocular allergy medications

Class	Drug	Indication	Comments
Vasoconstrictor/ antihistamine combinations	Naphazoline/ pheniramine	Rapid onset of action *SAC* *Episodic allergy*	Short duration of action Tachyphylaxis Mydriasis Ocular irritation Hypersensitivity Hypertension Potential for inappropriate patient use
Antihistamines	Levocabastine Emedastine Alcaftadine	Rapid onset of action Relief of itching Relief of signs/symptoms *SAC, PAC, AKC, VKC, GPC*	Short duration of action
Mast cell stabilizers	Cromolyn Nedocromil Lodoxamide NAAGA Pemirolast	Relief of signs and symptoms *SAC, PAC, AKC, VKC, GPC*	Long-term usage Slow onset of action Prophylactic dosing
Antihistamine/mast cell stabilizers (dual-acting)	Azelastine Bepotastine Epinastine Ketotifen Olopatadine	Treatment of signs and symptoms of SAC Rapid onset of action Long duration of action Excellent comfort *SAC, PAC, AKC, VKC, GPC*	Bitter taste (azelastine) No reported serious side effects Olopatadine once a day
Corticosteroids	Loteprednol Fluorometholone Desonide Rimexolone Dexamethasone	Treatment of allergic inflammation Use in severe forms of allergies *(PAC) AKC, VKC*	Risk for long-term side effects No mast cell stabilization Potential for inappropriate patient use Requires close monitoring

antihistamines, mast cell stabilizers, "dual-acting" agents (with antihistaminic and mast cell-stabilizing properties), and nonsteroidal anti-inflammatory agents. Corticosteroids, approved for use in the USA, are usually not needed in SAC and PAC and have potentially important side effects if used for periods longer than occasional short cycles to control severe recurrences, if any.

1.6.1 Non-pharmacological Management

The first treatment of ocular allergy should be avoidance of the offending allergens. This can be achieved usually for indoor, professional, or food allergens. Thus, the identification of allergens by skin or blood testing is necessary to allow for avoidance of precipitating factors. Non-pharmacological treatments include tear substitutes and lid hygiene for the washing out of allergens and mediators from the ocular surface and cold compresses for decongestion. Patients should be informed of the duration of the disease based on allergen diffusion and exposure.

1.6.2 Treatment of Allergic Conjunctivitis

Treatment of SAC and PAC includes topical ocular pharmacological treatment, topical ocular non-pharmacological treatments, topical non-ocular pharmacological treatment (see above), systemic pharmacological treatments, and immunotherapy.

1.6.2.1 Topical Ocular Pharmacological Treatment

Topical treatment is the first line of pharmacological treatment of allergic conjunctivitis. Decongestant/vasoconstrictors are alpha-adrenergic agonists approved topically for relief of conjunctival redness. They have little place in the pharmacological treatment of SAC and PAC except for the immediate removal of injection for cosmetic reasons but do have an adverse effect profile locally (glaucoma) and systemically (hypertension).

Topical antihistamines are H_1-receptor competitive antagonists of varying specificity, potency, and duration of action. The first-generation antihistamines, pheniramine and antazoline, are still available as over-the-counter products, particularly in association with vasoconstrictors. The newer antihistamines have a longer duration of action (4–6 h) and are better tolerated than their predecessors [9]. These include levocabastine hydrochloride and emedastine difumarate. Both drugs are effective and well tolerated also in pediatric subjects with allergic conjunctivitis.

Mast cell stabilizers inhibit degranulation by interrupting the normal chain of intracellular signals resulting from the cross-linking and activation of the high-affinity IgE receptor (FcεRI) by allergen [13]. These drugs inhibit the release of histamine and other preformed mediators and the arachidonic acid cascade of mediator synthesis. Several mast cell stabilizers are available for use in the eye: cromolyn sodium 4 %, nedocromil sodium 2 %, lodoxamide tromethamine ophthalmic solution 0.1 %, spaglumic acid 4 %, and pemirolast potassium ophthalmic solution 0.1 %. These drugs are approved for the treatment of allergic conjunctivitis, VKC, and GPC with four times daily dosing regimen. Both mast cell stabilizers and antihistamines have a good safety profile and may be used in treating seasonal and perennial allergic conjunctivitis.

The antihistamines, azelastine, epinastine, ketotifen, and olopatadine, which have mast cell-stabilizing and additional anti-inflammatory properties (called "double or multiple action"), are presently available and show evident benefits in treating all forms of ocular allergy. The advantage offered by these molecules is the rapidity of symptomatic relief given by immediate histamine-receptor antagonism, which alleviates itching and redness, coupled with the long-term disease-modifying benefit of mast cell stabilization [1]. All these medications are well tolerated and none are associated with significant acute ocular drying effects [54].

Bepotastine besilate 1.5 % topical ophthalmic solution is a selective histamine1-receptor antagonist and mast cell stabilizer with inhibitory effects on eosinophilic activity [31, 56]. Alcaftadine 0.25 % ophthalmic solution is approved in the USA for the treatment of itching from allergic conjunctivitis as a selective histamine1-receptor antagonist [55].

The use of nonsteroidal anti-inflammatory drugs (NSAIDs) can be considered, in some cases, for a short period of time, but NSAIDs have limited efficacy on ocular pruritus.

Corticosteroid formulations (including the so-called soft steroids) should be reserved for and carefully used only in the most severe cases that are refractive to other types of medications. Corticosteroids do not directly stabilize immune cell membranes and do not inhibit histamine release; however, they may modulate the mast cell response by inhibiting cytokine production and inflammatory cell recruitment and activation. Thus, they are not the ideal therapy of choice for inhibiting the acute allergic reaction, but however, clinically, are the most effective anti-inflammatory agents in active ocular allergy. Fluorometholone, medrysone, loteprednol, rimexolone, and desonide, called "soft" steroids, are considered to be those of choice when a mild, weakly penetrating drug is needed. In particular, loteprednol etabonate 0.2 % was more effective and had a safety profile than placebo in the treatment of seasonal allergic conjunctivitis [48].

1.6.2.2 Topical Non-ocular Pharmacological Treatment

The efficacy of intranasal corticosteroids in treating allergic nasal symptoms is well established. Recent data show a promising effect of intranasal corticosteroids on ocular symptoms of allergic rhinoconjunctivitis [40]. In SAC and PAC associated with allergic rhinitis, topical nasal steroids (and particularly new molecules with low systemic bioavailability, such as mometasone furoate and fluticasone furoate) have been shown to control the nasal-ocular reflex component of eye symptoms without increasing the risk of cataracts or of an increased ocular pressure. In fact, intranasal corticosteroids are considered safe due to their low systemic bioavailability. Analysis of an intranasal corticosteroid on individual ocular symptoms supported the positive impact of mometasone furoate on ocular symptoms [8]. Mometasone improved individual symptoms (eye itching, tearing, and redness) and subject-reported total ocular symptom scores compared with placebo, in addition to its established efficacy in reducing nasal symptoms of seasonal allergic rhinitis [8].

1.6.3 Systemic Pharmacological Treatment

Systemic antihistamines should be used in patients with concomitant major non-ocular allergic manifestations. In fact, allergic rhinoconjunctivitis is an equally frequent condition generally treated with systemic antihistamines that have been proven effective in relieving nasal and conjunctival signs and symptoms [9]. When allergic symptoms are isolated, focused therapy with topical (ophthalmic) antihistamines is often efficacious and clearly superior to systemic antihistamines, either as monotherapy or in conjunction with an oral or intranasal agent. First-generation H1-receptor antagonists may provide some relief of ocular itching but are sedating and have anticholinergic effects such as dry mouth, dry eye, blurred vision, and urinary retention. Second-generation antihistamines offer the same efficacy as their predecessors but with a low-sedating profile and lack of anticholinergic activity. These drugs include acrivastine, cetirizine, ebastine, fexofenadine, loratadine, and mizolastine. However, even their use has been associated with drying effects, particularly of the ocular surface [9]. Desloratadine and levocetirizine are considered a subsequent evolution of these second-generation agents.

1.6.4 Specific Immunotherapy

Allergen-specific immunotherapy (SIT) is indicated only when a clearly defined systemic hypersensitivity to identified allergens exists. The choice of the allergen to be employed for SIT should be made in accordance with the combination of clinical history and results of skin prick test. SIT is one of the cornerstones of allergic rhinoconjunctivitis treatment. Since the development of noninvasive formulations with better safety profiles, there is an increasing tendency to prescribe immunotherapy in youngsters. In these cases, sublingual immunotherapy (SLIT), which is better tolerated in children [46], can be considered since it is equally effective as traditional subcutaneous injections. Since the approval of SLIT by the World Health Organization in 1988, the efficacy and safety of SLIT have been confirmed in several new double-blind, placebo-controlled studies for mono-sensitized patients who are allergic to house-dust mites, grass pollens, ragweed, and birch pollen. Documented immunological responses to SLIT have included decreased serum eosinophilic cationic protein and interleukin-13 (IL-13) levels, an elevation in IL-12 levels, a reduction in late-phase responses, and increases in IgG4/IgE ratios [46]. However, successful treatment requires at least 2 years of therapy and adjustment of tolerated doses during the pollen season.

1.6.5 Treatment of GPC

Prevention is the most important management step in GPC. This involves prescription of the appropriate lens type and edge design and education on strict lens hygiene. Enzymatic cleaning of the lens is essential to minimizing the accumulation of lens coatings and removing protein buildup. The most essential treatment of early stage GPC is removal of the device that is causing the condition. In fact, patients are asymptomatic several days after discontinuation or removal of the contact lens, device, or suture. Re-initiation of lens wear with a clean lens or lens of a different type or design may be attempted within days of symptom resolution. Mild GPC symptoms may be alleviated by mast cell stabilizers or antihistamine agents. Tear substitutes can be used to minimize conjunctival trauma.

1.6.6 Treatment of VKC

Treatment of VKC requires multiple approaches to include conservative measures and the use of drugs. Patients and parents should be made aware of the long duration of disease, its chronic evolution, and possible complications. The potential benefits of frequent hand and face washing along with avoiding eye rubbing have to be emphasized. Exposure to nonspecific triggering factors such as sun, wind, and salt water should be avoided. The use of sunglasses, hats with visors, and swimming goggles is recommended.

The use of drugs should be well planned in patients with a history of the disease. Mast cell stabilizers, including disodium cromoglycate, nedocromil, spaglumic acid, and lodoxamide, and topical antihistamines are initially used and continued at a decreasing frequency if effective. However, there is a lack of evidence to support the recommendation of one specific type of medication for treating this disorder [33]. Newer topical formulations with combined mast cell-stabilizing properties and histamine-receptor antagonist, such as olopatadine and ketotifen, may be more effective. Nonsteroidal anti-inflammatory drugs such as ketorolac, diclofenac, and pranoprofen may be considered as steroid-sparing options. However, these drugs should be used for a limited period of time only. Oral aspirin at doses of 0.5–1 g/day may be beneficial. In VKC patients with extraocular allergies, systemic treatment with oral antihistamines or anti-leukotrienes can reduce the severity of ocular flare-ups.

Moderate to severe VKC may require repeated topical steroid treatment to downregulate conjunctival inflammation. "Soft corticosteroids" such as clobetasone, desonide, fluorometholone, loteprednol, and rimexolone may be considered preferentially as the first corticosteroid preparations to be used carefully. A "pulsed" corticosteroid treatment is recommended, in addition to the continuous use of mast cell stabilizers and/or

topical antihistamines. Doses are chosen based on the inflammatory state. Instillation frequency of four times per day for 5–10 days is recommended. The "harder" corticosteroid formulations of prednisolone, dexamethasone, or betamethasone have to be used as a second line and as a last resort for the management of the most severe cases [28]. If a systemic hypersensitivity to identified allergens exists, specific immunotherapy may be considered.

1.6.6.1 Cyclosporine and Other Immunosuppressive Treatments in VKC

Cyclosporine A is effective in controlling VKC-associated ocular inflammation by blocking Th2 lymphocyte proliferation and interleukin-2 production [57]. It inhibits histamine release from mast cells and basophils through a reduction in interleukin-5 production and may reduce eosinophil recruitment and effects on the conjunctiva and cornea. Cyclosporine is lipophilic and thus must be dissolved in an alcohol-oil base. Unavailability of a commercial preparation of topical cyclosporine, technical difficulties in dispensing cyclosporine eyedrops, and legal restrictions in many countries on its topical use preclude its widespread use in the treatment of VKC.

Cyclosporine A (CsA) 1 % or 2 % emulsion in castor or olive oil can be considered for treatment of severe VKC and can serve as a good alternative to steroids [7, 25, 43, 47, 49]. Cyclosporine 1 % was reported to be the minimum effective concentration in the treatment of vernal shield ulcer, with recurrence observed at lower concentrations [12]. In a randomized, controlled trial, the effects of 0.05 % topical cyclosporine were similar to placebo in the treatment of VKC [15]. Conversely, in another study, topical CsA 0.05 % decreased the severity of symptoms and clinical signs significantly after 6 months and the need for steroids was reduced, suggesting that CsA at low doses is an effective steroid-sparing agent in severe allergic conjunctivitis [41]. Frequent instillation may be inconvenient but no significant side effects of topical cyclosporine, except for a burning sensation during administration, have been reported. Thus, topical cyclosporine can control the symptoms of VKC, but further trials are required to establish the optimal concentration needed to treat the disease.

Short-term, low-dose, topical mitomycin-C 0.01 % has been considered for acute exacerbation periods of patients with severe VKC refractory to conventional treatment. A significant decrease in signs and symptoms compared with the placebo group was shown at the end of the 2-week treatment period [4]. Nevertheless, mitomycin-C is not approved for treatment of VKC.

Tacrolimus is a potent drug similar to cyclosporine in its mode of action, but chemically distinct. A skin ointment of tacrolimus has recently been licensed for the treatment of moderate to severe atopic eyelid diseases [60]. Treated patients may be at increased risk of folliculitis, acne, and herpes simplex. A recent study reported great efficacy of tacrolimus 0.1 % ointment in the treatment of severe VKC patients [19, 59]. Topical 0.005 % tacrolimus eyedrop seemed to be a safe and effective treatment for steroid-resistant refractory VKC; however, long-term use was needed to control the disease [24].

Severe cases that do not respond to any of these topical therapies may require treatment with systemic corticosteroids (prednisone 1 mg/kg a day) for a short period of time.

1.6.7 Treatment of AKC

The overall management of AKC involves a multidisciplinary approach. Identification of allergens by skin or blood testing is important for preventive measures. Cold compresses and regular lubrication may provide symptomatic relief. Tear substitutes help remove and reduce the effects of allergens and the release of mediators, thus reducing the potential for corneal involvement. Lid hygiene is essential: it prevents infectious blepharitis, improving meibomian gland function and tear film quality.

Prolonged use of topical anti-allergic drugs and mast cell stabilizers may be required. Topical antihistamines may be useful for the relief of itching, redness, and mucous discharge. Topical corticosteroids are effective, but should be used only when other topical treatments are not providing sufficient benefits. Brief periods of intensive topical corticosteroid therapy are often necessary to control the local inflammation in severe cases. Topical cyclosporine may improve the signs and symptoms in steroid-dependent patients, thus reducing the need for corticosteroids to control the ocular surface inflammation. Systemic antihistamines are often used to reduce itching and control widespread inflammation in patients with active skin involvement. Systemic corticosteroids may be necessary in severe cases.

1.6.7.1 Cyclosporine and Other Immunosuppressive Treatments in AKC

Topical CsA 2 % is an effective and safe steroid-sparing agent in AKC and, despite difficulties in patient tolerance, improves symptoms and signs [20]. The lower dose of topical CsA 0.05 % seems to be safe and has some effect in alleviating signs and symptoms of severe AKC refractory to topical steroid treatment [3]. In a multicentered randomized controlled trial, 0.05 % cyclosporine six times per day followed by four times per day was found to be effective in alleviating the signs and symptoms of AKC [3]. Although cyclosporine in a higher (1 %) concentration has been shown to be more effective, frequent instillations may compensate for the low concentration of cyclosporine in the currently available commercial preparations in the USA and South America.

Topical immunomodulators such as tacrolimus have revolutionized the treatment of atopic dermatitis. Application of topical tacrolimus on eyelid skin may be effective for treatment of severe atopic dermatitis of the eyelids and may have secondary benefits for AKC [36, 38, 45, 60]. Topical tacrolimus can be used for at least 1 year without apparent adverse reaction in some patients, although possible adverse reaction should be carefully monitored.

Systemic cyclosporine may be an alternative to systemic corticosteroids for treatment of AKC. Atopic dermatitis patients with and without keratoconus deteriorate graft prognosis statistically significantly.

In severe cases, systemic cyclosporine or tacrolimus may ameliorate both the dermatologic and ocular manifestations in severe patients who are refractory to conventional treatment ([14, 21, 44, 50]).

1.6.8 Surgical Treatment of Severe Allergic Keratoconjunctivitis

Corneal complications have to be carefully monitored and anti-inflammatory therapy adjusted accordingly. Secondary microbial infection can be prevented by prescription of antibiotics for a period of 1 week.

Surgical removal of corneal plaques is recommended to alleviate severe symptoms and to allow for corneal reepithelization. Giant papillae excision with or without combined cryotherapy may be indicated in cases of mechanical pseudoptosis or the presence of coarse giant papillae and continuous active disease. A combined treatment regime consisting of surgical removal of giant papillae and supratarsal corticosteroid injection followed by cyclosporine (0.05 %) and cromolyn sodium eyedrops applied five times daily has been proposed for the treatment of severe treatment-resistant shield ulcers [17, 52].

Amniotic membrane grafts following keratectomy have been described as a successful treatment in deep ulcers, in cases with slight stromal thinning [42]. The amniotic membrane patch may be enough to achieve epithelization. This procedure prevents the presence of membrane remains under the epithelium, which can affect postoperative corneal transparency.

Excimer laser phototherapeutic keratectomy and CO_2-assisted removal of giant papillae have been attempted in the treatment of shield ulcer with or without plaque [5].

More invasive procedures such as oral mucosal grafting or supratarsal corticosteroid injections should be avoided.

References

1. Abelson MB. A review of olopatadine for the treatment of ocular allergy. Expert Opin Pharmacother. 2004;5:1979–94.
2. Abu El Asrar AM, Al-Kharashi SA, Al-Mansouri S, et al. Langerhans' cells in vernal keratoconjunctivitis express the costimulatory molecule B7–2 (CD86) but not B7–1 (CD80). Eye. 2001;15:648–54.
3. Akpek EK, Dart JK, Watson S, et al. A randomized trial of topical cyclosporin 0.05% in topical steroid-resistant atopic keratoconjunctivitis. Ophthalmology. 2004; 111:476–82.
4. Akpek EK, Hasiripi H, Christen WG, et al. A randomized trial of low-dose, topical mitomycin-C in the treatment of severe vernal keratoconjunctivitis. Ophthalmology. 2000;107:263–9.
5. Belfair N, Monos T, Levy J, et al. Removal of giant vernal papillae by CO2 laser. Can J Ophthalmol. 2005;40:472–6.
6. BenEzra D. Classification of conjunctivitis and blepharitis. In: BenEzra D, editor. Blepharitis and conjunctivitis. Guidelines for diagnosis and treatment. Barcelona: Editorial Glosa; 2006.
7. BenEzra D, Pe'er J, Brodsky M, Cohen E. Cyclosporine eyedrops for the treatment of severe vernal keratoconjunctivitis. Am J Ophthalmol. 1986;101:278–82.
8. Bielory L. Ocular symptom reduction in patients with seasonal allergic rhinitis treated with the intranasal corticosteroid mometasone furoate. Ann Allergy Asthma Immunol. 2008;100:272–9.
9. Bielory L, Lien KW, Bigelsen S. Efficacy and tolerability of newer antihistamines in the treatment of allergic conjunctivitis. Drugs. 2005;65:215–28.
10. Bonini S, Bonini S, Lambiase A, et al. Vernal keratoconjunctivitis revisited. A case series of 195 patients with long-term follow up. Ophthalmology. 2000;107: 1157–63.
11. Bonini S, Micera A, Iovieno A, et al. Expression of Toll-like receptors in healthy and allergic conjunctiva. Ophthalmology. 2005;112:1548–9.
12. Cetinkaya A, Akova YA, Dursun D, et al. Topical cyclosporine in the management of shield ulcers. Cornea. 2004;23:194–200.
13. Cook EB, Stahl JL, Barney NP, et al. Mechanisms of antihistamines and mast cell stabilizers in ocular allergic inflammation. Curr Drug Targets Inflamm Allergy. 2002;1:167–80.
14. Cornish KS, Gregory ME, Ramaesh K. Systemic cyclosporin A in severe atopic keratoconjunctivitis. Eur J Ophthalmol. 2010;20:844–51.
15. Daniell M, Constantinou M, Vu HT, et al. Randomized controlled trial of cyclosporine A in steroid dependent allergic conjunctivitis. Br J Ophthalmol. 2006;90:461–4.
16. Foster CS, Calonge M. Atopic keratoconjunctivitis. Ophthalmology. 1990;97:992–1000.
17. Fujishima H, Fukagawa K, Satake Y, et al. Combined medical and surgical treatment of severe vernal keratoconjunctivitis. Jpn J Ophthalmol. 2000;44: 511–5.
18. Fukushima A, Yamaguchi T, Sumi T, et al. Roles of CD4+CD25+ T cells in the development of experimental murine allergic conjunctivitis. Graefes Arch Clin Exp Ophthalmol. 2007;245:705–14.
19. García DP, Alperte JI, Cristóbal JA, et al. Topical tacrolimus ointment for treatment of intractable atopic keratoconjunctivitis: a case report and review of the literature. Cornea. 2011;30:462–5.

20. Hingorani M, Calder VL, Buckley RJ, et al. The immunomodulatory effect of topical cyclosporin A in atopic keratoconjunctivitis. Invest Ophthalmol Vis Sci. 1999;40:392–9.

21. Hoang-Xuan T, Prisant O, Hannouche D, Robin H. Systemic cyclosporine A in severe atopic keratoconjunctivitis. Ophthalmology. 1997;104:1300–5.

22. Irkec MT, Orhan M, Erdener U. Role of tear inflammatory mediators in contact lens-associated giant papillary conjunctivitis in soft contact lens wearers. Ocul Immunol Inflamm. 1999;7:35–8.

23. Johansson SG, Hourihane JO, Bousquet J, et al. A revised nomenclature for allergy. An EAACI position statement from the EAACI nomenclature task force. Allergy. 2001;56:813–24.

24. Kheirkhah A, Zavareh MK, Farzbod F, Mahbod M, Behrouz MJ. Topical 0.005% tacrolimus eye drop for refractory vernal keratoconjunctivitis. Eye (Lond). 2011;25(7):872–80.

25. Kilic A, Gurler B. Topical 2% cyclosporine A in preservative-free artificial tears for the treatment of vernal keratoconjunctivitis. Can J Ophthalmol. 2006;41:693–8.

26. Kumagai N, Fukuda K, Fujitsu Y, et al. Role of structural cells of the cornea and conjunctiva in the pathogenesis of vernal keratoconjunctivitis. Prog Retin Eye Res. 2006;25:165–87.

27. Lambiase A, Normando EM, Vitiello L, et al. Natural killer cells in vernal keratoconjunctivitis. Mol Vis. 2007;13:1562–7.

28. Leonardi A. Vernal keratoconjunctivitis: pathogenesis and treatment. Prog Retin Eye Res. 2002;21:319–39.

29. Leonardi A, Brun P, Abatangelo G, et al. Tear levels and activity of matrix metalloproteinase (MMP)-1 and MMP-9 in vernal keratoconjunctivitis. Invest Ophthalmol Vis Sci. 2003;44:3052–8.

30. Leonardi A, Sathe S, Bortolotti M, Beaton A, Sack R. Cytokines, matrix metalloproteases, angiogenic and growth factors in tears of normal subjects and vernal keratoconjunctivitis patients. Allergy. 2009;64:710–7.

31. Macejko TT, Bergmann MT, Williams JI, et al. Multicenter clinical evaluation of bepotastine besilate ophthalmic solutions 1.0% and 1.5% to treat allergic conjunctivitis. Am J Ophthalmol. 2010;150:122–7. e125.

32. Maggi L, Santarlasci V, Liotta F, et al. Demonstration of circulating allergen-specific CD4 + CD25highFoxp3+ T-regulatory cells in both nonatopic and atopic individuals. J Allergy Clin Immunol. 2007;120:429–36.

33. Mantelli F, Santos MS, Petitti T, et al. Systematic review and meta-analysis of randomised clinical trials on topical treatments for vernal keratoconjunctivitis. Br J Ophthalmol. 2007;91:1656–61.

34. Manzouri B, Flynn T, Ohbayashi M, et al. The dendritic cell in allergic conjunctivitis. Ocul Surf. 2008;6:70–8.

35. Manzouri B, Ohbayashi M, Leonardi A, et al. Characterization of dendritic cell phenotype in allergic conjunctiva: increased expression of FcvarepsilonRI, the high-affinity receptor for immunoglobulin E. Eye. 2008;94:1662–7.

36. Miyazaki D, Tominaga T, Kakimaru-Hasegawa A, et al. Therapeutic effects of tacrolimus ointment for refractory ocular surface inflammatory diseases. Ophthalmology. 2008;115:988–99.

37. Nivenius E, Montan PG, Chryssanthou E, et al. No apparent association between periocular and ocular microcolonization and the degree of inflammation in patients with atopic keratoconjunctivitis. Clin Exp Allergy. 2004;34:725–30.

38. Nivenius E, van der Ploeg I, Jung K, et al. Tacrolimus ointment vs steroid ointment for eyelid dermatitis in patients with atopic keratoconjunctivitis. Eye. 2007; 21:968–75.

39. Ono SJ, Abelson MB. Allergic conjunctivitis: update on pathophysiology and prospects for future treatment. J Allergy Clin Immunol. 2005;115:118–22.

40. Origlieri C, Bielory L. Intranasal corticosteroids and allergic rhinoconjunctivitis. Curr Opin Allergy Clin Immunol. 2008;8:450–6.

41. Ozcan AA, Ersoz TR, Dulger E. Management of severe allergic conjunctivitis with topical cyclosporin a 0.05% eyedrops. Cornea. 2007;26:1035–8.

42. Pelegrin L, Gris O, Adán A, et al. Superficial keratectomy and amniotic membrane patch in the treatment of corneal plaque of vernal keratoconjunctivitis. Eur J Ophthalmol. 2008;18:131–3.

43. Pucci N, Novembre E, Cianferoni A, et al. Efficacy and safety of cyclosporine eyedrops in vernal keratoconjunctivitis. Ann Allergy Asthma Immunol. 2002;89:298–303.

44. Reinhard T, Möller M, Sundmacher R. Penetrating keratoplasty in patients with atopic dermatitis with and without systemic cyclosporin A. Cornea. 1999;18:645–51.

45. Rikkers SM, Holland GN, Drayton GE, et al. Topical tacrolimus treatment of atopic eyelid disease. Am J Ophthalmol. 2003;135:297–302.

46. Röder E, Berger MY, de Groot H, et al. Immunotherapy in children and adolescents with allergic rhinoconjunctivitis: a systematic review. Pediatr Allergy Immunol. 2008;19:197–207.

47. Secchi AG, Tognon MS, Leonardi A. Topical use of cyclosporine in the treatment of vernal keratoconjunctivitis. Am J Ophthalmol. 1990;110:137–42.

48. Shulman DG, Lothringer LL, Rubin JM, et al. A randomized, double-masked, placebo-controlled parallel study of loteprednol etabonate 0.2% in patients with seasonal allergic conjunctivitis. Ophthalmology. 1999;106:362–9.

49. Spadavecchia L, Fanelli P, Tesse R, et al. Efficacy of 1.25% and 1% topical cyclosporine in the treatment of severe vernal keratoconjunctivitis in childhood. Pediatr Allergy Immunol. 2006;17:527–32.

50. Stumpf T, Luqmani N, Sumich P, et al. Systemic tacrolimus in the treatment of severe atopic keratoconjunctivitis. Cornea. 2006;25:1147–9.

51. Sumi T, Fukushima A, Fukuda K, et al. Differential contributions of B7-1 and B7-2 to the development of

murine experimental allergic conjunctivitis. Immunol Lett. 2007;108:62–7.

52. Tanaka M, Takano Y, Dogru M, et al. A comparative evaluation of the efficacy of intraoperative mitomycin C use after the excision of cobblestone-like papillae in severe atopic and vernal keratoconjunctivitis. Cornea. 2004;23:326–9.

53. Toda M, Ono SJ. Genomics and proteomics of allergic disease. Immunology. 2002;106:1–10.

54. Torkildsen GL, Ousler 3rd GW, et al. Ocular comfort and drying effects of three topical antihistamine/mast cell stabilizers in adults with allergic conjunctivitis: a randomized, double-masked crossover study. Clin Ther. 2008;30:1264–71.

55. Torkildsen G, Shedden A. The safety and efficacy of alcaftadine 0.25% ophthalmic solution for the prevention of itching associated with allergic conjunctivitis. Curr Med Res Opin. 2011;27:623–31.

56. Torkildsen GL, Williams JI, Gow JA, et al. Bepotastine besilate ophthalmic solution for the relief of nonocular symptoms provoked by conjunctival allergen challenge. Ann Allergy Asthma Immunol. 2010; 105:57–64.

57. Utine CA, Stern M, Akpek EK. Clinical review: topical ophthalmic use of cyclosporin A. Ocul Immunol Inflamm. 2010;18:352–61.

58. Varadaradjalou S, Feger F, Thieblemont N, et al. Toll-like receptor 2 (TLR2) and TLR4 differentially activate human mast cells. Eur J Immunol. 2003;33: 899–906.

59. Vichyanond P, Tantimongkolsuk C, Dumrongkigchaiporn P, et al. Vernal keratoconjunctivitis: result of a novel therapy with 0.1% topical ophthalmic FK-506 ointment. J Allergy Clin Immunol. 2004;113: 355–8.

60. Virtanen HM, Reitamo S, Kari M, et al. Effect of 0.03% tacrolimus ointment on conjunctival cytology in patients with severe atopic blepharoconjunctivitis: a retrospective study. Acta Ophthalmol Scand. 2006;84:693–5.

61. Wilson FM. Allergy to topical medication. Int Ophthalmol Clin. 2003;43:73–81.

Immune Modulation in Ocular Mucous Membrane Pemphigoid

2

John Kenneth George Dart and Valerie P.J. Saw

Contents

J.K.G. Dart, MA, DM, FRCS, FRCOphth (✉)
V.P.J. Saw, MBBS (Hons), FRANZCO, PhD
Corneal and External Disease,
The National Institute of Health Research
Biomedical Research Centre (NIHR-BRC) at
Moorfields Eye Hospital NHS Foundation Trust and
the UCL Institute of Ophthalmology,
162 City Road, London EC1V 2PD, UK
e-mail: j.dart@ucl.ac.uk; v.saw@ucl.ac.uk

2.1 Definition

Mucous membrane pemphigoid (MMP) is a systemic autoimmune disease characterised by recurrent blistering of mucous membranes and the skin and healing with excessive scar tissue formation [1]. Ocular mucous membrane pemphigoid (OcMMP), without other signs of the disease, may occur in 50 % of cases referred to ophthalmologists [2–4] and is also known as ocular cicatricial pemphigoid (OCP). Ocular involvement occurs in 70 % of all cases, and blindness can develop in 27 % [5]. Although MMP is an uncommon condition, with an incidence of 1.16 per million population per year, ocular MMP remains one of the most difficult anterior segment conditions to manage for which appropriate treatment, started early, can prevent devastating

U. Pleyer et al. (eds.), *Immune Modulation and Anti-Inflammatory Therapy in Ocular Disorders*,
DOI 10.1007/978-3-642-54350-0_2, © Springer-Verlag Berlin Heidelberg 2014

irreversible blindness. Whilst the average age of onset is 65 years, it can occur in children and young adults, and the disease appears to be more aggressive in younger patients [2–4].

In this chapter, we summarise the pathogenesis, diagnosis and management of the ocular surface complications and focus on the role of immune modulation in managing the inflammatory component.

2.2 Pathogenesis

This is summarised in Fig. 2.1. An as-yet-unknown trigger, often in a genetically susceptible individual (the HLA-DQB*0301 allele presents antigen to T cells), provokes loss of tolerance to one or more components of the basement membrane zone (BMZ). Target antigens, components of the basement membrane, are

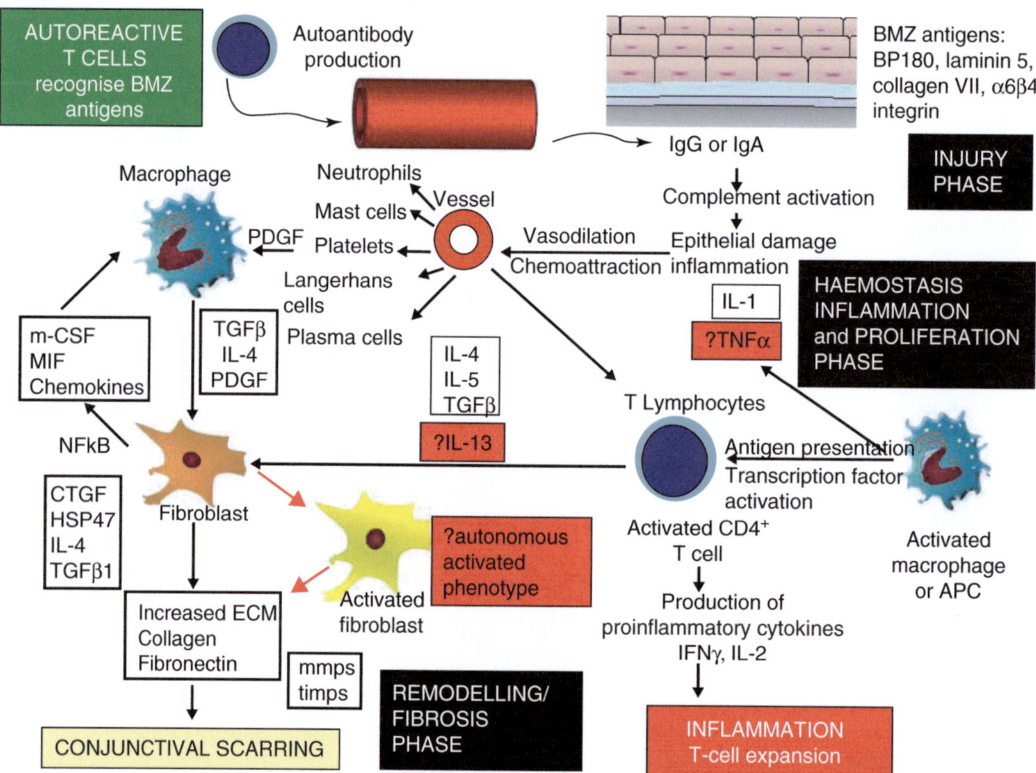

Fig. 2.1 Proposed pathogenesis of inflammation and fibrosis in ocular MMP
Injury phase: Autoreactive T cells recognise BMZ (basement membrane zone) antigens (BP180 bullous pemphigoid180 kDa antigen, laminin 5, collagen VII, α6β4 integrin) causing B cells in germinal centres to produce autoantibodies IgG (immunoglobulin G) and IgA. These bind to the BMZ and initiate a type II cytotoxic hypersensitivity reaction, activating the complement cascade to cause subepithelial bulla formation.
Inflammation and proliferation phase: Complement-mediated BMZ, epithelial and connective tissue damage causes vasodilation and release of blood cells and plasma proteins into the damaged site and attracts an acute inflammatory cell infiltrate consisting of neutrophils, activated macrophages, mast cells, platelets, Langerhans cells and lymphocytes, as well as acute inflammatory cytokine IL-1 (interleukin-1) production. T-cell activation and proliferation characteristic of a Th1 (type 1 helper T cell) response occur, with IFN-γ (interferon gamma) and IL-2 (interleukin-2) production. Th2 (type 2 helper T cell) cytokines IL-4 and IL-5 are also synthesised. Macrophages proliferate and play an important role in scar tissue formation and also contribute to production of the fibrogenic cytokines TGF-β (transforming growth factor beta) and PDGF (platelet-derived growth factor).
Fibrosis phase: Fibroblasts become activated, proliferate and synthesise increased extracellular matrix, CTGF (connective tissue growth factor), TGF-β and other cytokines. Endothelial cells may proliferate, forming fibrovascular granulation tissue. The scar tissue is then remodelled, becoming less cellular, and the final result is subconjunctival scarring. Other abbreviations in this figure: *APC* antigen-presenting cell, *m-CSF* macrophage colony-stimulating factor, *MIF* macrophage migration inhibitory factor, *NF-kB* nuclear factor-kappa B, *HSP47* heat-shock protein 47, *ECM* extracellular matrix, *MMPS* matrix metalloproteinases, *TIMPs* tissue inhibitors of matrix metalloproteinases

BP180 (subsets LAD1 and Nc16A), β4 integrin, laminin 5 and type 7 collagen, amongst others. These targets may differ when the disease affects different sites, e.g. β4 integrin may be important in the development of the ocular disease. The loss of tolerance may be due to failure of central tolerance (e.g. failure to delete or cause anergy in BP180 reactive thymocytes) or failure of peripheral tolerance (due to deficiency of regulatory T cells). Circulating T cells, autoreactive to the NC16A portion of BP180, have been detected in MMP [6]. These T cells generate specific B-cell clones, most likely in extraocular tissues, which produce circulating autoantibodies to BMZ glycoproteins. The autoantibodies generated (IgG and IgA) then bind to their specific antigen(s) in the BMZ, activating the complement cascade and initiating a type II cytotoxic hypersensitivity reaction. This in turn causes formation of subepithelial bullae in the skin and inflammatory infiltration of the substantia propria with predominance, in the acute stage, of neutrophils, macrophages and Langerhans antigen-presenting cells (APC), together with an increase in T cells. Further, T-cell expansion results from the production of proinflammatory cytokines such as interferon-γ resulting in further T-cell expansion. Macrophages are brought in by platelet-derived growth factor (PDGF), a potent chemoattractant for both macrophages and fibroblasts. Tumour necrosis factor alpha (TNF-α) and interleukin-1 (IL-1) are produced by macrophages, which in turn influence T-helper (T_H) cells by antigen processing and presentation [7, 8].

PDGF is also instrumental in upregulating thrombospondin which activates latent transforming growth factor beta (TGF-β) that is an important activator of fibroblasts, mediating extracellular matrix production and scarring. IL-13 is another major profibrotic mediator, which is produced by T_{H2} cells, mast cells and basophils and is also upregulated in the conjunctiva in MMP [8]. Activated fibroblasts increase extracellular matrix production influenced by connective tissue growth factor (CTGF), heat-shock protein (HSP), TGF-β and interleukin-4 (IL-4) [9].

2.3   Clinical Signs

Early diagnosis and initiation of appropriate treatment are essential to prevent the sight-threatening complications of mucous membrane pemphigoid. Ocular MMP typically presents with a red eye and persistent conjunctivitis that has not responded to topical therapy, or with recurrent cicatricial entropion and trichiasis, frequently following failed surgical repair. It may also present with ptosis. About 10 % of patients present with acute conjunctivitis and limbitis (Fig. 2.2a) leading to rapidly progressive scarring and surface failure if uncontrolled. However, the majority of patients present with subacute or low-grade chronic inflammation and slowly progressive scarring. The earliest clinical sign in patients with subacute disease is often medial canthal scarring, with loss of the plica and caruncle. Medial canthal scarring is usually an early sign of

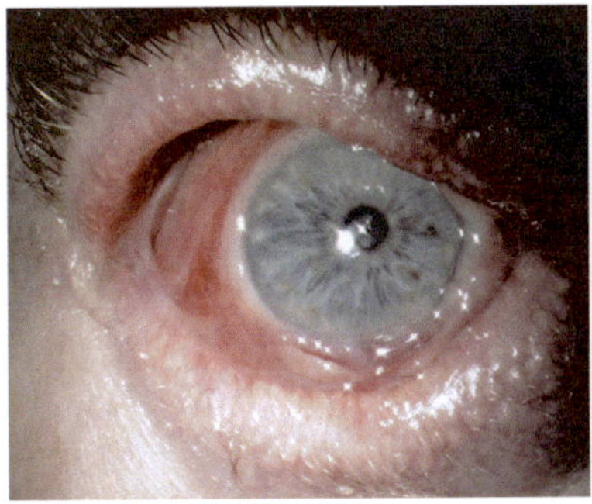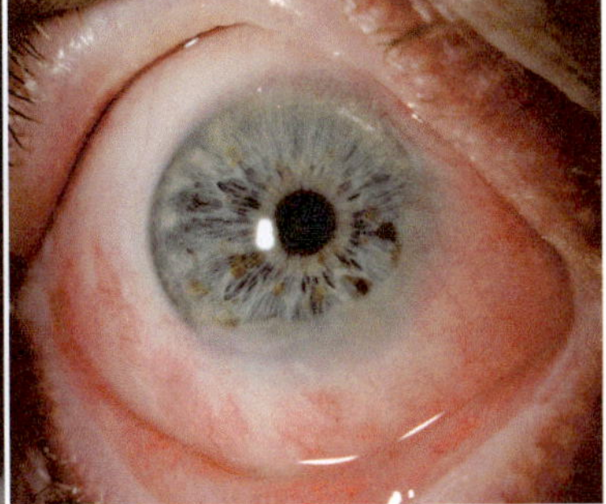

Fig. 2.2 Severe ocular MMP before and after treatment

MMP and not as frequent in conjunctival scarring due to other causes. Linear scarring in the marginal sulcus of the upper tarsus is sometimes present early in the disease. Other signs, in order of progression, are subepithelial reticular fibrosis; infiltration of the tarsal and bulbar conjunctiva; shortening of the fornices; symblepharon and cicatricial entropion, followed by ankyloblepharon; and, then, subsequent to scarring of the lacrimal ductules which usually occurs late in the disease, a totally dry "skinlike" eye. These signs are illustrated and described in a recent review by the authors [2–4].

## 2.4	Differential Diagnosis

Table 2.1 summarises many of the conditions that cause conjunctival scarring [2–4]. Progression of conjunctival scarring, including conjunctival scarring that is presumed to have progressed because of the absence of a previous history of eye disease, or the onset of cicatricial entropion, should alert the clinician to the possibility of MMP. This is complicated by a number of causes of chronic conjunctival inflammation that can induce fibrosis. Table 2.1a lists the disorders that are associated with conjunctival scarring that is either static, once the underlying disorder has been controlled or the precipitating drug withdrawn, or only very slowly progressive having no functional significance. A subset of patients with some of these disorders will develop severe progressive scarring similar to that in MMP.

Table 2.1b lists the disorders that more commonly cause progressive conjunctival scarring. Unilateral progressive scarring is uncommon and can be due to conjunctival tumours masquerading as MMP or secondary to drugs (usually given for the prolonged treatment of unilateral glaucoma or herpetic eye disease). The clinical progression that distinguishes most patients with MMP, and those subsets of the other mucocutaneous diseases that develop ocular disease like MMP, is that the scarring in these patients is rapidly progressive and functionally significant. In these groups of patients, and those with drug-induced pemphigoid, treatment with immunosuppressive

Table 2.1 Differential diagnosis of cicatrising conjunctivitis

1a. Static or very slowly progressive conjunctival scarring

1. Trauma

   Physical, chemical, thermal, radiation injury, artefacta

2. Infection

   Trachoma, membranous streptococcal and adenoviral conjunctivitis, *Corynebacterium diphtheriae*, chronic mucocutaneous candidiasis

3. Allergic eye disease

   Atopic keratoconjunctivitis

4. Drug-induced conjunctival cicatrisation[a]

5. Mucocutaneous disorders

   Stevens-Johnson syndrome and toxic epidermal necrolysis[a]

   Graft-versus-host disease

6. Immunobullous disorders

   Linear IgA disease[a], epidermolysis bullosa acquisita[a]

   Dermatitis herpetiformis, bullous pemphigoid

   Pemphigus vulgaris

   Discoid and systemic lupus erythematosus[b]

7. Systemic disease

   Rosacea, Sjögren's syndrome, inflammatory bowel disease, sarcoidosis, scleroderma, immune complex diseases, ectodermal dysplasia, porphyria cutanea tarda, erythroderma ichthyosiform congenita

1b. Progressive conjunctival scarring

1. Neoplasia

   Squamous cell carcinoma, sebaceous cell carcinoma, lymphoma

2. Mucous membrane pemphigoid (MMP)

   (a) MMP with ocular involvement

   (b) Ocular MMP associated with other disorders

      Linear IgA disease

      Epidermolysis bullosa acquisita

      Paraneoplastic MMP

      Drug-induced ocular MMP

      Stevens-Johnson syndrome

3. Other mucocutaneous and immunobullous disorders

   (a) Mucocutaneous disorders

      Lichen planus

   (b) Immunobullous disorders

      Paraneoplastic pemphigus

[a]A subset of patients with these diseases may develop autoantibody-positive progressive conjunctival scarring similar to MMP

[b]Rare cases can develop progressive scarring

therapy is usually necessary to control the underlying pathology that is causing progressive scarring.

The conjunctival signs in MMP may be identical to those observed in other mucocutaneous disorders (graft-versus-host disease, Stevens-Johnson syndrome, lupus erythematosus, lichen planus) and other immunobullous disorders (bullous pemphigoid, linear IgA disease, epidermolysis bullosa acquisita, dermatitis herpetiformis) although the conjunctival signs in the majority of patients with the latter disorders are mild. In many of these mucocutaneous and immunobullous disorders, the skin or oral disease precedes the eye disease so that there is rarely confusion about the diagnosis although clinicians may not be aware of the potential for progressive conjunctival scarring in a subset of this group and the fact that subgroups of patients with predominantly mucosal linear IgA disease and epidermolysis bullosa acquisita are currently recognised as a form of MMP. In Stevens-Johnson syndrome, major exacerbations of conjunctival inflammation can occur many years after the acute disease, leading to a condition indistinguishable from MMP, both in terms of the clinical signs and immunopathology.

Apart from topical medication-related disease, ocular MMP usually affects both eyes, but the signs and disease progression can be very asymmetric. It is said that the occasional patient presenting with unilateral ocular MMP typically develops fellow eye involvement within 2 years.

2.5 Immunopathological Investigations [2–4, 10, 11]

A clinical diagnosis of ocular mucous membrane pemphigoid can be made based on a history of progressive conjunctival scarring and the presence of typical clinical signs, after exclusion of other causes of conjunctival scarring. Most of the disorders in Table 2.1 can be identified or excluded by an accurate history, systemic examination and laboratory investigations including a connective tissue disease antibody screen and specialist referral for evaluation and biopsy of any skin and mouth lesions.

2.5.1 Histology

Ideally, the clinical diagnosis requires laboratory evidence of the presence of an autoimmune disease process with a biopsy from at least one site (skin, buccal, genital, nasopharyngeal or conjunctival mucosa) being positive on direct immunofluorescence (DIF) showing linear deposition of IgG, IgA and/or complement along the epithelial basement membrane zone (BMZ). This has been recommended as a mandatory requirement for the diagnosis of MMP [1]. DIF is almost always positive in MMP that involves tissues other than the eye. However, conjunctival DIF is positive in only 60–86 % cases of ocular MMP, and the results can be initially positive then subsequently negative, and vice versa, during the course of the disease, apparently unrelated to disease activity or treatment, so that ocular MMP cannot be excluded by a negative DIF result.

For these reasons, although a positive DIF result is useful and can also distinguish MMP from diseases such as lichen planus, lupus erythematosus or pemphigus vulgaris, which have characteristic immunopathological features of their own, a negative result is not conclusive. DIF is not a specific or sensitive test for MMP; although DIF for IgG, IgA and/or complement is characteristic of MMP, identical biopsy findings are found in bullous pemphigoid, which has to be distinguished by the clinical findings. In addition, a positive DIF result has been reported in ocular rosacea and ulcerative colitis. In effect, a positive DIF result is used as a surrogate to provide evidence for an autoimmune pathogenesis.

However, bulbar conjunctival biopsy is easy and safe providing the fornix is avoided and we recommend that both conjunctival and buccal biopsies (buccal biopsies are occasionally positive in patients without buccal symptoms when conjunctival biopsies are negative) are taken. They need to be processed in a laboratory that is experienced in this investigation.

Routine histopathology is of little value for the diagnosis of MMP because the conjunctiva is fragile and detection of basement membrane zone cleavage unreliable. However, it is mandatory to exclude neoplasia and can help diagnose atopic disease and sarcoidosis.

2.5.2 Serology

The potential value of indirect immunofluorescence (IIF) in MMP has been overlooked. Although often negative in MMP, positive indirect immunofluorescence showing circulating anti-basement membrane zone antibodies also provides evidence for an underlying autoimmune pathology and may be positive when DIF is negative. Research is underway to develop more sensitive and specific assays for detection of these autoantibodies. If antibody can be detected and a titre obtained, the titres correlate with disease activity.

2.6 Diagnostic Criteria for Ocular MMP

We propose three sets of criteria for the diagnosis of OcMMP:

(a) Patients with positive conjunctival DIF or positive DIF from another site meet currently agreed criteria [1].

(b) Patients with negative DIF from any site and positive indirect immunofluorescence can be diagnosed as having MMP.

(c) Patients with negative immunopathology can be diagnosed with OcMMP providing that they have a typical phenotype of progressive conjunctival scarring and that other diseases that may cause this phenotype have been excluded. When ocular cases are reported, the detailed immunopathology findings should be recorded so that the diagnosis can be interpreted in light of future modifications to diagnostic criteria.

2.7 Treatment

Disease progression is multifactorial (Fig. 2.3) and due to a combination of underlying immune-mediated inflammation, local ocular surface disease and scarring, each of which perpetuates inflammation leading to progressive scarring. Initial management is directed at treating the local ocular surface disorders that in themselves cause inflammation. These include blepharitis, dry eye, microbial infection, toxicity to topical

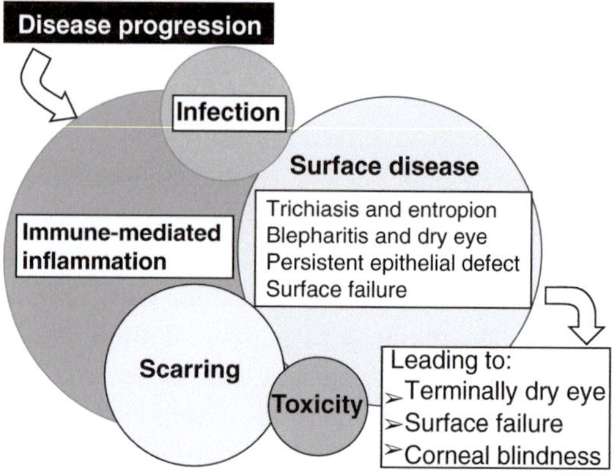

Fig. 2.3 Factors affecting disease progression in ocular MMP

medications, exposure secondary to lagophthalmos and ocular surface trauma secondary to entropion and trichiasis. The ocular surface disease management in OcMMP is described in detail in another review [2–4] and this chapter focuses on the role of immunosuppressive therapy described below.

2.7.1 When Is Inflammation due to Autoimmune Disease Activity?

Persisting inflammation, following optimal ocular surface disease treatment, is due to the underlying autoimmune disease and usually requires systemic immunosuppression. Whether the underlying autoimmune disease is active is best evaluated by examining the upper bulbar conjunctiva for inflammation, which is least likely to be affected by exposure, trichiasis and lid margin disease. There is no evidence that topical therapy alters the natural history of the disease [12, 13]. About 25 % of OcMMP patients do not require immunosuppression [14] as they have mild disease. In end-stage "burned out" disease, immunosuppression is also unnecessary as treatment can only arrest scarring, not reverse it; however, if conjunctival incision surgery, such as that required for fornix reconstruction, is planned in these patients, then immunosuppression must be started beforehand to prevent an exacerbation of postoperative inflammation and scarring leading to a poor surgical result and further progression of disease.

2.7.2 Evidence for the Use of Topical Immunosuppressive Therapy

Topical steroid treatment is ineffective in controlling progressive ocular MMP, offering only variable symptomatic relief [5, 12]. Its adverse effects of cataract and glaucoma generally outweigh the benefits. Subconjunctival steroids may be temporarily effective, but relapses occur when the injections are stopped [12] and prolonged use also leads to cataract and glaucoma. Topical ciclosporin has been used in only four reported cases of whom two had some response [15]; we have no experience with this and it is probable that the poor results reported for systemic therapy with ciclosporin may have inhibited further investigation of this modality.

2.7.3 Evidence for the Effect of Systemic Immunosuppression on Progression of Disease

The primary goals of treatment of ocular MMP are to control inflammation and arrest fibrosis, in order to prevent progression of disease to more advanced stages and blindness. Optimal management of inflammation in ocular MMP targets the inflammation due to systemic immunodysregulation with immunosuppressive agents, after treating inflammation due to local surface disease (blepharitis, trichiasis, dry eye), infection and toxicity [2–4]. Most cicatrisation is believed to occur during active inflammation [12], but despite control of inflammation in 70 % of patients with systemic immunosuppression, progressive fibrosis is still observed in 53 % [2–4]. Without treatment, conjunctival scarring in ocular MMP progresses in 64 % of patients over 10–53 months [16]. Progression is more frequent in the advanced stages of disease [17]. Use of immunosuppressive therapy has been shown to slow progression of disease in one case series [17] and control of inflammation has been shown to prevent progression in one RCT [13].

2.7.4 Evidence for the Efficacy of Different Immunosuppressive Regimens in Controlling Inflammation

Evidence for the effect of current immunosuppressive therapy in ocular MMP is summarised in Table 2.2 and comes from cohort studies [18, 19], interventional and retrospective case series [2–4, 11, 16, 20–29] and two randomised trials [13]. These have indicated a role for dapsone, sulphasalazine or sulphapyridine for mild to moderate inflammation; azathioprine, mycophenolate or methotrexate for moderate inflammation or for disease not responding to sulphonamide therapy; and cyclophosphamide together with a short course of prednisolone for severe inflammation. Interpretation of the results of the studies in this evidence base must be made with caution for several reasons.

Many of these reports are limited to a description of the relatively short-term effects of monotherapy, whereas, in many clinics, more than one drug is used and the outcomes vary from success, through qualified success (inflammation that was partially controlled, with some residual inflammation) [2–4], to failure. Three large case series, from centres with a special interest in MMP, place the studies in Table 2.2 in the context of the prolonged treatment required for this chronic lifelong disease. Of 61 patients with 12–264 months follow-up (FU) [30], the following drugs were used: dapsone in 51, methotrexate in 24, azathioprine in 23, cyclophosphamide in 15, prednisolone (always as adjunctive therapy) in 17, calcineurin antagonists in 6 and intravenous immunoglobulin in 8. Of the 61 patients, 22 % had one drug, 37 % had two drugs, 21 % had three drugs and 10 % had 4 drugs. Outcomes of therapy with individual drugs or combinations cannot be established from this paper; however, 90 % of patients had disease control using this approach. Of 78 patients [29] with 3 months to 17 years FU, 68 had initial combined therapy of which 63 had cyclophosphamide and prednisolone combination therapy. The success at 1 year, for all therapies, was 82.9 %. In a subset of 44 patients treated with cyclophosphamide and prednisolone, 91 % were in remission 2 years after initiation of therapy (reported in Table 2.2); the significant

Table 2.2 Results of studies reporting the efficacy of immunosuppressive agents in controlling inflammation in MMP

Immunosuppressive agent	Study	Severity of inflammation	% of patients or *eyes* responding to treatment
Nicotinamide and tetracycline	Reiche et al. [33]	Mild to moderate	63 ($n=8$) extraocular and ocular MMP
Dapsone	Rogers et al. [20]	Mild to moderate	83 ($n=24$) extraocular and ocular MMP
	Tauber et al. [11]	Mild to moderate	45 ($n=69$) ocular MMP
	Foster [13]	Mild to severe	70 ($n=20$) ocular MMP
Sulphapyridine	Elder et al. [25]	Mild to moderate	50 ($n=20$) ocular MMP
Sulphasalazine	Doan et al. [26]	Mild to moderate	45 ($n=9$) ocular MMP
Azathioprine	Tauber et al. [11]	Mild to moderate	33 ($n=11$) ocular MMP
Methotrexate	McCluskey et al. [28]	Mild to moderate	83 ($n=12$) ocular MMP
Cyclophosphamide and steroids	Thorne et al. [29]	Mild, moderate and severe	91 ($n=44$) ocular MMP
	Elder et al. [23]	Severe	15/19 *eyes* (79 %) ocular MMP
	Foster [13]	Severe	100 ($n=12$) ocular MMP
Cyclophosphamide	Tauber et al. [11]	Severe	89 ($n=9$) ocular MMP
Tacrolimus	Letko et al. [27]	Severe	33 ($n=6$) ocular MMP
Ciclosporin	Neumann et al. [21], Foster et al. [22][a]	Mild to moderate	2/22 patients (9 %) ocular MMP
Mycophenolate	Zurdel et al. [37]	Severe	9/10 eyes (90 %) ocular MMP
IVIG	Letko et al. [66], Sami et al. [42][b]	Moderate and severe	89 patients ($n=18$) ocular MMP
Infliximab, etanercept	John et al. [47], Prey et al. [49], Sacher et al. [31], Canizares et al. [43], Heffernan and Bentley [45]	Moderate and severe	100 ($n=7$)[c] ocular and extraocular MMP
Rituximab	Le Roux-Villet et al. [55], Taverna et al. [51], Ross et al. [52], Schumann et al. [53], Lourari et al. [54]	Severe	84 ($n=32$) ocular and extraocular MMP
IVIG and rituximab	Foster et al. [56]		100 ($n=6$) ocular MMP
Daclizumab	Papaliodis et al. [59]	Moderate	100 ($n=1$) ocular MMP
Oral corticosteroids	Hardy et al. [5], Mondino et al. [12], Foster [13]	Mild, moderate and severe	65 ($n=23$)[e] ocular MMP
Pentoxifylline + cyclophosphamide + steroids	El Darouti et al. [67]	Mild, moderate and severe	80 ($n=15$) ocular MMP
	Randomised trials		
Cyclophosphamide and short-term oral prednisolone versus oral prednisolone alone	Foster [13]	Severe	($n=24$) 12/12 responded to cyclophosphamide and oral prednisolone versus 5/12 to oral prednisolone. No progression of disease in cyclophosphamide group versus 7/12 progressing in prednisolone group
Dapsone versus cyclophosphamide	Foster [13]	Severe	($n=40$) 14/20 responded to dapsone versus 20/20 to cyclophosphamide

[a]Combined results of two case series
[b]Combined results of two case series
[c]Combined results of five case series
[d]Combined results of one series and four case reports
[e]Combined results of one large series and three case reports

complication rates associated with this therapy are described. Relapse rates for therapy were given at 0.04 % (95 % CI, 0.02–0.09) per person year. As for the previous series, it was not possible to establish the success rates for other individual combinations. Of 115 patients [2–4] with 6 months to 11 years FU, analysis of drug therapy is by treatment episode to take into account changing therapy over time. There were 388 episodes for 115 patients of whom 23 % had one episode, 26 % had two and 44 % had 3–10 episodes. Combination therapy was used in 47 % of episodes. Outcomes for the principal agents used in a treatment episode are given in Table 2.2.

Although effective at controlling acute disease activity because of their rapid onset of action, high-dose oral corticosteroids alone, without steroid-sparing immunosuppressants, are no longer used [5, 12]. This is because the high doses required to sustain disease control (greater than 40 mg prednisolone daily) lead to severe adverse effects including hypertension, diabetes, osteoporosis, peptic ulcer, myopathy and psychosis [13] in this elderly patient population. For severe disease, one randomised controlled trial found incomplete disease control with high-dose oral steroids, and in those with control, recurrence of disease activity recurred when corticosteroid doses were tapered, and the response was incomplete in 58 % of patients [13]. For these reasons, oral corticosteroids are useful in acutely inflamed eyes as a short 6- to 12-week course in combination with, and whilst awaiting the onset of effect of, immunosuppressive medication [1, 22].

The use of pulse intravenous methylprednisolone (IVMP) or dexamethasone to control active inflammation is mentioned in the management of ocular and extraocular MMP [28, 32]; however, there are no studies evaluating its efficacy specifically in ocular MMP. Equivalent doses of oral prednisolone have been shown to give similar clinical and immunological effects when compared with pulse IVMP in rheumatoid arthritis [33].

The calcineurin inhibitors, cyclosporin and tacrolimus, have failed to control inflammation in several studies [21, 22, 27], and their use in ocular MMP cannot be recommended on the basis of current evidence. Tetracycline and nicotinamide have been reported as safer alternatives to immunosuppression in mild to moderate extraocular and ocular MMP [34, 35], and mycophenolate mofetil has been described as being effective in extraocular MMP [36, 37] as well as ocular MMP [2–4, 38].

2.7.5 Does Control of Inflammation Prevent Fibrosis?

With current immunosuppressive regimens, progression of cicatrisation has still been observed in 10–53 % of ocular MMP patients [17, 25, 30]. There is also small subgroup of MMP patients with ocular involvement who appear to have ongoing conjunctival fibrosis without overt clinical signs of inflammation [39]. Despite the absence of clinical signs of inflammation, there may still be significant cellular infiltrate on histological evaluation ("white inflammation") [40, 41]. Further systemic immunosuppression with potential systemic toxicity may not necessarily be helpful in these cases, for whom more specific local therapy targeting the cellular infiltrate or fibrogenic process would be ideal. There is evidence for both ongoing residual subclinical inflammation [7, 8] and transformed profibrotic fibroblasts [9] as the putative drivers of scarring which progresses, despite apparent clinical control of inflammation with systemic immunosuppression. No current medical therapy is able to reverse the cicatrisation or ocular surface problems once they have developed.

2.7.6 How Is Immunosuppressive Therapy Given?

We recommend giving systemic immunosuppression using a stepladder strategy (Fig. 2.4) in which the risk of a poor initial response in mild and moderate disease is justified by less toxicity with undiminished prospects of later success with more toxic agents, whereas in severe disease, initial treatment with toxic agents, such as cyclophosphamide, is justified. Immunosuppressive therapy can be administered with the help of an

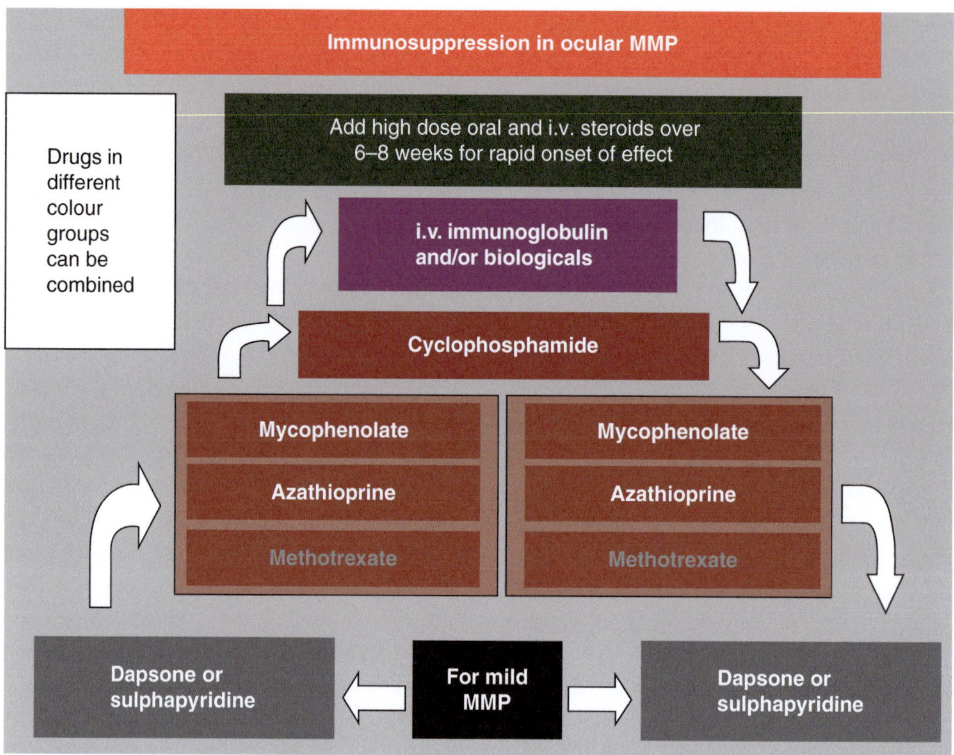

Fig. 2.4 Stepladder therapy for ocular MMP. Drugs in different *colour* groups can be combined. For example, a patient might be given steroids, cyclophosphamide and a biological or sulphonamide

experienced physician. We manage therapy with the myelosuppressives and sulphonamides ourselves and share the care of those few patients currently requiring biological therapy with physicians experienced in their use. Table 2.3 summarises the doses, side effects and strategies for identification and prevention of side effects for the immunosuppressives used in OcMMP.

Briefly, for "step-up" therapy, dapsone (diaminodiphenylsulfone, 25–50 mg bd) or sulphapyridine (500 mg od to 500 mg bd, given as sulphasalazine 500–1,000 mg bd when sulphapyridine is unavailable) or methotrexate is prescribed for mild or moderate inflammation. For disease not responding after 2–3 months of first-line therapy, azathioprine (1–2.5 mg/kg/day) is added (when there is some response) or substituted (if there is no response) for these first-line agents. For those intolerant of azathioprine, mycophenolate mofetil (500 mg–1 g bd) is effective [2–4]. Severe inflammatory disease is treated at the top of the stepladder with cyclophospha-

mide (1–2 mg/kg/day). As optimal effects with cyclophosphamide are not achieved until 8–12 weeks following the initiation of therapy, an adjunctive tapering 6–8-week course of oral corticosteroids (prednisolone commencing at 1–2 mg/kg/day) is employed, sometimes in conjunction with intravenous pulses of methylprednisolone (500 mg–1 g, up to three doses over three days). Due to an increased risk of bladder carcinoma, the safe duration of treatment with cyclophosphamide is limited to 12 months, so immunosuppression is "stepped down" to the less toxic medications azathioprine, mycophenolate, methotrexate or dapsone at the end of this period. Combination therapy is used for resistant cases and includes the combination of a sulpha (dapsone, sulphapyridine) and myelosuppressive agent (azathioprine, mycophenolate, cyclophosphamide) and/or the addition of prednisolone. High-dose oral corticosteroid does not have any role in long-term management, as the high doses required to control disease cannot be sustained due to adverse side effects [5], and the inflammation quickly recurs when the dose is reduced.

Once complete control of inflammation has been achieved (Fig. 2.2b), immunosuppression is continued for at least 12 months. Following this, the dose is slowly tapered and can be stopped if the patient wishes, providing they understand that it must be recommended if disease activity recurs. Lifelong follow-up is necessary, because disease recurs in up to one third of patients [22]. If the disease has been severe and resulted in loss of useful vision in one eye, lifelong therapy is recommended.

2.7.7 Side Effects of Treatment and Monitoring for Toxicity

Blood pressure, blood glucose and blood tests must be evaluated weekly upon the initiation of therapy, and thereafter two weekly or monthly in all patients on immunosuppression, to screen for drug-related toxic side effects. These agents should be used by physicians experienced in administering immunosuppressive agents and many ophthalmologists work with rheumatologists to achieve this. In patients taking cyclophosphamide, lymphopenia is universal and used to titrate treatment; the target lymphocyte count is $0.5-1.0 \times 10^9$ cells/ml [23, 24]. Table 2.3 summarises side effects and toxicity monitoring recommendations for the immunosuppressives used for the management of MMP.

2.7.8 Alternative Immunosuppressive Regimens

Alternatives to conventional immunosuppressive therapy have been sought where ocular MMP is resistant to treatment or in patients who have been unable to tolerate conventional immunosuppressants.

2.7.8.1 Intravenous Immunoglobulin

Severely active ocular MMP resistant to conventional immunosuppressive therapy has been treated with intravenous immunoglobulin (IVIg)

in several case series [41, 42, 66]. A major disadvantage of intravenous immunoglobulin therapy is its dependence on donated blood, an increasingly scarce and expensive resource. In one series, during a national blood shortage, patients received one fourth to one third of previous doses, and every one of the ten patients relapsed with dose reduction, albeit recovering full control within four cycles of full-dose IVIg [41]. Sudden discontinuation of IVIg therapy in two patients resulted in severe recurrence and loss of vision [42]. This is worrying because it is sometimes not possible for patients to present for therapy depending on emergencies and personal situations. Another disadvantage is the inconvenient and costly treatment regime. An infusion cycle of 4 h daily on 3 consecutive days is required every 2 weeks until clinical improvement and then every 3–4 weeks, increasing to 16-week intervals for a total of 25–43 months. The main benefits of IVIg appear to be its minimal side effects and effectiveness in disease refractory to conventional immunosuppression, although the studies are small and not randomised.

2.7.8.2 Tumour Necrosis Factor-α Antagonists

Case reports and small series of patients with MMP resistant to conventional immunosuppressive therapy have been described as improving after receiving the TNF-α antagonists etanercept ($n=6$) or infliximab ($n=1$) or adjuvant pentoxifylline ($n=15$) [31, 43–49]. This treatment was given either alone or in combination with dapsone or other immunosuppressive therapy. In some cases, continued TNF-α antagonist treatment was not necessary after achieving initial disease control, but in many cases, weekly etanercept treatment was ongoing at the time of reporting.

Conjunctival tissue expression of TNF-α has been demonstrated, with decreased but persistently elevated levels of expression in "white" eyes following immunosuppressive therapy [7]. Tissue expression appears to be important because in rheumatoid arthritis, whilst there is no evidence that plasma TNF-α levels can predict the clinical response to TNF-α antagonists,

Table 2.3 Guidelines for the use of immunomodulatory drugs

Drug and route of administration, dose and frequency	Principal side effects and differentiation from disease	Prevention of side effects
Myelosuppressives		
Cyclophosphamide oral 1–2 mg/kg/day [13] Once/day mane with 2 l fluid intake during day	Myelosuppression, lethargy, anorexia, nausea and vomiting, diarrhoea, abdominal discomfort, alopecia, headache, insomnia, myalgia, dyspnoea, dizziness, haemorrhagic cystitis, hepatotoxicity, opportunistic infections, cardiotoxicity, pulmonary fibrosis, azoospermia, teratogenic and risk of neoplasm. Common drug interaction: increased toxicity with allopurinol and other myelosuppressives such as azathioprine [3] *Differentiating side effects from disease*: temporarily discontinue medication to ascertain if side effects resolve. Consider secondary malignancy (or primary paraneoplastic pemphigoid) if persistent anorexia/weight loss despite discontinuing medication	Take concomitant oral clotrimazole as prophylaxis against pneumocystis pneumonia, exclude TB and hepatitis B and C prior to commencing therapy and educate patient regarding appropriate vaccinations and avoidance of infections. FBC, U+E, LFTs, blood sugar, lipids, BP and urinalysis and ± chest x-ray prior to commencing treatment. Monitor for oral candidiasis and use oral nystatin mouthwash. FBC and diff., liver and renal function and urinalysis weekly for 4 weeks, every 2 weeks during second month and then monthly. Target lymphocyte count (0.5–1.0 is target level) and aim for lymphopenia without neutropenia (WCC >3.0 neut. >2.0). If urinalysis positive for blood, send 3 urine samples (1 for cytology, 1 for microbiology culture, 1 for biochemistry analysis). Consider regular mammography and cervical smears (females). If elevated LFTs, stop therapy temporarily till normalises; can then recommence whilst maintaining normal LFTs. Pregnancy testing prior to commencing treatment. Concomitant gonadotropin-releasing hormone in females of childbearing age. Avoid cumulative dose greater than 300 mg/kg in males. Sperm banking
Cyclophosphamide i.v. 1 g/m² body surface area in 250 ml normal saline piggybacked onto 500 ml normal saline without [sodium 2-] mercaptoethane sulfonate, infused over a 2-h period [68] *Frequency*: once every 3–4 weeks depending on clinical response and nadir of leukocyte count	*Commonest*: fatigue, nausea, headache, alopecia, diarrhoea, respiratory tract infection, depression, dyspepsia, dizziness, dyspnoea *Potentially serious*: leukopenia, elevated LFTs, dehydration due to nausea, dyspnoea, opportunistic infections, gonadal failure, infection, haemorrhagic cystitis and bladder carcinoma	Fortnightly FBC incl. differential, U+E, LFTs and urinalysis until drug dosage, disease activity and haematologic parameters stabilised. Aim for WCC between 3,500 and 5,000 cells/ul, neutrophils ≥1,500 cells/ul and platelets ≥75,000 cells/ul. If elevated LFTs, stop therapy temporarily till normalises; can then recommence whilst maintaining normal LFTs. Pregnancy testing prior to commencing treatment. Concomitant gonadotropin-releasing hormone in females of childbearing age. Avoid cumulative dose greater than 300 mg/kg in males. Sperm banking. Pulse IV cyclophosphamide with careful adequate hydration during and post therapy minimises risk of haemorrhagic cystitis to near zero
Mycophenolate oral 1 g bd Morning and evening	GIT disturbance, leukopenia, sepsis, hepatotoxicity, hyperglycaemia and diabetes, dyspnoea, tremor, insomnia. Lymphoma and non-melanoma skin cancers rarely. Opportunistic infections, GIT haemorrhage and pulmonary oedema	FBC, U+E, LFTs, blood sugar, lipids, BP and urinalysis and ± chest x-ray prior to commencing treatment. Educate patient regarding appropriate vaccinations and avoidance of infections. Monitor for oral candidiasis and use oral nystatin mouthwash. Check FBC, liver and renal function and blood glucose weekly for 4 weeks, every 2 weeks for 2nd and 3rd months and then every 1–2 months thereafter

Azathioprine 1–2.5 mg/kg/day, titrate according to TPMT level Once daily	Myelosuppression, GIT disturbance, nausea and vomiting common, pancreatitis, headache, arthralgia, alopecia, hepatotoxicity, opportunistic infections. Common drug interactions: increased myelotoxicity with other immunosuppressants	Check TPMT (thiopurine methyltransferase) level and FBC, U+E, LFTs, blood sugar, lipids, BP and urinalysis and ± chest x-ray prior to commencing treatment. If TPMT <10 pmol/h/mgHb, should NOT receive azathioprine as pancytopenia is likely. If TPMT 10–25 pmol/h/mgHb, give 0.5–1 mg/kg azathioprine; if TPMT 26–50 pmol/h/mgHb, give 1–2 mg/kg; if TPMT >50 pmol/h/mgHb, give 1–2.5 mg/kg. Monitor FBC, liver and renal function and blood glucose weekly for 4 weeks, every 2 weeks for 2nd and 3rd months and then every 1–2 months thereafter. Educate patient regarding appropriate vaccinations and avoidance of infections. Monitor for oral candidiasis and use oral nystatin mouthwash
Methotrexate 10–15 mg once per week	Impaired liver function, hepatic fibrosis/cirrhosis (biopsy recommended every 1,500 mg cumulative dose), GIT disturbance, myelosuppression, interstitial pneumonitis/pulmonary fibrosis, opportunistic infections, ocular irritation and aggravation of seborrhoeic blepharitis. Teratogenic—no conception for 6 months after cessation for both males and females *Differentiating side effects from disease*: discontinue medication temporarily to see if ocular irritation resolves	Take with folic acid 5 mg alternate daily. Monitor FBC, liver function and renal function every month in the first 4 months and then 2 monthly thereafter. Consider lung function monitoring for pulmonary fibrosis. Educate patient regarding appropriate vaccinations and avoidance of infections. Monitor for oral candidiasis and use oral nystatin mouthwash
Sulphonamide		
Dapsone oral 50–150 mg/day	Dose-dependent haemolysis with anaemia and reticulocytosis, infectious mononucleosis-like syndrome, methaemoglobinaemia, GIT disturbance, elevated LFTs, blurred vision, peripheral neuropathy (reversible), psychosis, headache, diarrhoea *Differentiating side effects from disease*: discontinue medication temporarily to see if blurred vision resolves	Contraindicated if G6PD deficient. Check G6PD and FBC, U+E, LFTs, blood sugar, lipids and BP prior to commencing treatment. Monitor FBC and diff. and liver function monthly for 3 months and then 3 monthly. Stop temporarily or reduce dose if Hb <10 g/dl or symptomatic anaemia
Sulphasalazine or sulphapyridine oral Sulphasalazine 1 g bd, sulphapyridine 500 mg bd	GIT disturbance, myelosuppression, rash, reversible oligospermia; rarely: hepatitis, pancreatitis, photosensitisation, neurotoxicity, SLE-like syndrome, fibrosing alveolitis, proteinuria, haematuria, nephrotic syndrome, Stevens-Johnson syndrome, crystalluria	Check FBC, U+E, LFTs, blood sugar, lipids and BP prior to commencing treatment. Monitor FBC and liver and renal function 2 weeks after starting the drug and then monthly for 3 months, and then 3 monthly thereafter

(continued)

Table 2.3 (continued)

Drug and route of administration, dose and frequency	Principal side effects and differentiation from disease	Prevention of side effects
Calcineurin inhibitor		
Ciclosporin oral 3–5 mg/kg/day in two divided doses	Very nephrotoxic—reduce/stop CSA if creatinine >30 % above baseline or increases >20 µm. Also causes hypertension, hepatotoxicity, hirsutism, gingival hyperplasia, neurotoxicity incl. tremor, paraesthesia, hyperlipidaemia, hypomagnesaemia, opportunistic infections. Common drug interactions: enhanced effect—ketoconazole and other azoles, nicardipine, verapamil, diltiazem, erythromycin and the oral contraceptives. Reduced effect—rifampicin, phenytoin, carbamazepine, phenobarbitone. Increased nephrotoxicity—NSAIDS, gentamicin et al., amphotericin	Check FBC, U+E, LFTs, blood sugar, lipids, BP and urinalysis, and ± chest x-ray prior to commencing treatment. Monitor BP 2 weekly for the first 3 months and then 1–2 monthly thereafter. Monitor urinalysis every 1–2 months. Monitor U+E, FBC, LFTs, and blood glucose 2 weekly in the first 3 months and then every 2 months. Check lipids and Mg 3–6 monthly. Check trough levels (12–14 h post dose) monthly till stable in patients being given prophylaxis or if compliance or response is poor (therapeutic range: ciclosporin 100–225 µg/l, tacrolimus 8–12 µg/l). Educate patient regarding appropriate vaccinations and avoidance of infections. Monitor for oral candidiasis; use oral nystatin mouthwash
Steroid		
Prednisolone oral 1–1.5 mg/kg/day in one dose	Hyperglycaemia, mental disturbance (paranoia, psychosis or depression), opportunistic infections and, in the long term, obesity, adrenal suppression, dyspepsia, myopathy, hypertension, osteoporosis, osteonecrosis, elevated intraocular pressure, cataract. Common drug interactions: enhanced effect—ciclosporin, azathioprine, anticoagulants. Reduced effect—carbamazepine, rifampicin, phenytoin, phenobarbitone	Careful management of diabetes. Test vitamin D level. Test bone mineral density annually. BP and blood glucose each visit (weekly when on 40–80 mg). FBC, U+E, urinalysis (glycosuria) and lipids 3 monthly or if new symptoms develop. Take with 2 tabs Calcichew D3 daily ± Fosamax (alendronate) 70 mg weekly [if osteoporosis risk factors and dose ≥7.5 mg/day for ≥6 months] ± omeprazole 20 mg/day. Monitor for oral candidiasis and treat with nystatin mouthwash if necessary. Aim to discontinue steroids to avoid Cushing's syndrome in the long term
Methylprednisolone i.v. 0.5–1 g daily for 1–3 days	Cardiac arrhythmia, cardiac arrest, circulatory collapse, electrolyte disturbance, potassium depletion. Hyperglycaemia, mental disturbance (paranoia, psychosis or depression), opportunistic infections and, in the long term, obesity, adrenal suppression, dyspepsia, myopathy, hypertension, osteoporosis, elevated intraocular pressure, cataract. Common drug interactions: Care with digoxin electrolyte imbalance. Enhanced effect—ciclosporin, azathioprine, anticoagulants. Reduced effect—carbamazepine, rifampicin, phenytoin, phenobarbitone	Administer in hospital with monitoring of vital obs, BSL and urinalysis. Check ECG and electrolytes before infusion. Careful management of diabetes. Test vitamin D level. Test bone mineral density annually. Exclude TB prior to commencing therapy; educate patient regarding appropriate vaccinations and avoidance of infections. FBC, U+E, LFTs, blood sugar, lipids, BP and urinalysis and ± chest x-ray prior to commencing treatment. FBC, U+E, urinalysis (glycosuria), lipids 3 monthly or if new symptoms develop. Take with 2 tabs Calcichew D3 daily+Fosamax (alendronate) 70 mg weekly [if osteoporosis risk factors]+omeprazole 20 mg/day. Monitor for oral candidiasis and treat with nystatin mouthwash if necessary. Aim to discontinue long-term steroids to avoid Cushing's syndrome

Biologicals

Intravenous immunoglobulin (IVIG) 2–3 g/kg/cycle given in 3 equal doses on 3 consecutive days One cycle every 2–4 weeks until stabilised and then up to 2 cycles every 6, 8, 10, 12 or 16 weeks	Infusion reactions (fever, headache, myalgia, nausea, cardiovascular overload), haemolytic anaemia, hepatitis viral contamination, aseptic meningitis, renal failure, thrombotic stroke, alopecia	Contraindicated in presence of anti-IgA antibodies. Avoid/caution in renal failure and rheumatoid factor activity. Slow infusion. Administer under medically trained physician supervision
Infliximab i.v. 5 mg/kg infusions at zero, 2 weeks, 6 weeks and then 8 weekly (Heffernan 2006)	Infusion reactions (fever, headache, myalgia, nausea, hypotension), hepatotoxicity, lung or chest infections, dyspnoea, chest pain, GIT disturbance, lethargy, circulatory disturbance, multiple sclerosis-like disease, bacterial infections, arthralgia, anaemia, lymphoma, autoimmune disorders, meningitis	Administer under medically trained physician supervision
Etanercept subcut. 50 mg once weekly or 25 mg twice weekly	Infections, injection site reactions, autoantibody formation, allergic reactions, secondary malignancy, eye inflammation, psoriasis, nervous system disorders, congestive heart failure	Do
Rituximab i.v. 375 mg/m² body surface area once a week for 4 weeks or 2 infusions given 2 weeks apart. These cycles are repeated after 3–4 months for nonresponders or relapses	Infusion reactions (fever, headache, myalgia, nausea, hypotension), pancytopenia, hypogammaglobulinaemia and severe infections leading to death, cardiac events, autoimmune events, severe mucocutaneous reactions, progressive multifocal leukoencephalopathy	Administer under medically trained physician supervision. Detailed workup to exclude contraindicating conditions. CT neck, chest and pelvis to exclude pre-existing malignancy prior to treatment. Monitor lymphocyte counts and B cell levels during treatment

synovial expression of TNF-α appears to be a significant predictor of response to TNF-α antagonists [46]. Serum levels of TNF-α are elevated in MMP compared to normal controls [48].

Rituximab

There is currently a lot of interest in the use of rituximab, a monoclonal antibody directed against CD20-positive B cells, for the management of immunobullous disease in general as well as for the treatment of cases of ocular MMP refractory to treatment with *conventional* immunosuppression using nonbiological drugs. This therapy is likely to be useful in preventing pathogenic autoantibody production by B cells. Limitations in delivery of this biological have been the expense and lack of evidence from randomised controlled trials, which have proved impossible to conduct to date. The evidence available is from case series reporting the successful use of rituximab in 40 cases (25 with ocular involvement) of severe refractory MMP not responding to conventional immunosuppression [50–55] including a study of 6 patients with severe ocular MMP treated with rituximab and IVIg [56]. These results are given in detail in Table 2.4.

Serious Side Effects Probably due to Rituximab in These Series

Three patient in these series developed serious infections (two pulmonary and one renal), leading to two deaths [55]. These were attributed to pretreatment hypogammaglobulinaemia and the concomitant use of additional immunosuppressants. Lourari et al. reported a sudden death shortly after giving rituximab which may have been due to cardiac disease [54]. However, these severe side effects are uncommon except when combined with other immunosuppressants [57] and may also occur with conventional drugs like cyclophosphamide, such that a recent dermatology editorial has asked whether rituximab might be considered a drug of first choice in MMP [58].

Recommended Protocol for the Use of Rituximab

In the absence of clinical trials and studies comparing the use of 2 infusions (of 375 mg/m^2) given 2 weeks apart versus 4 infusions (of 375 mg/m^2) given weekly for 4 weeks, together with the reports of responders following a second cycle of infusions at 4 months [55], we have been recommending 2 infusions (of 375 mg/m^2) 2 weeks apart, repeated at 4 months if there is an inadequate response or a relapse. Because of the risk of life-threatening pulmonary infection attributed to the concomitant use of additional immunosuppressant's [55], we have discontinued all other immunosuppressants at the time of the first infusion of rituximab, apart from dapsone which has been continued, or started, unless otherwise contraindicated (Table 2.4).

Other Biological Drugs

Daclizumab, a monoclonal antibody which binds CD25 (Tac subunit) of the human IL-2 receptor which is expressed on activated T lymphocytes, has been used successfully in one patient with ocular MMP [59]. Its use in ocular MMP has not been investigated further.

Systemic administration of Campath-1H (alemtuzumab), a monoclonal antibody against CD52, which is the most prevalent cell-surface antigen on lymphocytes, particularly T cells, has been reported to induce long-lasting remission in patients with severe refractory noninfectious ocular inflammatory disease [60]. It has been given systemically by us to one patient with ocular MMP (unpublished data) but was unfortunately unsuccessful in controlling inflammation, and the patient developed atrial fibrillation.

2.8   Control of Fibrosis

Currently, the only demonstrated means of slowing the progression of scarring is good control of inflammation with systemic immunosuppression. Mondino et al. have previously reported success with systemic corticosteroids in suppressing acute disease activity and preventing the rapid shrinkage that accompanies active ocular MMP [16]. Therapy specifically targeted at fibrosis in MMP is limited. Local therapies for conjunctival scarring would be ideal. Mitomycin C, an alkylating agent which inhibits DNA synthesis and prevents fibroblast proliferation, has been injected subconjunctivally [61]

Table 2.4 Summary of reports of rituximab therapy of MMP with ocular involvement ($n=25$) and MMP with other sites involved ($n=15$)

Authors	Site of involvement by MMP	Number of infusions per course of treatment	Subsequent courses and interval between courses	Other immunosuppressants or not	Complications	Outcomes
Doan et al. [50]	4 ocular and laryngeal	4 infusions (of 375 mg/m^2) given weekly for 4 weeks	Unstated but 2 patients had further courses given	All discontinued except for dapsone	None reported	Responded in 4–8 weeks
Taverna et al. [51]	1 ocular, oral and skin	As above	Repeated at 3 months and then 4 maintenance infusions given every 3 months on 3 occasions	Mycophenolate and prednisolone	None reported	Responded after 16 weeks
Schumann et al. [53]	1 ocular, skin, perianal	4 infusions (of 375 mg/m^2) given weekly for 4 weeks	None required	Methylprednisolone and dexamethasone continued for 6 months	None	Responded within 6 months and remained quiescent 6 months after withdrawal of oral steroids
Ross et al. [52]	1 ocular, oral, skin and genital	2 infusions (of 375 mg/m^2) given 2 weeks apart	Not given	Uncertain	None reported	Responded after 6 weeks and in remission by 6 months
Foster et al. [56]	6 ocular (presence of disease at other sites not stated)	8 infusions (of 375 mg/m^2) given weekly for 8 weeks	1 infusion (of 375 mg/m^2) given monthly for months	In combination with IV immunoglobulin (IVIg) at 2 g/kg per course. Repeated monthly until B-cell levels normal and then at 6, 8, 10, 12, 14 and 16 weeks	None	All responded but time to response not reported
Lourari et al. [54]	2 ocular, oral, genital and nasal	4 infusions (of 375 mg/m^2) given weekly for 4 weeks	Not given	Oral prednisolone	None in ocular patients. 1 sudden death in a non-ocular probably due to heart disease and unrelated to therapy	1 complete remission and 1 partial remission
Le Roux-Villet et al. [55]	10 severe ocular or ocular/laryngeal AND 15 severe MMP at other sites	4 infusions (of 375 mg/m^2) given weekly for 4 weeks	Repeated at 4 months in 1 patient not responding to the first cycle	Dapsone	1 ocular and 2 other patients developed severe infections of whom 2 died	9/10 ocular cases responded at a median of 10 weeks. Overall, 22/25 responded fully after 2 cycles of therapy

or applied intraoperatively following division of symblephara in patients with ocular MMP [62] but no controlled treatment trials have been carried out. In the Donnenfeld study, absence of progression at a mean of 2 years was observed in 8/9 eyes receiving the subconjunctival mitomycin C injection, and there was no recurrence of symblephara at 19 months. Subconjunctival mitomycin C is not widely used in clinical practice for ocular MMP for several reasons, including variable efficacy, the adverse effect of tissue ischaemia which may affect the success of mucous membrane graft reconstructive surgery and the potential risk of damaging limbal stem cells. In Donnenfeld's series, all eyes receiving subconjunctival mitomycin C were Foster stage 3 with minimal or no inflammation. It may be that giving the injection at an earlier stage, whilst the disease is active, could prevent cicatrisation more effectively.

## 2.9	Surgery and Contact Lenses

Providing conjunctival inflammation is controlled beforehand both clear corneal incision cataract surgery and anterior lamellar reposition, or retractor plication surgery (that does not involve conjunctival incisions), for entropion is safe [23, 24] and does not require increased perioperative immunosuppression.

### 2.9.1	Fornix Reconstruction Surgery

Fornix reconstruction surgery, indicated for corneal exposure, carries a high risk of a severe disease exacerbation and requires increased systemic immunosuppression for a minimum of 2 months before surgery, with a perioperative course of oral corticosteroids [63]. Frequent monitoring after plastic surgery, to identify and manage the corneal epithelial defects that may complicate the surgery, is critical.

### 2.9.2	Rigid Contact Lenses

Rigid contact lenses can be useful for comfort and as treatment for irregular astigmatism in scarred corneas; MMP eyes are usually too dry for soft lens use.

### 2.9.3	Keratoplasty and Ocular Surface Reconstruction

Keratoplasty and ocular surface reconstruction are contraindicated in dry eyes and result in poor outcomes [64], due to the suboptimal corneal environment, causing poor epithelialisation, melt, infection, corneal vascularisation and disease reactivation.

### 2.9.4	Keratoprosthesis Surgery

Keratoprosthesis surgery is high risk and complications are frequent, but good visual outcomes can be achieved with the osteo-odonto keratoprosthesis for bilaterally blind patients [65].

## 2.10	Future Directions

As can be seen from this chapter, the major issues in the management of ocular MMP are several:

- There is little to offer patients who have reached the stage of dry eye, surface failure and ankyloblepharon apart from OOKP, which is costly and not widely available. Early diagnosis is critical in preventing this stage of the disease.
- Diagnosis is often delayed due to failure of clinicians to recognise early signs of what is a rare disease. The difficulty in diagnosis is compounded by the poor sensitivity of direct immunofluorescence, which is negative in 14–40 % of patients with typical signs of ocular MMP. Current studies into the autoantibody response to epithelial basement membrane epitopes are likely to lead both to improvements in diagnosis and to our understanding of disease pathogenesis. Genetic studies may help identify susceptible individuals leading to higher diagnostic certainty.
- Management of the inflammation in many patients requires toxic systemic therapies. The success of newer approaches using more targeted biological drugs may reduce toxicity and potentially provide local ocular therapies as opposed to systemic treatment. A better understanding of the pathogenesis of inflammation in this disease is key to making

use of available biologics and identifying potential new therapies.

- There have been very few treatments directed against the problem of scarring which probably progresses independently from inflammation once the disease has started. Developing antiscarring therapies is an exciting area of research in many body systems for which there are as yet no licensed drugs. This is an area that is likely to develop rapidly in the next decade.

References

1. Chan LS, Ahmed AR, Anhalt GJ, Bernauer W, Cooper KD, Elder MJ, Fine JD, Foster CS, Ghohestani R, Hashimoto T, Hoang-Xuan T, Kirtschig G, Korman NJ, Lightman S, Lozada-Nur F, Marinkovich MP, Mondino BJ, Prost-Squarcioni III C, Rogers RS, Setterfield JF, West DP, Wojnarowska F, Woodley DT, Yancey KB, Zillikens D, Zone JJ. The first international consensus on mucous membrane pemphigoid: definition, diagnostic criteria, pathogenic factors, medical treatment, and prognostic indicators. Arch Dermatol. 2002;138(3):370–9.
2. Saw VP, Dart JK. Ocular mucous membrane pemphigoid: diagnosis and management strategies. Ocul Surf. 2008;6(3):128–42.
3. Saw VP, Dart JK, Rauz S, Ramsay A, Bunce C, Xing W, Maddison PG, Phillips M. Immunosuppressive therapy for ocular mucous membrane pemphigoid strategies and outcomes. Ophthalmology. 2008;115:253–61.
4. Saw VPJ, Dart JKG, Reinhard LFT. Management of ocular mucous membrane pemphigoid. In: Kriegelstein GK, Weinreb RN, editors. Cornea and external eye disease. Berlin/Heidelberg: Springer; 2008. p. 154–75.
5. Hardy KM, Perry HO, Pingree GC, Kirby Jr TJ. Benign mucous membrane pemphigoid. Arch Dermatol. 1971;104(5):467–75.
6. Black AP, Wojnarowska F, Ogg GS. Role of T cells in the pathogenesis of mucous membrane pemphigoid. Expert Rev Dermatol. 2006;1(1):25–30.
7. Saw VP, Dart RJ, Galatowicz G, Daniels JT, Dart JK, Calder VL, Minassian D, Ramsay A, Henderson H, Poniatowski S, Warwick RM, Cabral S, Offiah I, Sitaru C, Zillikens D. Tumor necrosis factor-alpha in ocular mucous membrane pemphigoid and its effect on conjunctival fibroblasts. Invest Ophthalmol Vis Sci. 2009;50(11):5310–7.
8. Saw VP, Offiah I, Dart RJ, Galatowicz G, Dart JK, Daniels JT, Calder VL. Conjunctival interleukin-13 expression in mucous membrane pemphigoid and functional effects of interleukin-13 on conjunctival fibroblasts in vitro. Am J Pathol. 2009;175(6):2406–15.
9. Saw VP, Schmidt E, Offiah I, Galatowicz G, Zillikens D, Dart JK, Calder VL, Daniels JT, Dart RJ, Williams GP, Saeed T, Evans ST, Cottrell P, Curnow SJ, Nightingale P, Rauz S, Sitaru C. Profibrotic phenotype of conjunctival fibroblasts from mucous membrane pemphigoid. Am J Pathol. 2011;178(1):187–97.
10. Tauber J. Ocular cicatricial pemphigoid. Ophthalmology. 2008;115(9):1639–40; author reply 1640–31.
11. Tauber J, Sainz DLM, Foster CS. Systemic chemotherapy for ocular cicatricial pemphigoid. Cornea. 1991;10(3):185–95.
12. Mondino BJ, Brown SI, Lempert S, Jenkins MS. The acute manifestations of ocular cicatricial pemphigoid: diagnosis and treatment. Ophthalmology. 1979;86(4):543–55.
13. Foster CS. Cicatricial pemphigoid. Trans Am Ophthalmol Soc. 1986;84:527–663.
14. Elder MJ, Bernauer W, Leonard J, Dart JK. Progression of disease in ocular cicatricial pemphigoid. Br J Ophthalmol. 1996;80(4):292–6.
15. Holland EJ, Olsen TW, Ketcham JM, Florine C, Krachmer JH, Purcell JJ, Lam S, Tessler HH, Sugar J. Topical cyclosporin A in the treatment of anterior segment inflammatory disease. Cornea. 1993;12(5):413–9.
16. Mondino BJ, Brown SI. Ocular cicatricial pemphigoid. Ophthalmology. 1981;88(2):95–100.
17. Mondino BJ, Brown SI. Immunosuppressive therapy in ocular cicatricial pemphigoid. Am J Ophthalmol. 1983;96(4):453–9.
18. Foster CS, Wilson LA, Ekins MB. Immunosuppressive therapy for progressive ocular cicatricial pemphigoid. Ophthalmology. 1982;89(4):340–53.
19. Mondino BJ. Cicatricial pemphigoid and erythema multiforme. Ophthalmology. 1990;97(7):939–52.
20. Rogers III RS, Seehafer JR, Perry HO. Treatment of cicatricial (benign mucous membrane) pemphigoid with dapsone. J Am Acad Dermatol. 1982;6(2):215–23.
21. Neumann R, Tauber J, Foster CS. Remission and recurrence after withdrawal of therapy for ocular cicatricial pemphigoid. Ophthalmology. 1991;98(6):858–62.
22. Foster CS, Neumann R, Tauber J. Long-term results of systemic chemotherapy for ocular cicatricial pemphigoid. Doc Ophthalmol. 1992;82(3):223–9.
23. Elder MJ, Lightman S, Dart JK. Role of cyclophosphamide and high dose steroid in ocular cicatricial pemphigoid. Br J Ophthalmol. 1995;79(3):264–6.
24. Elder MJ, Dart JK, Collin R. Inferior retractor plication surgery for lower lid entropion with trichiasis in ocular cicatricial pemphigoid. Br J Ophthalmol. 1995;79(11):1003–6.
25. Elder MJ, Leonard J, Dart JK. Sulphapyridine: a new agent for the treatment of ocular cicatricial pemphigoid. Br J Ophthalmol. 1996;80(6):549–52.
26. Doan S, Lerouic JF, Robin H, Prost C, Savoldelli M, Hoang-Xuan T. Treatment of ocular cicatricial pemphigoid with sulfasalazine. Ophthalmology. 2001;108(9):1565–8.
27. Letko E, Ahmed AR, Foster CS. Treatment of ocular cicatricial pemphigoid with tacrolimus (FK 506).

Graefes Arch Clin Exp Ophthalmol. 2001;239(6): 441–4.

28. McCluskey P, Chang JH, Singh R, Wakefield D. Methotrexate therapy for ocular cicatricial pemphigoid. Ophthalmology. 2004;111(4):796–801.

29. Thorne JE, Woreta FA, Jabs DA, Anhalt GJ. Treatment of ocular mucous membrane pemphigoid with immunosuppressive drug therapy. Ophthalmology. 2008;115(12):2146–52 e2141.

30. Miserocchi E, Baltatzis S, Roque MR, Ahmed AR, Foster CS. The effect of treatment and its related side effects in patients with severe ocular cicatricial pemphigoid. Ophthalmology. 2002;109(1):111–8.

31. Sacher C, Rubbert A, Konig C, Scharffetter-Kochanek K, Krieg T, Hunzelmann N. Treatment of recalcitrant cicatricial pemphigoid with the tumor necrosis factor alpha antagonist etanercept. J Am Acad Dermatol. 2002;46(1):113–5.

32. Smith MD, Bertouch JV, Smith AM, Weatherall M, Ahern MJ, Brooks PM, Roberts-Thomson PJ, Needs CJ, Smith M, Boutagy J, Donovan S, Cosh D, McCredie M. The clinical and immunological effects of pulse methylprednisolone therapy in rheumatoid arthritis. I. Clinical effects. Comparison of methylprednisolone (1g i.v.) with prednisolone (1g orally) in rheumatoid arthritis: a pharmacokinetic and clinical study. J Rheumatol. 1988;15(2):229–32.

33. Reiche L, Wojnarowska F, Mallon E. Combination therapy with nicotinamide and tetracyclines for cicatricial pemphigoid: further support for its efficacy. Clin Exp Dermatol. 1998;23(6):254–7.

34. Dragan L, Eng AM, Lam S, Persson T. Tetracycline and niacinamide: treatment alternatives in ocular cicatricial pemphigoid. Cutis. 1999;63(3):181–3.

35. Megahed M, Schmiedeberg S, Becker J, Ruzicka T. Treatment of cicatricial pemphigoid with mycophenolate mofetil as a steroid-sparing agent. J Am Acad Dermatol. 2001;45(2):256–9.

36. Ingen-Housz-Oro S, Prost-Squarcioni C, Pascal F, Doan S, Brette MD, Bachelez H, Dubertret L. Cicatricial pemphigoid: treatment with mycophenolate mofetil. Ann Dermatol Venereol. 2005;132(1):13–6.

37. Zurdel J, Aboalchamat B, Zierhut M, Stubiger N, Bialasiewicz A, Engelmann K. Early clinical results with mycophenolate mofetil in immunosuppressive therapy of ocular pemphigoid. Klin Monatsbl Augenheilkd. 2001;218(4):222–8.

38. Elder MJ, Dart JK, Lightman S. Conjunctival fibrosis in ocular cicatricial pemphigoid: the role of cytokines. Exp Eye Res. 1997;65(2):165–76.

39. Bernauer W, Wright P, Dart JK, Leonard JN, Lightman S. The conjunctiva in acute and chronic mucous membrane pemphigoid. An immunohistochemical analysis. Ophthalmology. 1993;100(3):339–46.

40. Elder MJ. The role of cytokines in chronic progressive conjunctival cicatrisation. Dev Ophthalmol. 1997; 28:159–75.

41. Foster CS, Ahmed AR. Intravenous immunoglobulin therapy for ocular cicatricial pemphigoid: a preliminary study. Ophthalmology. 1999;106(11):2136–43.

42. Sami N, Letko E, Androudi S, Daoud Y, Foster CS, Ahmed AR. Intravenous immunoglobulin therapy in patients with ocular-cicatricial pemphigoid: a long-term follow-up. Ophthalmology. 2004;111(7): 1380–2.

43. Canizares MJ, Smith DI, Conners MS, Maverick KJ, Heffernan MP. Successful treatment of mucous membrane pemphigoid with etanercept in 3 patients. Arch Dermatol. 2006;142(11):1457–61.

44. Sacher C, Hunzelmann N. Cicatricial pemphigoid (mucous membrane pemphigoid): current and emerging therapeutic approaches. Am J Clin Dermatol. 2005;6(2):93–103.

45. Heffernan DD, Bentley DD. Successful treatment of mucous membrane pemphigoid with infliximab. Arch Dermatol. 2006;142(10):1268–70.

46. Wijbrandts CA, Dijkgraaf MG, Kraan MC, Vinkenoog M, Smeets TJ, Dinant H, et al. The clinical response to infliximab in rheumatoid arthritis is in part dependent on pretreatment tumour necrosis factor alpha expression in the synovium. Ann Rheum Dis. 2008;67(8):1139–44.

47. John H, Whallett A, Quinlan M. Successful biologic treatment of ocular mucous membrane pemphigoid with anti-TNF-alpha. Eye (Lond). 2007;21(11): 1434–5.

48. Lee SJ, Li Z, Sherman B, Foster CS. Serum levels of tumor necrosis factor-alpha and interleukin-6 in ocular cicatricial pemphigoid. Invest Ophthalmol Vis Sci. 1993;34(13):3522–5.

49. Prey S, Robert PY, Drouet M, Sparsa A, Roux C, Bonnetblanc JM, Bedane C. Treatment of ocular cicatricial pemphigoid with the tumour necrosis factor alpha antagonist etanercept. Acta Derm Venereol. 2007;87(1):74–5.

50. Doan S, Roux-Villet C, Prost-Squarcioni C, Caux F, Hoang-Xuan T. Rituximab in severe ocular cicatricial pemphigoid. ARVO Meeting Abstr. 2006;47(5):594.

51. Taverna JA, Lerner A, Bhawan J, Demierre MF. Successful adjuvant treatment of recalcitrant mucous membrane pemphigoid with anti-CD20 antibody rituximab. J Drugs Dermatol. 2007;6(7):731–2.

52. Ross A, Jaycock HP, Cook SD, Dick AD, Tole DM. The use of rituximab in refractory mucous membrane pemphigoid with severe ocular involvement. Br J Ophthalmol. 2009;93(4):421–2, 548.

53. Schumann T, Schmidt E, Booken N, Goerdt S, Goebeler M. Successful treatment of mucous membrane pemphigoid with the anti-CD-20 antibody rituximab. Acta Derm Venereol. 2009;89(1):101–2.

54. Lourari S, Herve C, Doffoel-Hantz V, Meyer N, Bulai-Livideanu C, Viraben R, Maza A, Adoue D, Bedane C, Paul C. Bullous and mucous membrane pemphigoid show a mixed response to rituximab: experience in seven patients. J Eur Acad Dermatol Venereol. 2010;25:1238–40.

55. Le Roux-Villet C, Prost-Squarcioni C, Alexandre M, Caux F, Pascal F, Doan S, Brette MD, Soued I, Gabison E, Aucouturier F, Letestu R, Laroche L, Bachelez H. Rituximab for patients with refractory

mucous membrane pemphigoid. Arch Dermatol. 2011;147(7):843–9.

56. Foster CS, Chang PY, Ahmed AR. Combination of rituximab and intravenous immunoglobulin for recalcitrant ocular cicatricial pemphigoid: a preliminary report. Ophthalmology. 2010;117(5):861–9.

57. Edwards JC, Szczepanski L, Szechinski J, Filipowicz-Sosnowska A, Emery P, Close DR, Stevens RM, Shaw T. Efficacy of B-cell-targeted therapy with rituximab in patients with rheumatoid arthritis. N Engl J Med. 2004;350(25):2572–81.

58. Hertl M, Bernard P, Borradori L. Rituximab for severe mucous membrane pemphigoid: safe enough to be drug of first choice? Arch Dermatol. 2011;147(7):855–6.

59. Papaliodis GN, Chu D, Foster CS. Treatment of ocular inflammatory disorders with daclizumab. Ophthalmology. 2003;110(4):786–9.

60. Dick AD, Meyer P, James T, Forrester JV, Hale G, Waldmann H, Isaacs JD. Campath-1H therapy in refractory ocular inflammatory disease. Br J Ophthalmol. 2000;84(1):107–9.

61. Donnenfeld ED, Perry HD, Wallerstein A, Caronia RM, Kanellopoulos AJ, Sforza PD, D'Aversa G. Subconjunctival mitomycin C for the treatment of ocular cicatricial pemphigoid. Ophthalmology. 1999;106(1):72–8.

62. Secchi AG, Tognon MS. Intraoperative mitomycin C in the treatment of cicatricial obliterations of conjunctival fornices. Am J Ophthalmol. 1996;122(5):728–30.

63. Heiligenhaus A, Shore JW, Rubin PA, Foster CS. Long-term results of mucous membrane grafting in ocular cicatricial pemphigoid. Implications for patient selection and surgical considerations. Ophthalmology. 1993;100(9):1283–8.

64. MacLeod JD, Dart JK, Gray TB. Corneal and cataract surgery in chronic progressive conjunctival cicatrisation. Dev Ophthalmol. 1997;28:228–39.

65. Falcinelli G, Falsini B, Taloni M, Colliardo P. Modified osteo-odonto-keratoprosthesis for treatment of corneal blindness: long-term anatomical and functional outcomes in 181 cases. Arch Ophthalmol. 2005;123(10):1319–29.

66. Letko E, Miserocchi E, Daoud YJ, Christen W, Foster CS, Ahmed AR. A nonrandomized comparison of the clinical outcome of ocular involvement in patients with mucous membrane (cicatricial) pemphigoid between conventional immunosuppressive and intravenous immunoglobulin therapies. Clin Immunol. 2004;111(3):303–10.

67. El Darouti MA, Fakhry Khattab MA, Hegazy RA, Hafez DA, Gawdat HI. Pentoxifylline (anti-tumor necrosis factor drug): effective adjuvant therapy in the control of ocular cicatricial pemphigoid. Eur J Ophthalmol. 2011;21(5):529–37.

68. Durrani K, Papaliodis GN, Foster CS. Pulse IV cyclophosphamide in ocular inflammatory disease: efficacy and short-term safety. Ophthalmology. 2004 May;111(5):960–5.

Claire Hooper and Peter McCluskey

Contents

C. Hooper, MBBS
Department of Ophthalmology,
Liverpool Hospital, 23/45-47 Goulburn Street,
Liverpool, NSW 2170, Australia
e-mail: cy_hooper@hotmail.com

P. McCluskey, MD, FRANZCO, FRACS (✉)
Department of Ophtalmology,
Save Sight Institute, South Block
Sydney Hospital & Sydney Eye Hospital,
8 Macquarie Street, Sydney, NSW 2000, Australia
e-mail: peter.mccluskey@sydney.edu.au

3.1 Immune Modulation and Anti-inflammatory Therapy of Scleritis

3.1.1 Definition and Classification

Scleritis is defined as inflammation of the sclera, with dilatation or closure of the deep episcleral vascular plexus being its hallmark clinical sign. The most widely used classification system is that developed by Watson and Hayreh which divides scleritis into anterior and posterior types. Anterior scleritis is further subclassified into diffuse, nodular and necrotising scleritis, with or without inflammation (scleromalacia perforans) [1]. Anatomical classification is useful in that it correlates well with severity, with diffuse anterior scleritis being generally the most benign, nodular scleritis being of intermediate severity and necrotising scleritis being the most severe and difficult to treat [2]. The majority of patients remain in the same clinical category throughout the course of their disease. In a study of 290 patients, of the 104 (35.9 %) patients who experienced a recurrence, only 12 progressed from diffuse to nodular anterior scleritis, and 10 patients who originally had nodular scleritis developed necrotising scleritis [2].

Posterior scleritis is defined as involvement of the sclera posterior to the insertion of the rectus muscles and may occur in the presence or absence of anterior scleritis. In a study of 99 patients with posterior scleritis, 36 patients had anterior scleritis at the time of presentation and 59 patients

U. Pleyer et al. (eds.), *Immune Modulation and Anti-Inflammatory Therapy in Ocular Disorders*,
DOI 10.1007/978-3-642-54350-0_3, © Springer-Verlag Berlin Heidelberg 2014

developed anterior scleritis at some time during follow-up [3]. Diffuse and nodular forms of posterior scleritis can be identified either clinically or on B-scan ultrasonography. Necrotising posterior scleritis has been reported on histopathologic examination of enucleated eyes but currently cannot be differentiated either clinically or on B-scan ultrasonography [3].

3.1.2 Clinical Features

The mean age of onset of scleritis is around 50 years, with females accounting for 56–71 % of patients. Scleritis is frequently unilateral initially, but bilateral disease develops in 35–51 % of patients [3–9]. The characteristic feature of scleritis is the subacute onset of boring, deep, periocular pain which may radiate to the temple and jaw. The pain is typically worse at night, interfering with sleep and waking the patient early in the morning [10]. It may be exacerbated by eye movement or accommodation and can be so severe as to interfere with normal activities – particularly in patients with necrotising scleritis with inflammation. However, in some patients pain may not be a prominent feature – particularly patients with posterior scleritis or those who are already taking anti-inflammatory medications. Other symptoms related to anterior scleritis include photophobia and watering. Approximately 30 % of patients with posterior scleritis present with reduced vision [3]. Scleromalacia perforans may also present with blurred vision due to high astigmatism from loss of scleral rigidity, or may be asymptomatic [11].

The clinical signs of scleritis vary according to the location of the scleritis and its severity. In addition, complications of scleritis, such as keratitis, uveitis, raised intraocular pressure, cataract, exudative retinal detachment and optic disc oedema, may be present due to spillover of the scleral inflammation into adjacent structures.

Diffuse anterior scleritis is the most common form of scleritis and manifests as an intense violaceous vascular congestion, often best appreciated in natural light, which may be localised to a patch of the sclera or may involve the entire anterior

sclera. Slit lamp examination reveals scleral oedema with oedema of the overlying episcleral tissue and disruption of the normal radial pattern of the superficial episcleral vessels. Use of the red-free light aids visualisation of the engorged deep episcleral vascular plexus. Application of phenylephrine 10 %, which blanches the superficial episcleral and conjunctival plexuses, can also aid detection of deep episcleral vascular plexus involvement. Following an acute episode, the sclera may assume a grey-blue discolouration, which is due to rearrangement of the scleral collagen fibres and should not be confused with scleral thinning [10].

Nodular anterior scleritis is characterised by the development of discrete nodules of scleral oedema which are a deep red in colour, immobile and extremely tender and quite separate from the overlying oedematous episclera. They may be multiple and may become confluent [10].

Necrotising anterior scleritis with inflammation is an uncommon form of scleritis. It is characterised by poor or absent perfusion of the episcleral vascular plexuses resulting in a white avascular thinned area of sclera with intense inflammation at the edge of the lesion. There may also be yellow-white avascular areas of episcleral, and sometimes conjunctival, tissue overlying an area of scleral oedema. Scleral necrosis may result in exposure of the underlying dark grey-black uvea, covered by only a thin layer of conjunctiva [10]. Associated keratitis, anterior uveitis and elevated intraocular pressure are common, and staphyloma formation may occur [11].

Necrotising anterior scleritis without inflammation (scleromalacia perforans) is a very rare form of scleritis. Areas of sclera and episclera become white, avascular and thinned and may become sequestered from surrounding normal tissue [10]. Large areas of underlying uvea may become exposed, but staphylomas do not occur in the absence of raised intraocular pressure. There is no associated keratitis but peripheral corneal thinning may occur [11].

Posterior scleritis is more common than previously recognised. It may occur in association with anterior scleritis, in which case the hallmark features of scleral oedema and congestion of the deep episcleral vascular plexus will be present. If it occurs in isolation, the eye may appear white, but inflamed posterior sclera may sometimes be visualised at the extremes of gaze [11]. In a large series of posterior scleritis [3], serous retinal detachment was the most common posterior segment finding. Other signs included optic disc swelling, subretinal localised granuloma, choroidal effusion and folds, RPE changes, retinal vasculitis, low-grade uveitis and raised intraocular pressure. In 17 % of cases there were no signs. B-scan ultrasonography is the key to diagnosis and can demonstrate increased thickness of the ocular coats (greater than 2.0 mm is considered abnormal), fluid in the Tenon capsule (T-sign), optic disc swelling, retinal detachment and scleral nodules [3].

3.1.3 Differential Diagnosis

Episcleritis is the main differential diagnosis and must be distinguished from scleritis because it is a benign condition in which complications are more likely to result from aggressive management than from the disease itself. The onset of episcleritis is usually acute, and the patient's chief complaint is redness and mild discomfort, in contrast to scleritis in which pain is usually the prominent feature. In episcleritis, only the superficial episcleral vascular plexus is engorged, resulting in a pinkish-red colour, as opposed to the violaceous hue seen with deep episcleral vascular plexus involvement in scleritis. These subtle colour differences are often best appreciated in natural light. Slit lamp examination with red-free light reveals congestion and outward displacement of the conjunctival and superficial episcleral vascular plexuses, but their radial configuration is preserved, there are no areas of capillary non-perfusion and the deep episcleral vascular plexus is uninvolved, lying flat against non-oedematous scleral tissue. Application of phenylephrine 10 % will blanch the conjunctival and superficial episcleral vascular plexuses, but will not blanch the deep episcleral vascular congestion of scleritis. Occasionally, episcleritis may progress to scleritis so careful examination of each recurrence of inflammation is required.

Other differential diagnoses of anterior scleritis include conjunctival squamous cell carcinoma, in which corneal and scleral invasion may occur, and lymphoma which classically presents with a salmon pink, elevated, solid mass [11]. These tumours typically obscure the normal vascular architecture. A biopsy is required if the diagnosis is in doubt. Carotico-cavernous fistula causes vascular congestion which does not blanch with phenylephrine, but the corkscrew vessels are diagnostic. Intraocular tumours, in particular choroidal melanoma, may mimic posterior uveitis, but features on B-scan ultrasonography should differentiate between them [11].

3.1.4 Aetiology

Scleritis may be idiopathic in origin, associated with a systemic autoimmune disorder or associated with local or systemic infection. Other causes include postoperative, traumatic, metabolic (gout) and drug-induced, in particular bisphosphonates. Scleritis can also be associated with intraocular and orbital neoplasms.

3.1.4.1 Systemic Autoimmune Associations

A US tertiary referral centre found an associated systemic autoimmune disorder in 50 % of patients [12, 13]. In contrast, a non-tertiary referral centre identified an associated systemic autoimmune disorder in only 31 % of cases [7]. Japanese studies have revealed even lower incidences of 15–22 % [6]. A UK tertiary referral centre series of posterior scleritis reported 29 % of patients as having an associated systemic disease. Patients older than 50 years of age and those who developed an associated anterior scleritis had a significantly increased risk of associated systemic autoimmune disorders [3]. Scleritis is most commonly associated with rheumatoid arthritis (RA) and Wegener granulomatosis (WG). Seronegative spondyloarthropathies, relapsing polychondritis and systemic lupus erythematosus (SLE) are less frequent associations. Uncommon and rare associations include polyarteritis nodosa, Takayasu disease, giant cell arteritis, juvenile idiopathic arthritis, Vogt-Koyanagi-Harada disease, sarcoidosis, lymphoma, carcinoma of the lung, Cogan syndrome, congenital erythropoietic porphyria and graft-versus-host disease following allogenic bone marrow transplantation [11].

Scleritis occurs in 0.15–6.3 % of patients with RA; conversely up to 30 % of patients presenting with scleritis will have RA [10]. The most common phenotype is diffuse anterior scleritis; however, there are no clinical features to distinguish the scleritis seen in RA from that in other conditions except that scleromalacia perforans virtually only occurs in RA. In addition, keratoconjunctivitis sicca or corneal changes ('contact lens cornea') may be present which occur more commonly in RA than other conditions [10]. Patients with RA-related scleritis are older and are more likely to develop necrotising scleritis, decreased vision and peripheral ulcerative keratitis compared with patients with idiopathic scleritis [12, 13].

Scleritis occurs in approximately 10 % of WG patients [14]. The clinical features of scleritis can be diagnostically useful in WG; there may be a raised granulomatous mass, and the inflammatory changes involve the conjunctiva, episclera and sclera. If the lesion is adjacent to the limbus, the limbal arcade of vessels will be broken and the vessels leak profusely. Destruction of both the cornea and sclera occurs and a gutter appears that involves limbal tissue. This transgression of the limbus by a destructive change is only seen in WG and polyarteritis nodosa [10]. Patients with WG-related scleritis are more likely to develop necrotising scleritis, decreased vision and peripheral ulcerative keratitis compared with patients with scleritis associated with any other systemic vasculitic disease [15].

Scleritis occurs in approximately 40 % of patients with relapsing polychondritis [16]. The most common phenotype is diffuse anterior scleritis, but it can be of any type. Along with RA-related scleritis, it is considered a disease of intermediate severity [15]. Although the inflammation rarely causes destruction of the globe or decreased vision, the pain is very severe and very resistant to treatment [10]. Scleritis occurs uncommonly in patients with systemic lupus erythematosus. It is virtually always of the diffuse

or nodular subtype and is therefore, along with scleritis associated with the spondyloarthropathies, considered the most benign, although it can be quite resistant to treatment until the systemic disease is brought under control [10, 15].

3.1.4.2 Infectious Scleritis

Approximately 5–10 % of cases of anterior scleritis are infectious [17, 18]. Viruses, bacteria, fungi and parasites can all cause infectious scleritis, either by direct invasion of organisms or via an immune response induced by the organism [11]. Infectious scleritis should be suspected in patients with a history of ocular trauma or surgery, recurrent attacks of herpes zoster or simplex, systemic review consistent with infection or progression of disease whilst on immunomodulatory therapy [17, 19]. Unifocal or multifocal scleral abscesses and contiguous corneal infiltration may be present [20]. The most common causative pathogens include varicella zoster virus (VZV), herpes simplex virus (HSV), *Treponema pallidum*, *Mycobacterium* spp., *Pseudomonas aeruginosa* and *Aspergillus* spp. [11].

VZV-related scleritis occurs in up to 8 % of patients with a history of herpes zoster ophthalmicus, often manifesting months after an episode [21]. Active herpetic scleral disease is typically diffuse or nodular in subtype, whereas immune-mediated is usually of the necrotising subtype [21]. There is a high risk of scleral thinning, staphyloma formation and globe perforation [19]. HSV-related scleritis is probably an underrecognised clinical entity. A retrospective case series reported on nine patients (10 eyes) with biopsy-proven HSV-related scleritis [19]. No patient had a past or concurrent history of herpetic keratitis or eyelid disease or genital herpes. The mean duration of symptoms prior to tissue diagnosis was 3.2 years. Acyclovir treatment led to a rapid and complete resolution of inflammation in all cases. A retrospective study compared 35 cases of herpetic scleritis with 321 cases of idiopathic scleritis from the same two institutions [18]. It found that no patient with herpetic scleritis presented with posterior scleritis or scleromalacia perforans. Compared with idiopathic scleritis, patients with herpetic scleritis were more likely to have necrotising scleritis (8.6 vs 1.2 %; $P<0.05$), unilateral disease (80 vs 56.7 %; $P<0.05$) and vision loss (34.3 vs 11.5 %; $P<0.001$). Corneal involvement, anterior uveitis and more severe pain were also more commonly seen in herpetic scleritis, although the differences were not statistically significant [18].

Pseudomonas aeruginosa is the most common pathogen associated with postsurgical scleritis, particularly pterygium surgery with or without adjunctive beta irradiation or mitomycin C [22]. Syphilis has also been reported to be a common bacterial pathogen associated with scleritis [11], and a recent study from Japan attributed the cause of scleritis to tuberculosis (TB) in 6 of 83 (7.2 %) cases [6]. Fungal scleritis is generally a rare entity; however, it may be more common in hot and humid climates such as in India [20]. A recent series of infectious scleritis from India found fungi to be the most common pathogen, occurring in 8 of 21 (38 %) eyes, with *Aspergillus flavus* being the most common fungus isolated in these cases [20].

3.1.4.3 Surgically Induced Scleritis

Surgically induced necrotising scleritis (SINS) occurs most commonly after extracapsular cataract extraction, particularly through a limbal incision, but also occurs following scleral buckling, pars plana vitrectomy, trabeculectomy and strabismus surgery [23]. In a large series of 43 patients (52 eyes) with surgically induced scleritis, scleral inflammation developed adjacent to the surgical wound in all cases, with 94 % having necrotising anterior scleritis and 6 % nodular anterior scleritis [23]. In 75 % of cases, patients had undergone two or more surgical procedures prior to the onset of the scleritis. The mean time to the development of scleritis was 5.7 months (range 1 day to 3.5 years), excluding five patients who had a single strabismus correction procedure in childhood with onset of scleral disease many years later (mean 21.7 years, range 6.5–40 years). Systemic disease was present in 63 % of patients, with 39 % of these having a connective tissue disease. Surgically induced diffuse scleritis has also been reported following extracapsular cataract extraction [11].

3.1.5 Immunopathology

Understanding of the immunopathogenesis of scleritis is hampered by a limited availability of tissue for pathological examination, resulting in small series with most specimens being obtained from necrotising scleritis cases, often late in the course of the disease. A report of 25 specimens of necrotising scleritis and 5 specimens of non-necrotising scleritis found the presence of vasculitis and vascular immunodeposits in a high proportion of cases, suggesting that immune complex-mediated vasculitis with subsequent activation of complement and neutrophil enzyme release (type III hypersensitivity reaction) plays a pivotal role in the development of scleritis [24]. However, a subsequent series of eight cases (only one of which had necrotising scleritis) did not identify primary vasculitis in any of the specimens [25]. In keeping with previous investigators, the study found that cellular infiltrate consisted largely of lymphocytes and to a lesser extent macrophages, plasma cells and giant cells. More than 90 % of lymphocytes were T cells with a predominance of CD4+ cells, and there was a marked increase in MHC II-expressing cells capable of presenting local antigens to these infiltrating CD4+ cells. These findings, in addition to signs of a granulomatous process with activated macrophages, suggest a T-cell-mediated disease (delayed hypersensitivity reaction) at some stage of scleritis [25].

A large clinicopathologic study of 55 cases of necrotising scleritis identified distinct histopathologic patterns which may reflect different mechanisms of immunopathogenesis [26]. In cases with an associated systemic autoimmune disorder, the histopathologic finding of vasculitis with zonal granulomatous inflammation surrounding a central necrotic sclera was reported to be consistent with a type III hypersensitivity reaction. In idiopathic cases, the pattern of nonzonal diffuse scleritis in the absence of vasculitis, often in the absence of granulomatous inflammation and in the presence of a reactive connective tissue proliferation was reported to be consistent with a delayed hypersensitivity reaction or type IV hypersensitivity.

Utilising this histopathologic grading system, Usui and colleagues selected three enucleated eyes with necrotising zonal scleral inflammation associated with RA (autoimmune group) and three enucleated eyes with necrotising diffuse nongranulomatous scleral inflammation without an associated systemic disorder (idiopathic group) [27]. Immunohistochemical staining was performed for CD3 (pan T lymphocytes), CD4 (helper T lymphocytes), CD8 (cytotoxic-suppressor T lymphocytes), CD20 (B lymphocytes), CD68 (macrophages) and DRC (dendritic reticulum cells). Within the autoimmune group, about 43 % of inflammatory cells stained positive with CD20, 35 % with CD68, 17 % with CD3, 8 % with CD8, 4 % with DRC and less than 1 % with CD4. Within the idiopathic group, about 43 % stained positive with CD68, 23 % with CD3, 17 % with CD20, 7 % with CD8, 1 % with DRC and less than 1 % with CD4. The authors concluded that these findings suggest that B cells may drive the inflammatory process in necrotising scleritis associated with a systemic autoimmune disease and that macrophages may also play a role in the necrotising process in both autoimmune and idiopathic groups [27].

More recently, T-helper type 17 (Th 17) cells have been implicated in the pathogenesis of scleritis [28]. The number of peripheral blood Th 17 cells was noted to increase during active scleritis and decrease following treatment in eight patients. Th 17 cells were expanded by interleukin (IL)-2 and inhibited by interferon (IFN)-γ [28]. IL-2 is a proinflammatory cytokine produced by CD4+ cells which activates macrophages to produce other proinflammatory cytokines such as tissue necrosis factor (TNF)-α and interleukin (IL)-1. Local production of proinflammatory cytokines by infiltrating inflammatory cells not only propagates the inflammatory response but is also thought to play an important role in the destruction of extracellular matrix components in scleritis. TNF-α and IL-1 have been demonstrated to induce matrix metalloproteinases (MMPs) which can cause scleral remodelling and destruction [29]. Plasma cells have also been shown to produce MMPs, in addition to releasing TNF-α [29].

3.1.6 Management

Management of scleritis involves clinical assessment of the type of scleritis, the severity of disease and the presence of any complications. A careful history and examination and targeted investigations are critically important to determine if there is an underlying systemic autoimmune disease or a local or systemic infectious cause. Treatment of scleritis usually requires systemic therapy and involves a stepped approach.

3.1.6.1 Investigations

In every patient with scleritis, it is essential to exclude an associated systemic disease, particularly a primary vasculitic disease such as WG or PAN as these are more likely to present initially as scleritis and if left untreated are potentially fatal [7, 30]. In a large series of 107 scleritis patients with an associated systemic disease, 78 % had a pre-existing diagnosis, 14 % were diagnosed as a result of the initial evaluation and 8.4 % developed a systemic disease during follow-up. Systemic vasculitis was less likely to have been previously diagnosed than other rheumatic diseases (59 vs 84 %) and more likely to be diagnosed as a result of the initial evaluation (27 vs 9 %) [30]. Subsequent studies have reported similar results and have recommended a work up to exclude primary vasculitic disease even in scleritis patients with a known non-vasculitic systemic disease [7].

Initial evaluation involves a comprehensive history with a detailed systems review, thorough examination, B-scan ultrasonography if posterior scleritis is suspected and targeted investigations. Blood pressure measurement and urine analysis should be performed on the day of presentation, and all patients should undergo a chest X-ray and anti-neutrophil cytoplasmic antibody (ANCA) testing. Other relevant blood tests include renal function, syphilis serology, rheumatoid factor and anti-nuclear antibodies (ANA). A positive ANCA titre in the presence of a positive ANA result is inaccurate and requires specific anti-myeloperoxidase and anti-proteinase 3 ANCA titres to determine the presence of ANCA antibodies. Additional investigations, such as acute phase response reactant levels, Lyme serology, HLA-B27, serum angiotensin-converting enzyme, sinus imaging and biopsies of other organs, are determined by clinical assessment and abnormalities detected on the initial blood tests.

Diagnosis of infectious scleritis is of utmost importance as the management is completely different, and systemic immunosuppressive therapy alone will worsen the condition. If bacterial, fungal or acanthamoeba infection is suspected, scleral scraping or biopsy should be performed. If an ulcerative lesion is present, scleral scrapings are taken from the base of the active lesion. If a biopsy is planned, it is often best undertaken in the operating theatre, where adequate anaesthesia enables a sterile, pain-free procedure. If there is a non-ulcerative lesion, episcleral and scleral specimens are collected following careful dissection of the overlying conjunctiva. Specimens should be plated for microscopy and culture on blood and chocolate agar, brain-heart infusion broth, thioglycollate broth, non-nutrient agar with an overlay of *Escherichia coli* and Sabouraud's dextrose agar [20]. If a herpes infection is suspected, conjunctival or scleroconjunctival biopsy is required for PCR testing and immunofluorescence studies [19]. Specimens should also be collected for histopathology and immunopathology.

3.1.6.2 Treatment Overview

In a large retrospective series [4, 5], data on treatment and response to treatment was available for 69 patients with scleritis. Overall, approximately 30 % of patients were treated with NSAIDs, 32 % required oral prednisolone and 26 % needed additional immunosuppressive drugs. This series, in addition to an earlier analysis of therapeutic failure for initial regimens in 132 patients with noninfectious anterior scleritis [31], has provided useful treatment guidelines for the various subtypes of scleritis.

Sainz de la Maza and colleagues recommended that, in patients with diffuse and nodular anterior scleritis, NSAIDs should be the initial choice, oral corticosteroids should be second-line therapy and immunosuppressive agents should be third-line therapy. However, in patients with necrotising anterior scleritis,

additional immunosuppressive agents should be commenced at the outset, as therapeutic failure for initial regimens occurred in 100 % of patients treated with oral NSAIDs and in 91 % of patients treated with oral corticosteroids [31]. Jabs and colleagues also determined that patients with nodular and diffuse anterior scleritis were more likely to respond to oral NSAIDs but found that a smaller proportion (70 %) of patients with necrotising anterior scleritis required additional immunosuppressive agents. Posterior scleritis was treated most often with oral corticosteroids (83 %), with immunosuppressive agents being needed less frequently (17 %) [4, 5]. An associated systemic autoimmune disorder has also been found to increase the likelihood of needing more aggressive immunosuppressive therapy [3].

3.1.6.3 Topical Corticosteroids

Aside from treating any associated anterior uveitis, topical corticosteroids play a limited role as adjunctive therapy in the management of non-necrotising anterior scleritis in patients who are not steroid responders.

3.1.6.4 Subconjunctival Corticosteroid Injection

There has been renewed interest in the use of subconjunctival corticosteroid injection for the treatment of non-necrotising, noninfectious anterior scleritis, particularly in patients who fail to respond to initial systemic therapy. Historically, the injection of corticosteroids has been contraindicated in scleritis due to concerns regarding efficacy and case reports from the 1970s of scleral necrosis and perforation [32]. More recent case series [33] have questioned these concerns, and there are now several published series reporting the use of subconjunctival corticosteroid injection in non-necrotising, noninfectious anterior scleritis [34].

A recent retrospective, interventional, non-comparative multicenter study [35, 36] represents the largest series to date on the use of subconjunctival corticosteroid injection for the treatment of non-necrotising, noninfectious anterior scleritis. Sixty-eight eyes of 53 patients with diffuse or nodular anterior scleritis with at least 6 months follow-up were included. Patients with a history of glaucoma, ocular hypertension or steroid response were excluded. Median follow-up was 28 months (mean 33.6, range 6–100 months). Signs and symptoms improved in 66 (97 %) eyes and completely resolved in 61 (89.7 %) eyes after one injection. Kaplan-Meier estimates found 68 and 50 % of eyes were recurrence-free after one injection, at 24 and 48 months respectively. Repeated injections did not result in loss of treatment effect. Subconjunctival corticosteroid injection reduced the requirement for systemic therapy from 96 to 43 %.

The technique of subconjunctival corticosteroid injection involves topical anaesthesia and then administration of triamcinolone acetonide (Kenalog 40 mg/ml) via subconjunctival injection using a 25- or 27-gauge needle under direct vision with the slit lamp. For nodular scleritis, 0.05–0.1 ml is injected under the conjunctiva immediately adjacent to the nodule. For diffuse scleritis, 0.05–0.2 ml is injected per inflamed quadrant [35, 36]. Patients need to be warned of the risk of raised intraocular pressure, and those with a history of ocular hypertension, glaucoma or steroid response should be excluded. In the series by Sohn and colleagues, transient ocular hypertension not requiring treatment developed in 14 (20.6 %) eyes, and ocular hypertension or glaucoma requiring medical management or surgical management occurred in 2 (2.9 %) eyes each. Other adverse events included subconjunctival haemorrhage (7 eyes) and cataract (6 eyes) [35, 36]. Patients also need to be warned about the possibility of scleral necrosis and perforation. There were no cases of scleral necrosis in this series or other recent series [34–36]. This may be because of better patient selection due to increased recognition of the early subtle signs of scleral necrosis or it may be due to the use of triamcinolone acetonide rather than methylprednisolone acetate. Alternatively, it may simply be that there are inadequate numbers of patients at present to detect this rare event [34].

3.1.6.5 Oral NSAIDs

Oral NSAIDs are considered first-line therapy in the management of non-necrotising anterior scleritis.

However, success rates differ greatly, whereas one series reported control of inflammation in 91 % of nodular and 93 % of diffuse anterior scleritis cases [31], and another series documented success rates of only 57 % for nodular and 33 % for diffuse anterior scleritis [4, 5]. A recent study identified younger age, unilateral disease, anterior nodular scleritis and without associated disease as factors associated with successful response to oral NSAIDs [8, 9]. Oral NSAIDs have been determined to be ineffective for necrotising anterior scleritis with one series finding a 100 % therapeutic failure rate in patients initially treated with NSAIDs [31]. Some success has been reported in treating idiopathic posterior scleritis with NSAIDs [3]. However, patients with loss of vision, evidence of optic nerve involvement or associated systemic disease are unlikely to respond and should be commenced on systemic corticosteroids at the outset.

Several NSAID agents are available but flurbiprofen and indomethacin have anecdotally been found to be most effective [4, 5, 10]. The initial dosage for flurbiprofen is usually 50–100 mg three times daily. The initial dosage for indomethacin is 25–50 mg three times daily. Jabs and colleagues typically started patients on indomethacin 25 mg four times daily. If the scleritis improved, the dose was reduced to 25 mg three times daily until the scleritis was completely quiet, at which stage the indomethacin was discontinued. If the scleritis did not initially improve, the dose was increased to 150 mg daily. Approximately 50 % of patients who responded to NSAIDs did so at the lower dose (100 mg daily or less) and 50 % required the higher dose (150 mg daily). The median duration of therapy was 7.5 weeks [4]. A small study of 24 patients with diffuse anterior scleritis found 95 % were treated successfully with celecoxib 200–800 mg daily in divided doses [37]. Celecoxib is a selective cyclooxygenase (COX)-2 inhibitor. Whereas COX-1 is constitutively expressed in the gastrointestinal (GI) tract, kidneys, platelets and vascular endothelium, COX-2 is an inducible enzyme that is primarily upregulated during inflammatory responses. However, although COX-2 inhibitors may reduce gastrointestinal toxicity, they appear to have equivalent nephrotoxicity to conventional NSAIDs, and there are concerns regarding cardiovascular side effects [38].

Gastrointestinal side effects are common with oral NSAIDs and patients need to be warned of the possibility of gastric irritation, peptic ulceration and bleeding. Renal impairment, particularly when used in combination with ACE inhibitors and diuretics, and CNS side effects are uncommon but serious. Other NSAID-related side effects include haematologic toxicity, hepatic toxicity, dermatologic reactions and hypersensitivity responses including rashes, bronchospasm and anaphylactoid reactions. Oral NSAIDs are contraindicated in pregnancy because they can cause premature closure of the fetal ductus arteriosus and fetal renal impairment [38]. In the study by Jabs and colleagues, indomethacin was well tolerated in over 70 % of patients with only two patients (4.1 %) discontinuing the drug due to side effects [4].

3.1.6.6 Systemic Corticosteroids

Oral corticosteroids are considered first-line therapy for patients with necrotising scleritis or posterior scleritis and second-line therapy in patients with non-necrotising anterior scleritis who do not respond to, or are intolerant of, oral NSAIDs. The standard starting dose is prednisolone 1 mg/kg/day and tapering is individualised. A typical tapering schedule is to reduce the oral prednisolone by 10–20 mg weekly until a dose of 40 mg/day is reached, then reduce by 5–10 mg weekly until a dose of 10–20 mg/day is reached and then reduce by 2.5–5 mg increments thereafter until cessation or an acceptable maintenance dose is reached. In some patients with long-standing disease, reduction below 10 mg/day requires 1 mg increments [4, 10]. Patients whose eyes are not completely quiet after 1 month of high-dose oral prednisolone or patients who relapse at doses of prednisolone greater than 7.5 mg/day should be commenced on adjunctive immunosuppressive therapy.

Intravenous methylprednisolone is primarily reserved for situations in which rapid control of inflammation is required, usually in cases of necrotising scleritis with threatened scleral or corneal perforation. A small retrospective case series [39]

reported an improvement in the scleritis score of all 14 patients who were treated with pulsed intravenous methylprednisolone. Intravenous methylprednisolone (0.5–1.0 g/day) is typically given for up to three consecutive days prior to commencing high-dose oral prednisolone therapy.

All patients should be warned of the side effects of systemic corticosteroids. These are dose- and duration-dependent and occur more frequently in the elderly, diabetics, hypoalbuminaemic states, psychiatric patients and in pregnancy [11]. A common serious adverse effect is hyperglycaemia, which developed in 10 % of scleritis patients treated with oral prednisolone in the study by Jabs and colleagues [4]. Cushingoid habitus is also a common occurrence and hypertension may also occur. All patients should have their weight, blood pressure and blood sugar level monitored regularly. Mild mood disturbances, particularly insomnia and anxiety, are common, and severe psychiatric disturbances may develop in up to 7 % [4]. Osteoporosis is an uncommon but serious complication. A baseline bone densitometry scan should be performed in patients over the age of 65, those with a family or personal history of osteoporosis or those in whom it is anticipated that oral prednisolone therapy will be required for more than 3 months.

3.1.6.7 Immunosuppressive Agents

Non-biologic immunosuppressive agents can be grouped into antimetabolites, T-cell inhibitors and alkylating agents. The antimetabolites include azathioprine, methotrexate and mycophenolate mofetil; the T-cell inhibitors include cyclosporine and tacrolimus; and the alkylating agents include cyclophosphamide and chlorambucil. Comprehensive guidelines, based on recommendations of an expert panel, for the use of these agents in patients with ocular inflammatory diseases have been published [4]. Immunosuppressive agents may be indicated at the outset in patients with a known systemic autoimmune disease requiring such treatment (usually WG), if there is a failure to control inflammation despite 1 month of high-dose prednisolone, if there are frequent recurrences on attempting to taper the oral prednisolone to a safe

Table 3.1 Treatment success rates of various agents, derived from the Systemic Immunosuppressive Therapy for Eye Diseases Cohort Study

Immunosuppressive agent	AZA	MTX	MMF	CsA	CYP
Controlled inflammation (no activity) within 6 months (%)	20	56	49	62	53
Controlled inflammation and ≤10 mg/day prednisolone within 6 months (%)	22	37	26	53	30
Controlled inflammation (no activity) within 12 months (%)	73	72	86	62	82
Controlled inflammation and ≤10 mg/day prednisolone within 12 months (%)	35	58	49	53	61

Adapted from Daniel et al. [42], Gangaputra et al. [43], Kacmaz et al. [44], Pasadhika et al. [45], Pujari et al. [46]

AZA azathioprine, *CsA* cyclosporine, *CYP* cyclophosphamide, *MMF* mycophenolate mofetil, *MTX* methotrexate

long-term daily dose or if intolerable corticosteroid side effects develop.

The largest reported series relating to the use of non-biologic immunosuppressive agents in scleritis are derived from the Systemic Immunosuppressive Therapy for Eye Diseases (SITE) Cohort Study. This retrospective study compiled data from four tertiary ocular inflammatory centres across the USA to evaluate the safety and efficacy of various types of monotherapy in the treatment of noninfectious ocular inflammation [40, 41]. The main outcome measures were successful control of inflammation, corticosteroid-sparing benefit and incidence of and reason for discontinuation of therapy. Successful control of inflammation was evaluated by the time to transition from active or slightly active disease at initiation of monotherapy (with or without corticosteroids) to inactive disease over at least two visits spanning at least 28 days. Successful corticosteroid-sparing benefit was evaluated by the time to successful tapering of corticosteroids to ≤10 mg/day, ≤5 mg/day and 0 mg while maintaining control of inflammation over at least two visits spanning at least 28 days (5 refs). Table 3.1 provides a summary of the main treatment success outcome measures, but it is important to note that the SITE Cohort Study is an observational study, and it is therefore not possible to directly compare success of the various agents; for example, cyclophosphamide is likely to have been reserved for more severe cases associated with systemic vasculitic disease, and therefore, cyclophosphamide outcomes will appear less favourable.

Azathioprine

Azathioprine is a purine nucleoside analogue which interferes with DNA replication and RNA transcription. It decreases the numbers of peripheral T and B lymphocytes and reduces mixed lymphocyte reactivity, IL-2 synthesis and IgM production. Azathioprine is well absorbed orally, but there is an up to fourfold individual variation in the rate of metabolism due to variable thiopurine-S-methyltransferase activity. The usual dose is 1–3 mg/kg/day but should be reduced when used with allopurinol. The most common serious adverse effects are reversible bone marrow suppression and hepatotoxicity. A full blood count (FBC) should be performed every 4–6 weeks, and liver function tests (LFTs) should be performed every 12 weeks to assess aspartate aminotransferase and alanine aminotransferase levels. If these enzyme levels are >1.5 times the upper limit of normal, the dose should be decreased by 25–50 mg/day and the LFTs rechecked in 2 weeks. If there is a marked enzyme elevation, azathioprine should be discontinued, at least temporarily (Category D evidence) [5].

In the SITE Cohort Study, azathioprine therapy was evaluated in 27 eyes of 16 patients with scleritis (Category C evidence) [45]. The Kaplan-Meier estimate of the proportion achieving sustained control of inflammation within 6 and 12 months was 20.0 and 73.3 % respectively. Of those patients on >10 mg/day prednisolone initially, an estimated 22.2, 18.2 and 0 % succeeded in tapering their prednisolone dosage to ≤10, ≤5 and 0 mg daily respectively within the first 6 months of therapy. By 12 months of therapy, 35.2, 29.9 and 11.1 % of patients achieved these outcomes. Discontinuation data was available for 123 patients overall with 24.1 % of patients stopping therapy within 1 year due to adverse drug effects. The most common side effect leading to cessation of azathioprine was gastrointestinal upset (9 %) followed by bone marrow suppression (5 %), elevated liver enzymes

(4 %) infection (2 %) and allergy (1 %). Advantages of azathioprine include that it is relatively inexpensive and there is extensive experience in its use.

Methotrexate

Methotrexate is a folic acid analogue which inhibits DNA replication, affecting rapidly dividing cells such as leukocytes. Methotrexate is completely absorbed if administered parentally, but if taken orally up to 35 % may be metabolised by intestinal flora before absorption. The usual dose is 7.5–25 mg once weekly, and folic acid (1 mg/day) is administered concurrently to minimise nausea and bone marrow suppression effects. The most common serious adverse effects are hepatotoxicity, bone marrow suppression and interstitial pneumonia. Methotrexate is also teratogenic. Baseline FBC, LFTs and hepatitis B and C serology are obtained and an FBC and LFTs should be performed every 4–8 weeks. If liver enzymes are >2 times normal on two separate occasions, the dose should be reduced, and a liver biopsy should be performed if abnormal LFTs persist after discontinuation of the drug. Patients should be advised to abstain from alcohol consumption whilst on methotrexate (Category D evidence) [5].

In the SITE Cohort Study, methotrexate was evaluated in 84 eyes of 56 patients with scleritis (Category C evidence) [43]. The proportion achieving sustained control of inflammation within 6 and 12 months was 56.4 and 71.5 % respectively. Of those patients on >10 mg/day prednisolone initially, an estimated 37.3, 26.3 and 6.2 % succeeded in tapering their prednisolone dosage to ≤10, ≤5 and 0 mg daily respectively within the first 6 months of therapy. By 12 months of therapy, 58.3, 55.6 and 17.5 % of patients achieved these outcomes. Discontinuation data was available for 345 patients overall with an estimated 17.5 % of patients stopping therapy within 1 year due to adverse drug effects. The most common side effects leading to discontinuation were gastrointestinal upset (2.9 %), bone marrow suppression (2.6 %) and elevated liver enzymes (2.3 %). There was one case of cirrhosis of the liver. Malaise, allergy, mouth ulcers and alopecia were other reasons for discontinuation. Advantages of methotrexate include that it is relatively inexpensive; there is extensive experience in its use, particularly in children; and it appears to be well tolerated.

Mycophenolate Mofetil

Mycophenolate mofetil is a selective inhibitor of inosine monophosphate dehydrogenase that interferes with guanosine nucleotide synthesis. It prevents T- and B-cell proliferation, suppresses antibody synthesis, interferes with cellular adhesion to vascular endothelium and decreases leukocyte recruitment. It has high oral bioavailability, and its active metabolite is excreted renally so it should be used with caution in patients with renal impairment. The usual dose is 1 g twice daily with doses of 3 g daily being associated with increased toxicity. The most common serious adverse effect is bone marrow suppression. High rates of opportunistic infections and nonmelanoma skin cancers have been reported with 3 g daily doses in transplant patients receiving other immunosuppressive agents (Category D evidence) [5]. Mycophenolate mofetil may also be associated with an increased risk of progressive multifocal leukoencephalopathy (PML), due to reactivation of JC virus, in patients with underlying conditions independently associated with PML who are using concomitant immunosuppressive therapy (Category D evidence) [47]. Mycophenolate mofetil is also teratogenic [48]. An FBC should be performed weekly for 4 weeks then fortnightly for 2 months and then monthly thereafter. It is also recommended that LFTs be performed 12 weekly (Category D evidence) [5].

In the SITE Cohort Study, mycophenolate mofetil was evaluated in 51 eyes of 33 patients with scleritis (Category C evidence) [42]. The proportion achieving sustained control of inflammation within 6 and 12 months was 48.7 and 85.7 % respectively. Of those patients on >10 mg/day prednisolone initially, an estimated 25.5, 20.5 and 7.1 % succeeded in tapering their prednisolone dosage to ≤10, ≤5 and 0 mg daily respectively within the first 6 months of therapy. By 12 months of therapy, 49.4, 44.7 and 7.1 % of patients achieved these outcomes. Discontinuation data was available for 209 patients overall with an estimated 12 % of patients stopping therapy within 1 year due to adverse drug effects. The most common side effects leading to discontinuation were gastrointestinal upset (2.5 %), bone marrow suppression (1.7 %) and elevated liver enzymes (1.3 %). Malaise and allergy were other reasons for discontinuation. There were no cases of opportunistic infection or progressive multifocal leukoencephalopathy. Mycophenolate mofetil appears to be safe and well tolerated in patients with ocular inflammation, and there is some evidence that it may be more effective than the other antimetabolites (Category D evidence) [49].

Cyclosporine A

Cyclosporine A is a natural metabolite of some fungi and is thought to inhibit transcription in immunocompetent T cells, blocking their replication and ability to produce cytokines such as IL-2, by inhibiting calcineurin. Two oral preparations are available; the microemulsion preparation (Neoral) has greater bioavailability than the gelatine capsule (Sandimmune), and hence, the two cannot be used interchangeably. Cyclosporine A is metabolised in the liver and excreted in bile. The usual dose is 2–5 mg/kg/day in two divided doses. The most common serious adverse effects are dose-related nephrotoxicity and hypertension with hepatotoxicity occurring less frequently. Blood pressure should be checked at every visit and no less frequently than monthly initially and then three monthly thereafter. Serum creatinine should be checked fortnightly initially and then monthly once the dosage is stabilised (Category D evidence) [5].

In the SITE Cohort Study, cyclosporine A was evaluated in 23 eyes of 15 patients with scleritis (Category C evidence) [44]. The proportion achieving sustained control of inflammation within 6 and 12 months was 62.3 %. Of those patients on >10 mg/day prednisolone initially, an estimated 52.8, 40.8 and 16.7 % succeeded in tapering their prednisolone dosage to ≤10, ≤5 and 0 mg daily respectively within the first 6 months of therapy. By 12 months of therapy, 52.8, 50.6 and 25.0 % of patients achieved these outcomes. A systemic autoimmune disease was present in 53.3 %, suggesting that cyclosporine A is a good treatment option in young patients who may otherwise require alkylating agents and wish to avoid the risk of sterility associated with these agents. Discontinuation data was available for 312 patients overall with an estimated 10.7 % of patients stopping therapy within 1 year due to adverse drug effects. The most common side effects leading to discontinuation were nephrotoxicity (4.3 %), hypertension (3.2 %) and elevated liver enzymes (1.1 %). Gingival hyperplasia, hirsutism, malaise, opportunistic infection and bone marrow suppression were other reasons for discontinuation. Compared with 18–39 year olds, patients aged 55–64 years and those aged 65 years or older were more likely to cease treatment due to side effects (relative risk (RR) 3.2 and 5.7 respectively).

Tacrolimus

Tacrolimus is a macrolide antibiotic produced by *Streptomyces tsukubaensis* which inhibits the activation of T lymphocytes in a manner similar to that of cyclosporine A. Oral bioavailability is incomplete and variable, and monitoring of blood concentrations may be necessary. An initial dose of 0.10–0.15 mg/kg/day is recommended for adult liver transplant patients, but in ocular inflammation, an initial dose of 0.05 mg/kg/day may suffice. The most common serious adverse effects are nephrotoxicity, neurological symptoms and hyperglycaemia. Serum creatinine and electrolytes, blood urea nitrogen, LFTs, blood glucose, lipid profile and FBC should be performed weekly initially and three monthly thereafter (Category D evidence) [5].

There is limited reported experience with the use of tacrolimus in scleritis. A single case report detailed successful prevention of a recurrence of necrotising scleritis in a scleral patch graft for SINS after two previous scleral patch grafts had failed within 1 month of surgery despite the use of cyclophosphamide and azathioprine (Category D evidence) [50].

Cyclophosphamide

Cyclophosphamide is a nitrogen mustard-alkylating agent which alkylates purines in DNA and RNA, ultimately resulting in cell death. It is cytotoxic to both resting and dividing lymphocytes, decreasing the numbers of B lymphocytes and activated T lymphocytes. Delayed-type hypersensitivity, mixed lymphocyte reactions, mitogen-induced and antigen-induced blastogenesis and cytokine production are all suppressed. Cyclophosphamide can be administered both orally (1–3 mg/kg/day) and intravenously (750–1,000 mg/m^2 body surface area every 3–4 weeks). It is metabolised by the liver and excreted primarily by the kidney. Doses need to be reduced by 30–50 % in patients with renal failure (Category D evidence) [5]. Jabs and colleagues have provided detailed guidelines regarding their use of oral cyclophosphamide in scleritis patients. The typical starting dose was 2 mg/kg/day in conjunction with prednisolone 1 mg/kg/day. The prednisolone was then tapered and could often be discontinued over the first 4–8 weeks of therapy. The goals of treatment were to achieve complete suppression of the inflammation (whilst maintaining the white blood cell (WBC) count between 3,000 and 4,000 cells/ml), maintain quiescence for 1 year and then taper and discontinue the cyclophosphamide with a total duration of therapy of less than 18 months (Category D evidence) [4].

Due to a high incidence of serious side effects, cyclophosphamide is reserved for cases of refractory necrotising scleritis, and patients should be comanaged by a rheumatologist, immunologist or other medical physician. The most common serious adverse effect is dose-dependent, reversible bone marrow suppression, which is more common in patients older than 65 years. Severe granulocytopenia (neutrophil count <1,000 cells/ml) is associated with an increased risk of bacterial infections. Lymphopenia is associated with opportunistic infections, particularly *Pneumocystis carinii* pneumonia (PCP), and primary prophylaxis with trimethoprim/sulfamethoxazole is recommended. Haemorrhagic cystitis is a serious but infrequent adverse effect, primarily occurring in individuals with bladder stasis or insufficient fluid intake. Patients should be encouraged to drink two or more litres of fluid a day. Intravenous pulsed cyclophosphamide with concomitant 2-mercaptoethane sulphonate also reduces the risk of bladder toxicity and cancer. There is a high incidence of sterility, and cryopreservation of oocytes or sperm prior to commencement of therapy may be considered (Category D evidence) [5]. Cyclophosphamide is also teratogenic and there is a potential concern regarding the development of late malignancy (Category D evidence) [40, 41]. For oral therapy, an FBC and urinalysis should be obtained weekly initially and at least 4 weekly thereafter. If mild bone marrow suppression occurs, the dose should be reduced by 25 from 50 mg/day and the FBC rechecked in 2 weeks. If the WBC count falls below 2,500 cells/ml, cyclophosphamide is discontinued until the WBC counts have recovered and it can then be reinstituted at a lower dose. If haematuria occurs, cyclophosphamide should be discontinued (unless an associated life-threatening systemic vasculitis dictates otherwise) and a urologist consulted if the haematuria persists after 3–4 weeks (Category D evidence) [5].

In the SITE Cohort Study, cyclophosphamide was evaluated in 76 eyes of 48 patients with scleritis (Category C evidence) [46]. The proportion achieving sustained control of inflammation within 6 and 12 months was 53.3 and 82.2 % respectively. Of those patients on >10 mg/day prednisolone initially, an estimated 30.2, 17.9 and 0 % succeeded in tapering their prednisolone dosage to ≤10, ≤5 and 0 mg daily respectively within the first 6 months of therapy. By 12 months of therapy, 60.5, 37.8 and 15.9 % of patients achieved these outcomes. Discontinuation data was available for 195 patients overall with an estimated 33.5 % of patients stopping therapy within 1 year due to adverse drug effects, usually of a reversible nature. The most common side effects leading to discontinuation were low WBC count (18 %), haematuria or haemorrhagic cystitis (6.5 %), anaemia or low platelet count (4.7 %) and opportunistic infection (2.8 %) including one death due to PCP. No patient developed a malignancy. Cyclophosphamide therapy resulted in a high rate of drug-free disease remission, with 63 % of patients overall being able to discontinue therapy within 2 years of initiation of treatment.

Chlorambucil

Chlorambucil is an alkylating agent which substitutes an alkyl group for hydrogen ions in organic compounds resulting in interference in DNA replication, DNA transcription and nucleic acid function. Oral bioavailability is variable. Chlorambucil is metabolised in the liver before being excreted by the kidney. It has a slower onset of action than cyclophosphamide. There are two approaches in its use in patients with ocular inflammatory disease. The first is similar to that of cyclophosphamide therapy, with a dose of 0.1–0.2 mg/kg/day (6–12 mg daily) given for 1 year after quiescence of disease before tapering. The second method is short-term (usually 3–6 months) high-dose therapy which involves an initial dose of 2 mg daily for 1 week, followed by escalation by 2 mg/day each week until complete suppression of the inflammation is achieved or until the WBC drops below 2,400 cells/ml or the platelet count drops below 125,000 cells/ml (Category D evidence) [5, 51].

Similar to cyclophosphamide, a high incidence of serious side effects means chlorambucil is reserved for cases of refractory necrotising scleritis, and patients should be comanaged by a rheumatologist, immunologist or other medical physician. The most common serious adverse effect is bone marrow suppression, which is usually reversible but may be prolonged. Opportunistic infections may occur and primary PCP prophylaxis is recommended. Sterility usually occurs in men and older women, and cryopreservation of oocytes or sperm prior to commencement of therapy may be considered. Chlorambucil is also teratogenic and there is a potential concern regarding the development of late malignancy. Gastrointestinal upset is uncommon and alopecia and bladder toxicity do not occur. An FBC should be performed weekly initially and during dose escalation and at least 4 weekly thereafter (Category D evidence) [5].

Jabs and colleagues substituted chlorambucil for cyclophosphamide in two patients with necrotising scleritis who developed bladder toxicity. The initial dose was 0.1 mg/kg/day and a dosing method similar to that of cyclophosphamide was utilised. One patient developed reversible leukopenia and one patient developed PCP (Category D evidence) [4]. Goldstein and colleagues treated 53 patients with sight-threatening ocular inflammation, of whom 6 had scleritis, with short-term high-dose chlorambucil therapy for a mean duration of 16 weeks. Five scleritis patients had

adequate follow-up of 24 months or more. All achieved drug-free disease remission, with only 1 patient requiring retreatment for 1 week. Among all the patients, the most common side effect seen was premature ovarian failure in females (26 %) and testicular dysfunction in males (12.5 %). Six patients (12 %) developed nonophthalmic cutaneous herpes zoster and two patients (4 %) required a platelet transfusion. No patient developed a malignancy (Category D evidence) [51].

3.1.6.8 Biologic Immunosuppressive Agents

Biologics are a novel class of agents comprising recombinant fusion proteins and monoclonal antibodies directed against proinflammatory cytokines, their receptors and other selected cell surface markers. Biologic agents reported in the treatment of scleritis include the TNF-α inhibitors etanercept, infliximab and adalimumab; the IL-1 receptor antagonist anakinra; and the IL-2 receptor antagonist daclizumab and the anti-CD20 (B cell) antibody rituximab. Administration and monitoring of biologic therapy should be performed by a rheumatologist or immunologist.

TNF-α Inhibitors

TNF-α is a proinflammatory cytokine produced primarily by cells of the macrophage-monocyte lineage, which exists in both soluble and cell membrane-bound forms. Its biologic effects include adhesion molecule expression, synthesis of proinflammatory cytokines and chemokines, activation of macrophages and other immune cells and inhibition of regulatory T cells. Etanercept is a dimeric fusion protein consisting of the extracellular ligand-binding portion of the human p75 TNF receptor linked to the Fc portion of human immunoglobulin (Ig) G1. Etanercept inhibits the activity of TNF-α by acting as a decoy receptor and competitively binding to soluble TNF-α. Infliximab is a chimeric monoclonal antibody composed of the human IgG1 constant region fused with the murine variable region recognising TNF. Adalimumab has a similar composition but is fully humanised. Infliximab and adalimumab bind to both soluble and cell membrane-bound TNF and can also induce apoptosis in cells expressing TNF [52].

Etanercept is administered subcutaneously. The usual dose used in ocular inflammation is 25 mg twice weekly or 50 mg weekly. Infliximab is administered via intravenous infusion. Typically a loading dose of 3–5 mg/kg is given at weeks 0, 2 and 6 and then infusions are continued every 6–8 weeks thereafter. Scleritis patients may require the interval to be reduced to 4 weekly to maintain control of inflammation (Category D evidence) [53]. Adalimumab is administered subcutaneously. The usual dose is 40 mg fortnightly, which may be increased to 40 mg weekly if inflammation is not controlled. TNF-α inhibitors have a rapid onset of action and are therefore well suited for rescue therapy. Serious adverse effects reported with TNF-α inhibitors include reactivation of latent tuberculosis, new onset of autoimmune disease and demyelinating disease and congestive cardiac failure. However, generally TNF-α inhibitors are well tolerated with infusion reactions, upper respiratory tract infections and headache being the most common side effects seen. TNF-α inhibitors are classified as FDA Category B (no definite harm but insufficient evidence) in pregnancy [54, 55].

The use of TNF-α inhibitors in RA patients has been shown to confer a four- to sevenfold increased risk of reactivation of latent tuberculosis (Category A evidence) [54, 55]. The risk is greater for infliximab and adalimumab, as compared with etanercept (Category B evidence) [54, 55]. Screening and treatment for latent TB prior to commencement of a TNF-α inhibitor reduces the risk of reactivation in these patients (Category B evidence) [54, 55]. Therefore, every patient should be thoroughly assessed for the possibility of TB prior to initiating TNF-α therapy. Repeat screening should be performed in the event of TB exposure and should be considered in patients who are at an ongoing risk for TB exposure (Category C evidence) [54, 55]. There is also an approximately two- to fourfold increased risk of serious and nonserious bacterial infections (Category B evidence) [54, 55]. The most common associated infections are upper respiratory tract infections, cellulitis, urinary tract infections and pneumonia [54, 55]. TNF-α inhibitors should not be given if an active infection is present (Category C evidence) [54, 55]. TNF-α inhibitors do not appear to significantly increase the risk of reactivating chronic viral infections (Category C evidence) [54, 55].

Autoantibody formation is common following TNF-α inhibitor therapy, but development of antiphospholipid and lupus-like clinical syndromes is rare (Category C evidence) [54–56]. TNF-α inhibitors should be discontinued in the case of a new onset of a clinical picture suggestive of SLE, lupus-like syndrome or vasculitis [56]. There are also rare reports of new-onset multiple sclerosis, optic neuritis and peripheral neuropathies occurring in patients being treated with any of the three TNF-α inhibitors (Category C evidence) [54, 55]. Accordingly, these agents are contraindicated in patients with a history of demyelinating disease and should be discontinued if new neurological symptoms develop [56].

Studies examining the risk of congestive cardiac failure in RA patients with TNF-α inhibitors have shown inconsistent results [54, 55]. However, a pilot RCT investigating the use of infliximab in congestive heart failure found an increased risk of death or hospitalisation in the group treated with infliximab (Category B evidence) [57]. In addition, the FDA's MedWatch program reported 47 cases of new onset or exacerbation of heart failure in patients treated with infliximab or etanercept for a variety of systemic autoimmune conditions (Category C evidence) [58]. Hence, TNF-α inhibitors are contraindicated in class III/IV heart failure and should probably be avoided in patients with any class of heart failure. Initial meta-analyses reported a higher rate of solid malignancies in RA patients, but subsequent analyses with greater patient numbers did not demonstrate an increased incidence (Category A evidence) [54, 55]. However, in a study of WG patients, some of whom had scleritis, combined treatment with etanercept and cyclophosphamide had a significantly greater risk of developing solid tumours compared with those treated with cyclophosphamide alone ($p = 0.01$) (Category B evidence) [59].

Most studies regarding the use of TNF-α inhibitors in ocular inflammatory disease have revealed very little toxicity. However, one small prospective trial of 23 patients treated with infliximab therapy for refractory uveitis reported a high incidence of serious adverse events, including 1 case of new-onset congestive cardiac failure, 2 possible cases of lupus-like syndrome and 1 patient who developed endometrial cancer but had, unbeknownst to the investigators, an abnormal Papanicolaou test result before entering the study (Category D evidence) [60].

- *Etanercept*

  In a small retrospective study [61], seven RA patients with refractory articular disease were treated with etanercept ($n=6$) or infliximab ($n=1$). Of the six patients treated with etanercept, one patient achieved complete quiescence of scleritis, one patient had minimally active scleritis and in one patient etanercept was ineffective for the scleritis; the other three patients developed bilateral scleritis for the first time, 1, 2 and 6 months after commencing etanercept. These results mirror the reported experience of etanercept in the treatment of uveitis in ankylosing spondylitis patients, in which etanercept has variously been found to have some benefit, no effect or be linked with onset or recurrence of uveitis [62]. In contrast, a retrospective study by Hernandez-Illas and colleagues reported resolution of diffuse or necrotising anterior scleritis in all eight patients, seven of whom had an associated systemic autoimmune disease. However, data regarding concomitant immunosuppressive therapy and length of follow-up were not provided [63]. There were no recorded systemic adverse effects in the patients taking etanercept in either study [61, 63].

- *Infliximab*

  In a retrospective study by Sobrin and colleagues, 27 patients with refractory ocular inflammatory disease, of whom 10 had scleritis, were treated with infliximab with a mean follow-up of 25.6 months. Of the scleritis patients, 9 (90 %) achieved complete resolution of inflammation and 6 (60 %) were able to discontinue or decrease the dose of their concomitant immunosuppressive therapy. Three patients, all with scleritis, were able to achieve drug-free remission. The authors noted that

scleritis patients may be a subgroup who responds well to infliximab therapy (Category D evidence) [64]. In a more recent report from the same institution [53], 10 patients with refractory scleritis, 7 of whom had received prior therapy with an alkylating agent, were treated with infliximab with a mean follow-up of 16.4 months. Infliximab 5 mg/kg was given at weeks 0 and 2 as a loading dose and then continued 4–8 weekly thereafter. Nine (90 %) patients achieved complete resolution of inflammation with 6 (60 %) being able to discontinue all concomitant immunosuppressive therapy. The mean time to a clinical response was 13 weeks with most patients requiring 4 weekly infusions to maintain quiescence. One patient (10 %) developed a lupus-like reaction necessitating discontinuation of infliximab and two patients developed streptococcal upper respiratory tract infections.

Sen and colleagues conducted a prospective open label pilot study in five patients with refractory, non-necrotising anterior scleritis. Infliximab 5 mg/kg was administered at weeks 0 and 2 and then 4 weekly through to week 30 after which the infusion interval was increased. All patients initially achieved quiescence by week 14, but this could not be sustained in 1 patient. Three (60 %) patients were able to taper prednisolone to <10 mg/day, but none achieved drug-free remission. Two patients developed nonserious adverse effects, including urinary tract infection, upper and lower respiratory tract infections, ear infection, facial rash and headache, all of which resolved spontaneously or with appropriate treatment [65].

- *Adalimumab*

  There is a single case report of a patient with RA-associated nodular anterior scleritis, who was intolerant of oral corticosteroids, being successfully treated with adalimumab [66]. At 3 months after commencement of subcutaneous adalimumab 40 mg fortnightly, in addition to methotrexate 20 mg weekly, the inflammation had virtually resolved, and the scleritis remained quiescent at 6 months follow-up.

Anakinra

Anakinra is a recombinant IL-1 receptor antagonist, an imitation of the naturally occurring IL-1 receptor antagonist, which blocks the activity of IL-1. IL-1 is a proinflammatory cytokine which has also been implicated in scleral destruction through the induction of MMPS. The usual dose in RA patients is 100 mg/day subcutaneously, either alone or in combination with methotrexate. There is no evidence to date that anakinra is associated with an increased risk of tuberculosis (Category D evidence) [54, 55]. However, there is an increased risk of serious bacterial infection, particularly in patients who are also receiving corticosteroids, and anakinra should not be commenced if a serious infection is present (Category A evidence) [54, 55]. There is a high rate (up to 70 % of patients) of injection-site reactions, but these reactions often do not require treatment and seem to be moderated with continued use in most patients (Category A evidence) [54, 55]. Anakinra is classified as FDA Category B (no definite harm but insufficient evidence) in pregnancy [54, 55].

There is a single case report of two patients with RA-associated diffuse anterior scleritis who were successfully treated with anakinra [67]. In one patient infliximab was ineffective and the other patient developed scleritis while on etanercept treatment for her arthritis. Both were commenced on subcutaneous anakinra 100 mg/day in combination with methotrexate 10 mg/week. The first patient noted a dramatic improvement after 8 weeks and the scleritis remained quiescent, over a period of 3 years, with tapering of prednisolone to 5 mg/day and methotrexate to 7.5 mg/week. The second patient noted remission of symptoms and signs after 6 weeks, and the scleritis remained quiescent, over a period of 1 year, on anakinra alone.

Daclizumab

Daclizumab is a humanised monoclonal antibody that exerts its immunosuppressive effect through competitive antagonism of the alpha (Tac/CD25) subunit of the IL-2 receptor on activated T cells, effectively preventing the IL-2-mediated stimulation of lymphocytes. Daclizumab was primarily used in the prevention of rejection in transplant patients, but some success had been reported in its use in patients with scleritis and other ocular inflammatory diseases. However, it has recently been withdrawn from the European market due to manufacturing costs not being met by demand [68].

Rituximab

Rituximab is a chimeric monoclonal antibody directed against CD20, a B cell surface antigen expressed by pre-B cells through memory B cells but not by stem cells or plasma cells. Rituximab is proposed to deplete CD20+ B cells by several mechanisms including antibody-dependent cellular cytotoxicity, complement-dependent toxicity and induction of apoptosis. Rituximab can deplete peripheral B cells for up to 9 months or longer after a single course of therapy. B cells not only produce autoantibodies but also produce proinflammatory cytokines, present antigens to T cells and provide costimulatory signals essential for T-cell activation, clonal expansion and effector function [69]. In patients with scleritis, the usual dose is two 1 g intravenous infusions (given with 100 mg IV methylprednisolone or equivalent) separated by an interval of 2 weeks. In RA patients, repeated treatment courses have been shown to be effective in initial responders (Category C evidence) [54, 55]. Serious adverse events reported with rituximab include viral reactivation, type III hypersensitivity reactions (more common in patients with an underlying autoimmune condition) and a severe, life-threatening condition known as cytokine release syndrome (seen in non-Hodgkin lymphoma (NHL) patients) [69]. However, generally rituximab is well tolerated with mild to moderate infusion reactions being the most common adverse event. Rituximab is classified as FDA Category C (no human studies and animal studies either show risk or are lacking; however, potential benefits may justify potential risks) in pregnancy [54, 55].

There is an increased risk of certain viral infections, including cytomegalovirus, HSV, VZV, hepatitis B virus and JC virus in patients treated with rituximab. Fatal hepatitis B reactivation has been reported in NHL patients treated with rituximab. Hence, rituximab is contraindicated in patients with hepatitis B, and hepatitis B status should be checked before treatment. Rituximab appears safe in patients with hepatitis C (Category D evidence) [54, 55]. Cases of PML have been reported in patients treated with rituximab who have underlying disorders that independently carry a risk for PML [47]. There is a small increased risk of serious bacterial infections which does not appear to increase further with repeated courses (Category A and D evidence) [54, 55]. There is no evidence of an increased incidence of tuberculosis in NHL patients treated with rituximab [54, 55]. Rituximab should not be given in the presence of serious or opportunistic infection [54, 55]. Infusion reactions are most common with the first infusion of the first course (up to 35 %) and are reduced with the second and subsequent infusions (5–10 %). Concurrent administration of intravenous corticosteroids reduces the incidence and severity of infusion reactions by about 30 % without impacting on efficacy (Category A evidence) [54, 55].

The reported use of rituximab in the treatment of scleritis is limited to single case studies and a few small case series. Chauhan and colleagues presented three cases of RA-associated scleritis which were successfully treated with rituximab. A cycle of 2 rituximab infusions (1 g/infusion 2 weeks apart) resulted in remission of joint and eye disease in all three patients at a follow-up of 6 months (two patients) or 2 years (one patient) [70]. Taylor and colleagues retrospectively reviewed data from ten consecutive patients with refractory ophthalmic WG who were treated with rituximab. Of the ten patients, there were three cases in which refractory scleritis was the primary reason for treatment. Of these, all three were either on cyclophosphamide or had been previously treated with cyclophosphamide at the time of commencement of rituximab therapy. Remission was achieved after a single cycle of 2 rituximab infusions (1 g/infusion 2 weeks apart) in all three patients within 7 months. One patient was retreated at 6 months due to a return of B cells and proteinase 3, but remained in clinical remission throughout this period. All three patients were able to taper prednisolone to $\leq$7.5 mg/day, with only one requiring a concomitant second-line agent (azathioprine 100 mg/day) at 12 months follow-up. Rituximab was well tolerated in all ten patients with no significant adverse effects [71].

Preliminary results from a phase I/II prospective randomised dose-ranging pilot study [72] of the use of rituximab in the treatment of refractory scleritis and noninfectious orbital inflammation have also been encouraging. Patients were randomised to receive either 500 mg or 1 g infusions of rituximab on study days 1 and 15. Retreatment was permitted after week 24 for initial responders. Primary endpoints of the study, measured at weeks 24 and 48, were corticosteroid tapering by at least 50 % and a two step decrease in disease activity grading score. Of the 10 patients with scleritis, 3 (30 %) achieved corticosteroid tapering and 8 (80 %) had improvement in disease activity score at week 24. Seven patients (70 %) required retreatment at a mean of 32 weeks. Of the 20 patients overall, 6 of the first 7 enrolled had early post-infusion inflammatory exacerbations, but peri-infusional corticosteroids decreased the incidence to 2 of the last 13 (15 %) patients. Four patients (20 %) had an infusion reaction, and to date there has been 1 case each of cellulitis, recurrent genital herpes and exacerbation of psoriasis.

3.1.7 Future Directions

Scleritis is a rare disease and collecting data on its clinical features and treatment outcomes is difficult. Conducting randomised clinical trials to evaluate new therapies is also not feasible at this time. Collaborative studies using standardised activity scoring systems, photographic documentation and Internet-based databases (www.scleritisonline.com) offer the best approach at present to gather useful prospective data on scleritis and its management. Such studies are being established at present. Studies using this technology should allow clinicians to establish the safety and efficacy of current treatments such as subconjunctival triamcinolone and other potential new local and systemic therapies.

References

1. Watson PG, Hayreh SS. Scleritis and episcleritis. Br J Ophthalmol. 1976;60(3):163–91.
2. Tuft SJ, Watson PG. Progression of scleral disease. Ophthalmology. 1991;98(4):467–71.

3. McCluskey PJ, Watson PG, Lightman S, Haybittle J, Restori M, Branley M. Posterior scleritis: clinical features, systemic associations, and outcome in a large series of patients. Ophthalmology. 1999;106(12):2380–6.

4. Jabs DA, Mudun A, Dunn JP, Marsh MJ. Episcleritis and scleritis: clinical features and treatment results. Am J Ophthalmol. 2000;130(4):469–76.

5. Jabs DA, Rosenbaum JT, Foster CS, Holland GN, Jaffe GJ, Louie JS, et al. Guidelines for the use of immunosuppressive drugs in patients with ocular inflammatory disorders: recommendations of an expert panel. Am J Ophthalmol. 2000;130(4):492–513.

6. Keino H, Watanabe T, Taki W, Nakashima C, Okada AA. Clinical features and visual outcomes of Japanese patients with scleritis. Br J Ophthalmol. 2010;94(11):1459–63.

7. Raiji VR, Palestine AG, Parver DL. Scleritis and systemic disease association in a community-based referral practice. Am J Ophthalmol. 2009;148(6):946–50.

8. Sainz de la Maza M, Molina MP, Gonzalez-Gonzalez L, Doctor P, Tauber J, Foster CS. Clinical characteristics of a large cohort of patients with scleritis and episcleritis. Ophthalmology. 2012;119:43–50.

9. Sainz de la Maza M, Molina MP, Gonzalez-Gonzalez L, Doctor P, Tauber J, Foster CS. Scleritis therapy. Ophthalmology. 2012;119:51–8.

10. Hakin KN, Watson PG. Systemic associations of scleritis. Int Ophthalmol Clin. 1991;31(3):111–29.

11. Okhravi N, Odufuwa B, McCluskey P, Lightman S. Scleritis. Surv Ophthalmol. 2005;50(4):351–63.

12. Sainz de la Maza M, Foster CS, Jabbur NS. Scleritis associated with rheumatoid arthritis and with other systemic immune-mediated diseases. Ophthalmology. 1994;101(7):1281–6; discussion 1287–88.

13. Sainz de la Maza M, Jabbur NS, Foster CS. Severity of scleritis and episcleritis. Ophthalmology. 1994;101(2):389–96.

14. Hoffman GS, Kerr GS, Leavitt RY, Hallahan CW, Lebovics RS, Travis WD, et al. Wegener granulomatosis: an analysis of 158 patients. Ann Intern Med. 1992;116(6):488–98.

15. Sainz de la Maza M, Foster CS, Jabbur NS. Scleritis associated with systemic vasculitic diseases. Ophthalmology. 1995;102(4):687–92.

16. Hoang-Xaun T, Foster CS, Rice BA. Scleritis in relapsing polychondritis. Response to therapy. Ophthalmology. 1990;97(7):892–8.

17. Albini TA, Rao NA, Smith RE. The diagnosis and management of anterior scleritis. Int Ophthalmol Clin. 2005;45(2):191–204.

18. Gonzalez-Gonzalez L, Molina-Prat N, Doctor P, Tauber J, Sainz de la Maza M, Foster CS. Clinical features and presentation of infectious scleritis from herpes viruses. A report of 35 cases. Ophthalmology. 2012;119:1460–4.

19. Bhat PV, Jakobiec FA, Kurbanyan K, Zhao T, Foster CS. Chronic herpes simplex scleritis: characterization of 9 cases of an underrecognized clinical entity. Am J Ophthalmol. 2009;148(5):779–789.e772.

20. Jain V, Garg P, Sharma S. Microbial scleritis-experience from a developing country. Eye. 2009;23(2):255–61.

21. Liesegang TJ. Diagnosis and therapy of herpes zoster ophthalmicus. Ophthalmology. 1991;98(8):1216–29.

22. Lin CP, Shih MH, Tsai MC. Clinical experiences of infectious scleral ulceration: a complication of pterygium operation. Br J Ophthalmol. 1997;81(11):980–3.

23. O'Donoghue E, Lightman S, Tuft S, Watson P. Surgically induced necrotising sclerokeratitis (SINS)–precipitating factors and response to treatment. Br J Ophthalmol. 1992;76(1):17–21.

24. Fong LP, Sainz de la Maza M, Rice BA, Kupferman AE, Foster CS. Immunopathology of scleritis. Ophthalmology. 1991;98(4):472–9.

25. Bernauer W, Watson PG, Daicker B, Lightman S. Cells perpetuating the inflammatory response in scleritis. Br J Ophthalmol. 1994;78(5):381–5.

26. Riono WP, Hidayat AA, Rao NA. Scleritis: a clinicopathologic study of 55 cases. Ophthalmology. 1999;106(7):1328–33.

27. Usui Y, Parikh J, Goto H, Rao NA. Immunopathology of necrotising scleritis. Br J Ophthalmol. 2008;92(3):417–9.

28. Amadi-Obi A, Yu C-R, Liu X, Mahdi RM, Clarke GL, Nussenblatt RB, et al. TH17 cells contribute to uveitis and scleritis and are expanded by IL-2 and inhibited by IL-27/STAT1. Nat Med. 2007;13(6):711–8.

29. Di Girolamo N, Lloyd A, McCluskey P, Filipic M, Wakefield D. Increased expression of matrix metalloproteinases in vivo in scleritis tissue and in vitro in cultured human scleral fibroblasts. Am J Pathol. 1997;150(2):653–66.

30. Akpek EK, Thorne JE, Qazi FA, Do DV, Jabs DA. Evaluation of patients with scleritis for systemic disease. Ophthalmology. 2004;111(3):501–6.

31. Sainz de la Maza M, Jabbur NS, Foster CS. An analysis of therapeutic decision for scleritis. Ophthalmology. 1993;100(9):1372–6.

32. Jabs DA. Discussion of a prospective evaluation of subconjunctival injection of triamcinolone acetonide for resistant anterior scleritis. Ophthalmol 2002;109:806–8.

33. Zamir E, Read RW, Smith RE, Wang RC, Rao NA. A prospective evaluation of subconjunctival injection of triamcinolone acetonide for resistant anterior scleritis. Ophthalmology. 2002;109(4):798–805; discussion 805–797.

34. Roufas A, Jalaludin B, Gaskin C, McCluskey P. Subconjunctival triamcinolone treatment for non-necrotising anterior scleritis. Br J Ophthalmol. 2010;94(6):743–7.

35. Sohn E, Wang R, Read R, Roufas A, Teo L, Moorthy R, et al. Long-term, multicenter evaluation of subconjunctival injection of triamcinolone for non-necrotizing, noninfectious anterior scleritis. Ophthalmology. 2011;118:1932–7.

36. Sohn EH, Wang R, Read R, Roufas A, Moorthy R, Albini T, et al. Long-term, multi-center evaluation of

subconjunctival injection of triamcinolone for non-necrotizing, non-infectious anterior scleritis. Ophthalmol 2011;118:1932–7.

37. Bauer AM, Fiehn C, Becker MD. Celecoxib, a selective inhibitor of cyclooxygenase 2 for therapy of diffuse anterior scleritis. Am J Ophthalmol. 2005;139(6):1086–9.

38. Kim SJ, Flach AJ, Jampol LM. Nonsteroidal anti-inflammatory drugs in ophthalmology. Surv Ophthalmol. 2010;55(2):108–33.

39. McCluskey P, Wakefield D. Intravenous pulse methylprednisolone in scleritis. Arch Ophthalmol. 1987;105(6):793–7.

40. Kempen JH, Daniel E, Gangaputra S, Dreger K, Jabs DA, Kacmaz RO, et al. Methods for identifying long-term adverse effects of treatment in patients with eye diseases: the Systemic Immunosuppressive Therapy for Eye Diseases (SITE) Cohort Study. Ophthalmic Epidemiol. 2008;15(1):47–55.

41. Kempen JH, Gangaputra S, Daniel E, Levy-Clarke GA, Nussenblatt RB, Rosenbaum JT, et al. Long-term risk of malignancy among patients treated with immunosuppressive agents for ocular inflammation: a critical assessment of the evidence. Am J Ophthalmol. 2008;146(6):802–812.e801.

42. Daniel E, Thorne JE, Newcomb CW, Pujari SS, Kacmaz RO, Levy-Clarke GA, et al. Mycophenolate mofetil for ocular inflammation. Am J Ophthalmol. 2010;149(3):423–432.e421–422.

43. Gangaputra S, Newcomb CW, Liesegang TL, Kacmaz RO, Jabs DA, Levy-Clarke GA, et al. Methotrexate for ocular inflammatory diseases. Ophthalmology. 2009;116(11):2188–2198.e2181.

44. Kacmaz RO, Kempen JH, Newcomb C, Daniel E, Gangaputra S, Nussenblatt RB, et al. Cyclosporine for ocular inflammatory diseases. Ophthalmology. 2010;117(3):576–84.

45. Pasadhika S, Kempen JH, Newcomb CW, Liesegang TL, Pujari SS, Rosenbaum JT, et al. Azathioprine for ocular inflammatory diseases. Am J Ophthalmol. 2009;148(4):500–509.e502.

46. Pujari SS, Kempen JH, Newcomb CW, Gangaputra S, Daniel E, Suhler EB, et al. Cyclophosphamide for ocular inflammatory diseases. Ophthalmology. 2010;117(2):356–65.

47. Berger JR. Progressive multifocal leukoencephalopathy and newer biological agents. Drug Saf. 2010;33(11):969–83.

48. Ostensen M, Lockshin M, Doria A, Valesini G, Meroni P, Gordon C, et al. Update on safety during pregnancy of biological agents and some immunosuppressive anti-rheumatic drugs. Rheumatology. 2008;47 Suppl 3:iii28–31.

49. Galor A, Jabs DA, Leder HA, Kedhar SR, Dunn JP, Peters 3rd GB, et al. Comparison of antimetabolite drugs as corticosteroid-sparing therapy for noninfectious ocular inflammation. Ophthalmology. 2008;115(10):1826–32.

50. Young AL, Wong SM, Leung ATS, Leung GYS, Cheng LL, Lam DSC. Successful treatment of surgically induced necrotizing scleritis with tacrolimus. Clin Experiment Ophthalmol. 2005;33(1):98–9.

51. Goldstein DA, Fontanilla FA, Kaul S, Sahin O, Tessler HH. Long-term follow-up of patients treated with short-term high-dose chlorambucil for sight-threatening ocular inflammation. Ophthalmology. 2002;109(2):370–7.

52. Cush J, Kavanaugh A. TNF-alpha blocking therapies. 4th ed. Philadelphia: Mosby Elsevier; 2008.

53. Doctor P, Sultan A, Syed S, Christen W, Bhat P, Foster CS. Infliximab for the treatment of refractory scleritis. Br J Ophthalmol. 2010;94(5):579–83.

54. Furst DE. The risk of infections with biologic therapies for rheumatoid arthritis. Semin Arthritis Rheum. 2010;39(5):327–46.

55. Furst DE, Keystone EC, Braun J, Breedveld FC, Burmester GR, De Benedetti F, et al. Updated consensus statement on biological agents for the treatment of rheumatic diseases, 2010. Ann Rheum Dis. 2010;70 Suppl 1:i2–36.

56. Caramaschi P, Bambara LM, Pieropan S, Tinazzi I, Volpe A, Biasi D. Anti-TNFalpha blockers, autoantibodies and autoimmune diseases. Joint Bone Spine. 2009;76(4):333–42.

57. Chung ES, Packer M, Lo KH, Fasanmade AA, Willerson JT, Anti TNFTACHFI. Randomized, double-blind, placebo-controlled, pilot trial of infliximab, a chimeric monoclonal antibody to tumor necrosis factor-alpha, in patients with moderate-to-severe heart failure: results of the anti-TNF Therapy Against Congestive Heart Failure (ATTACH) trial. Circulation. 2003;107(25):3133–40.

58. Kwon HJ, Cote TR, Cuffe MS, Kramer JM, Braun MM. Case reports of heart failure after therapy with a tumor necrosis factor antagonist. Ann Intern Med. 2003;138(10):807–11.

59. Wegener's Granulomatosis Etanercept Trial Research Group. Etanercept plus standard therapy for Wegener's granulomatosis. N Eng J Med. 2005;352(4):351–61.

60. Suhler EB, Smith JR, Wertheim MS, Lauer AK, Kurz DE, Pickard TD, et al. A prospective trial of infliximab therapy for refractory uveitis: preliminary safety and efficacy outcomes. Arch Ophthalmol. 2005;123(7):903–12.

61. Smith JR, Levinson RD, Holland GN, Jabs DA, Robinson MR, Whitcup SM, et al. Differential efficacy of tumor necrosis factor inhibition in the management of inflammatory eye disease and associated rheumatic disease. Arthritis Rheum. 2001;45(3):252–7.

62. Hooper C, Taylor S, Lightman S. Uveitis in rheumatic diseases. Curr Rheum Rev. 2011;7(1):24–38.

63. Hernandez-Illas M, Tozman E, Fulcher SFA, Jundt JW, Davis J, Pflugfelder SC. Recombinant human tumor necrosis factor receptor Fc fusion protein (Etanercept): experience as a therapy for sight-threatening scleritis and sterile corneal ulceration. Eye Contact Lens. 2004;30(1):2–5.

64. Sobrin L, Kim EC, Christen W, Papadaki T, Letko E, Foster CS. Infliximab therapy for the treatment of refractory ocular inflammatory disease. Arch Ophthalmol. 2007;125(7):895–900.

65. Sen HN, Sangave A, Hammel K, Levy-Clarke G, Nussenblatt RB. Infliximab for the treatment of active scleritis. Can J Ophthalmol. 2009;44(3):e9–12.

66. Restrepo JP, Molina MP. Successful treatment of severe nodular scleritis with adalimumab. Clin Rheumatol. 2010;29(5):559–61.

67. Botsios C, Sfriso P, Ostuni PA, Todesco S, Punzi L. Efficacy of the IL-1 receptor antagonist, anakinra, for the treatment of diffuse anterior scleritis in rheumatoid arthritis. Report of two cases. Rheumatology. 2007;46(6):1042–3.

68. Campara M, Tzvetanov IG, Oberholzer J. Interleukin-2 receptor blockade with humanized monoclonal antibody for solid organ transplantation. Expert Opin Biol Ther. 2010;10(6):959–69.

69. Lee S, Ballow M. Monoclonal antibodies and fusion proteins and their complications: targeting B cells in autoimmune diseases. J Allergy Clin Immunol. 2010;125(4):814–20.

70. Chauhan S, Kamal A, Thompson RN, Estrach C, Moots RJ. Rituximab for treatment of scleritis associated with rheumatoid arthritis. Br J Ophthalmol. 2009;93(7):984–5.

71. Taylor SRJ, Salama AD, Joshi L, Pusey CD, Lightman SL. Rituximab is effective in the treatment of refractory ophthalmic Wegener's granulomatosis. Arthritis Rheum. 2009;60(5):1540–7.

72. Butler NJ, Lim LL, Giles TR, de Saint Sardos A, Ali A, Lee ST, et al. Rituximab in the treatment of refractory scleritis and non-infectious orbital inflammation: 24 week outcomes from a phase I/II prospective, randomized study. Paper presented at The Association for Research in Vision and Ophthalmology. Fort Lauderdale, Florida, USA, 2011.

Noninfectious Inflammation in Cataract Surgery

4

Nick Mamalis and Stanley R. Fuller

Contents

N. Mamalis, MD (✉)
Department of Ophthalmology,
John A. Moran Eye Center, University of Utah,
65 Mario Capechhi Dr., Salt Lake City
84132, UT, USA
e-mail: nick.mamalis@hsc.utah.edu

S.R. Fuller, MD
Department of Ophthalmology, John A. Moran Eye
Center, University of Utah,
65 Mario Capechhi Dr., Salt Lake City
84132, UT, USA
e-mail: srfuller@geisinger.edu

4.1 Introduction

Intraocular Inflammation following cataract surgery is a well-recognized aspect of cataract extraction, with severity ranging from transient and mild to chronic and severe. While a majority of cataract cases are associated with mild and transient inflammation with no lasting sequelae, postoperative inflammation that is persistent and/or moderate to severe can result in major sequelae including corneal decompensation, chronic uveitis, cystoid macular edema, and glaucoma. The end result may be poor visual outcomes. There are several causes of anterior segment inflammation following cataract surgery including surgical trauma, infectious agents, retained lens material, mechanical trauma associated with the implanted artificial lens, sterile toxic substances, and exacerbation of preexisting uveitis. The main subject to be covered in this chapter will be noninfectious causes of post-cataract surgery inflammation, although infectious etiologies will be briefly mentioned as they are an important part of the differential in both acute and chronic cases of postoperative inflammation. Recognizing and accurately diagnosing the cause(s) of inflammation following cataract surgery can lead to early appropriate treatment and better outcomes.

U. Pleyer et al. (eds.), *Immune Modulation and Anti-Inflammatory Therapy in Ocular Disorders*, DOI 10.1007/978-3-642-54350-0_4, © Springer-Verlag Berlin Heidelberg 2014

4.2 Noninfectious, Acute Postoperative Intraocular Inflammation

4.2.1 Inflammation Secondary to Surgery and Surgical Complications

While modern cataract surgery using phacoemulsification is much less invasive and harmful to ocular tissues than historical methods, there still remains an element of inflammation that is directly related to the surgery itself. Incisional and manipulative trauma triggers the inflammatory cascade and the conversion of arachidonic acid to prostaglandins and thromboxanes (cyclooxygenase pathway) and leukotrienes (lipoxygenase pathway). The release of these inflammatory mediators, along with histamine and various kinins, leads to a breakdown of the blood-aqueous barrier [1]. Longer surgeries and those in which extensive manipulations are involved can lead to a more pronounced postoperative inflammation. Postsurgical inflammation is evident on exam in the form of aqueous cells, flare, fibrin, and occasionally engorged iris vessels. This inflammation, while usually transient, can be exacerbated by retained lens material or mechanical damage to the intraocular structures from an implanted intraocular lens (IOL).

Perioperative topical NSAID and corticosteroid use has become commonplace in an attempt to reduce surgically induced inflammation, although opinions on the proper usage differ among ophthalmologists. The anti-inflammatory properties of NSAIDs lie in blocking the cyclooxygenase (COX) enzymes, which play an important role in the synthesis of prostaglandins from arachidonic acid, whereas corticosteroids block both the cyclooxygenase and lipoxygenase pathways. By inhibiting prostaglandin production, NSAIDs reduce the intraocular effects of prostaglandins including vasodilation, leukocyte migration, and breakdown of the blood-aqueous barrier [2]. NSAIDs have been shown to be beneficial in the prevention of surgically induced miosis, reducing postoperative inflammation, preventing and treating cystoid macular edema, and

decreasing postoperative discomfort and pain. Corticosteroids are commonly used postoperatively in a 1- to 6-week course and perform well in reducing postoperative inflammation, although they carry a risk of increasing intraocular pressure (IOP) and complications if used long term [2, 3].

When used appropriately, studies support the efficacy of the suprofen 1 %, flurbiprofen 0.03 %, diclofenac 0.1 %, ketorolac 0.4 and 0.5 %, indomethacin 1 %, nepafenac 0.1 %, and bromfenac 0.09 % in decreasing postoperative inflammation after cataract surgery without significant toxicity. With the exception of the indomethacin, nepafenac, and bromfenac, all have been found to also be effective in preventing miosis during cataract surgery. In addition, studies have shown that perioperative topical NSAID use has a measurable beneficial effect on visual acuity after cataract surgery and that using NSAIDs in addition to corticosteroids has an additive effect [2].

The use of heparin in the irrigating solution also has been evaluated as a method to decrease post-cataract surgery inflammation. Although traditionally an anticoagulant, heparin has also been found to possess anti-inflammatory effects as well [4]. Several studies have shown a decrease in inflammatory markers on exam in the early postoperative period [5, 6]. There is some evidence that heparin should be used with caution in patients with a blood-aqueous barrier disturbance such as patients with diabetes or uveitis, as it can predispose to bleeding and postoperative hyphema [7]. Heparin has been shown to be safe and effective in pediatric cataract surgery as well [8]. Low-molecular-weight heparin, which carries less of a risk of bleeding complications but still retains its anti-inflammatory properties, has shown similar reductions in early postoperative inflammation when added to the irrigating solution [9].

4.2.2 TASS

4.2.2.1 Introduction/Pathophysiology

Toxic anterior segment syndrome (TASS), a term first coined in 1992 by Monson et al. [10], is a sterile inflammation of the anterior segment, most commonly seen following anterior segment surgery. Occurrences of TASS are rare in general, with cases often occurring in groups or clusters, but also seen in individual cases. It is important to distinguish TASS from infectious cases of postoperative inflammation as their presentations can be somewhat similar but their treatments are significantly different.

The pathophysiology of TASS involves the common end point of damage to the corneal endothelial cell layer, iris, and trabecular meshwork from toxic insult and widespread breakdown of the blood-aqueous barrier. The possible causative agents of the damage are many, and possible suspects include any substance that enters the eye either during or immediately after surgery. A thorough and detailed investigation is often required to find the cause. Two broad categories for common etiologic causes of TASS include (1) instrument cleaning and sterilization and (2) the concentration and composition of any liquids and medications used intraocularly. In addition, there are many other avenues in which the sensitive corneal endothelial cells and intraocular tissue can come in contact with damaging chemicals or substances, many of which will be detailed in the following discussion.

It is difficult to accurately determine the true incidence of TASS, as the reporting of cases by surgical centers and physicians is not mandatory and many may feel that mild cases are not of enough significance to report. Adding to the difficulty is the sporadic nature of the occurrences, with a surgeon or surgical center often having hundreds to thousands and even tens of thousands of surgeries without a TASS case, and then having multiple cases on the same day. While not indicating incidence, a recent report summarizing the data from all the cases reported to the ASCRS-supported TASS Task Force over a 3-year period showed that at 68 centers that had experienced TASS cases, 909 cases of TASS were seen out of 50,114 cataract surgeries performed concurrently at the centers [11].

4.2.2.2 Patient Presentation

The most common clinical symptom seen in TASS patients is significant blurred vision. The eye can also be irritated and injected. On slit lamp exam,

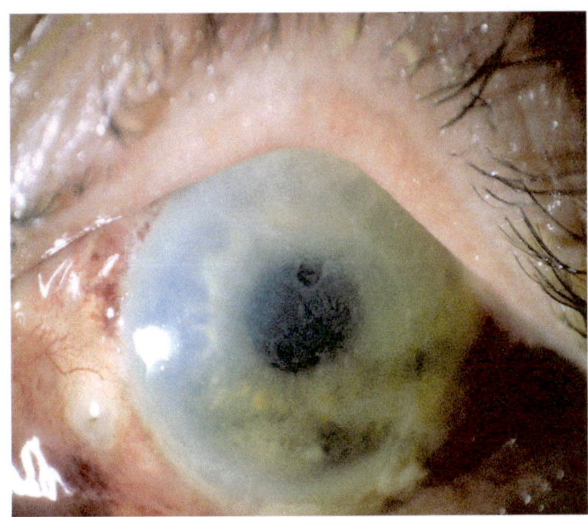

Fig. 4.1 TASS syndrome – diffuse or "limbus to limbus" corneal edema from widespread endothelial damage (Reprinted from Mamalis et al. [12], copyright ©2006, with permission from Elsevier)

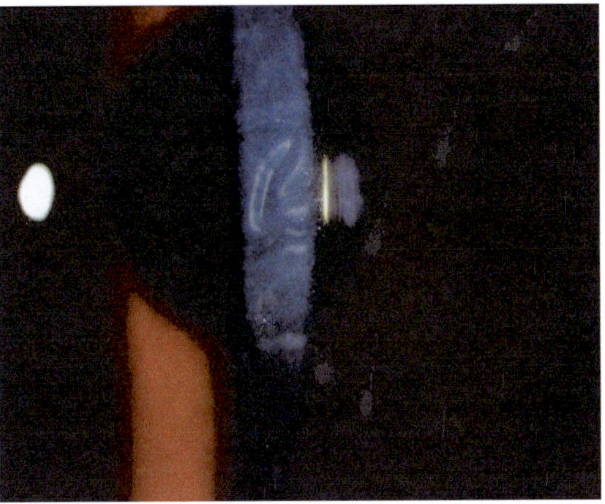

Fig. 4.2 TASS syndrome – slit lamp photomicrograph showing Descemet's folds and corneal thickening secondary to edema (Reprinted from Mamalis [13], copyright ©2009, with permission from American Academy of Ophthalmology)

the blurred vision is confirmed to be secondary to cornea edema. This edema is diffuse and is often described as being "limbus to limbus," helping the clinician to distinguish between TASS and postoperative focal edema with difficult cataract surgeries (Figs. 4.1 and 4.2). The second most striking feature of TASS is the anterior segment inflammation, seen as fibrin, inflammatory cells, and aqueous flare in the anterior chamber. This inflammation is a result of prostaglandin production and release,

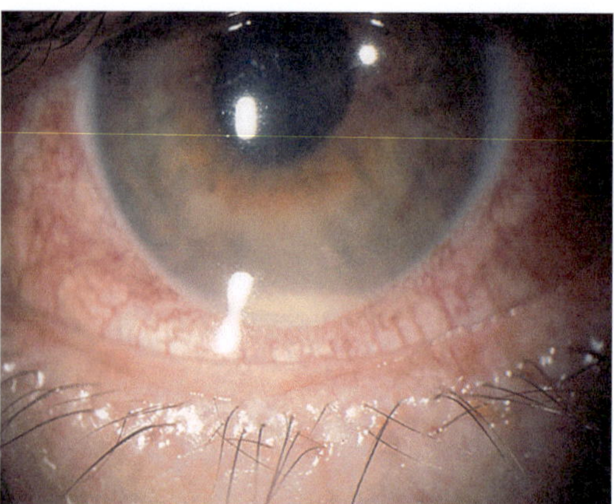

Fig. 4.3 TASS syndrome – anterior segment inflammation with hypopyon (Reprinted from Mamalis et al. [12], copyright ©2006, with permission from Elsevier)

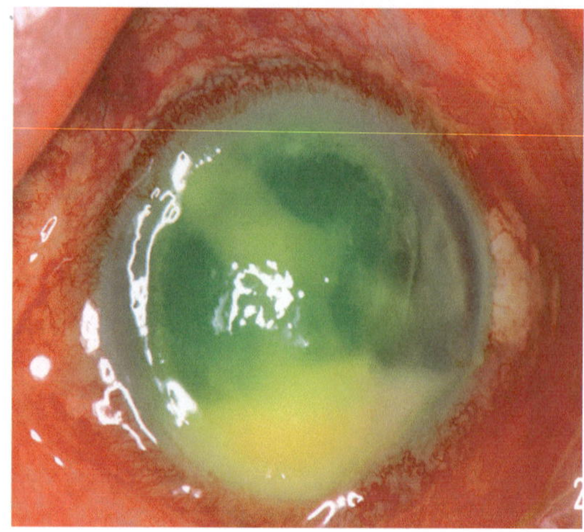

Fig. 4.5 Acute infectious endophthalmitis

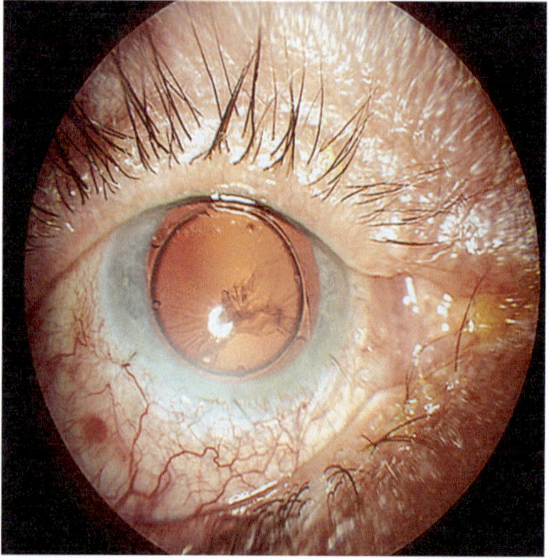

Fig. 4.4 TASS syndrome – dilated, atrophic iris with irregular pupil (Reprinted from Mamalis et al. [12], copyright ©2006, with permission from Elsevier)

which facilitates disruption of the blood-ocular barrier and leukocyte migration [2]. Secondary to the inflammation, an inferior hypopyon is often seen, as are strands of fibrin which can extend from the wound or side-port incisions and/or between the intraocular lens and iris (Fig. 4.3). Iris and pupillary abnormalities can be seen, such as transillumination of a thinned iris or a permanently dilated iris or pupil (Fig. 4.4). In addition, significant damage to the trabecular meshwork can lead to a secondary glaucoma [12, 13].

A patient presenting with acute postoperative anterior segment inflammation should be closely examined and a brief history taken in order to distinguish between infectious and non-infectious causes. While it is sometimes difficult to discern between the two causes as they often share the signs of blurry vision, eye redness, and in some cases pain, the following generalities in the presentation of patients with TASS and infectious endophthalmitis can help the clinician determine the etiology of the inflammation. TASS patients characteristically present earlier, anywhere from 12 to 48 h postoperatively but typically within 24 h, are always gram stain and culture negative, have diffuse corneal edema, have inflammatory cells and fibrin in the anterior chamber and/or a hypopyon, and can show pupil/iris changes. Infectious endophthalmitis cases characteristically present later, usually 2–7 days postoperatively with the exception of highly virulent strains of bacteria, can have a positive gram stain or culture and do not typically have diffuse corneal edema or pupil/iris changes (Fig. 4.5). In addition, TASS cases tend to be limited to the anterior chamber, with rare spillover into the vitreous, whereas infectious endophthalmitis cases commonly involve the vitreous. Patients with endophthalmitis are also more likely to have pain, whereas pain is usually absent in patients with TASS unless the inflammation is severe. If treatment with steroids is begun, TASS patients will generally improve, whereas acute infectious endophthalmitis patients will not [12, 13].

4.2.2.3 Etiology/Causes

The etiologies of TASS are many and one must often evaluate all surgical procedures and protocols to discover possible causes and reduce the risk of future occurrences. Proper instrument cleaning and sterilization plays a key role in the prevention of TASS. Since the phaco- and I/A handpieces enter and spend time within the eye, they can potentially act as a conduit to allow toxic materials to enter the eye. Residual OVD or cortex from previous cataract surgery, detergent or enzyme residue from cleaning solutions, endotoxin from ultrasound baths, and condensates from impure cleaning water used by sterilization equipment [14] all can gain access to the anterior chamber during surgery and cause TASS.

Ophthalmic instruments used in cataract surgery differ from most other general surgical instruments in that they accumulate very little bioburden during their use. As such, their cleaning and sterilization processes should not be assumed to be the same as other surgical instruments. Two methods commonly used to remove bioburden from surgical instruments are washing with detergents and/or enzymes and putting the instruments in an ultrasound bath. Both of these methods should be used with caution in ophthalmic instrument cleaning. Detergents and enzymes can remain on the instruments if not well flushed with sterile water following their cleaning, and autoclaving will not cause them to be fully inactivated [15]. Ultrasound baths can become contaminated with bacteria that produce heat-stable endotoxins if not cleaned often (at least daily) and properly [16]. The bacteria will be killed by autoclaving, but the endotoxin can remain active, attach to the instruments, and cause toxicity if injected into the eye [12, 13].

A key step in proper cleaning and sterilization of instruments is to flush the handpieces and any reusable cannulas immediately after use with at least 120 cm^3 of sterile deionized or sterile distilled water per port [11]. If immediate flushing is not available, the instruments can be set in a ster-

ile water bath until flushed to prevent the drying of material on their surfaces or within the lumens, as once OVD or cortex has dried, it can be significantly more difficult to remove. This flushing will serve to remove any small amount of OVD or cortex that may have attached to the instruments and will make unnecessary the use of enzymes, detergents, or an ultrasound bath as the bioburden will have been removed. Further guidelines of cleaning and sterilizing ophthalmic instruments can be found in the special report by ASCRS and ASORN entitled "Recommended Practices for Cleaning and Sterilizing Intraocular Surgical Instruments" [17].

In addition to improper instrument cleaning and sterilization, improper concentration and/or composition of any solution that has access to the anterior chamber during cataract surgery can lead to inflammation and TASS. Preservatives and stabilization agents have been found to be toxic to corneal endothelium; thus, all fluids that enter the eye should be preservative-free. Lidocaine used for intraocular anesthesia should be ensured to be methylparaben-free (MPF), as methylparaben is a preservative linked to endothelial toxicity. Epinephrine that is added to BSS during surgery should be free of stabilizing agents such as bisulphites and metasulphites [18]. OVD that contains the preservative benzalkonium chloride should be avoided [19]. All of the offending agents can lead to toxicity of the corneal endothelium, corneal edema, and postoperative inflammation [12, 13, 20].

The concentration and composition of solutions used intraocularly should also be closely monitored for adherence to guidelines. Antibiotics, such as gentamicin or vancomycin, if bought as a concentrate, must be diluted properly or they can cause cornea toxicity. Lidocaine at a level of 2.0 % or higher has caused significant corneal thickening and opacification postoperatively [21]. Any abnormality in the composition of BSS used for surgical irrigation (i.e., incorrect pH, osmolarity, ionic composition, or contaminants) can be a source of cell damage and subsequent TASS [22–24]. Even solutions that would otherwise be harmless can cause inflammation and TASS if in contact with the anterior chamber tissues for an extended period of time. One example of this phenomenon is cases of TASS caused by significant amounts of OVD left in the anterior segment at the conclusion of surgery.

Even after surgery, a poorly constructed wound or wounds that are not watertight can allow access to the anterior chamber of the eye. Many drops and ointments, as they are not manufactured for use inside the eye, contain preservatives that are toxic to corneal endothelial cells. The application of ointment to the postsurgical eye should not be done under a tight pressure patch, as this has been shown to facilitate ingress of ointment into the anterior chamber with resulting inflammation [25]. Patients should be counseled to avoid rubbing the eye during the immediate postoperative period, as anecdotal evidence has suggested that this may contribute to a temporary decrease in wound integrity which allows access to the anterior chamber for toxic and possibly infectious agents.

As there are many people, procedures, products, and variables involved in bringing about a single cataract surgery, there are many places where seemingly small missteps or mistakes can lead to an end result of TASS for the patient. Thus, proper training and continuing education for surgeon and staff and review of pertinent procedures and protocols are crucial parts of TASS prevention. All individuals involved should remain vigilant in their respective duties to ensure all precautions are taken to prevent TASS. A TASS outbreak is a serious problem and requires a complete analysis of all cleaning and sterilization protocols and all medications and fluids used during surgery.

4.2.2.4 Treatment

The most effective way to deal with TASS is to prevent it from happening, as once the offending agent is in the eye and has caused damage, there is little that can be done other than attempt to suppress the inflammatory response. As maximal damage has presumably already occurred, anterior chamber washout is not routinely recommended and often deemed unhelpful. The treatment of TASS should begin immediately after diagnosis has been established and infectious etiology ruled out. If there is uncertainty

regarding a patient's diagnosis but TASS is most likely according to the patient's presentation and symptoms, treatment for TASS should begin and the patient followed closely. A low threshold should be maintained for vitreous tap and antibiotic injection if there is no clinical improvement.

The mainstay of treatment is topical corticosteroids, aimed at decreasing the inflammatory response to the toxic insult and limiting damage to intraocular tissue. Prednisone acetate 1 % drops should be used topically every 1–2 h and the patient followed carefully for the first several days to monitor for improvement. Slit lamp exams should be used often to monitor for the resolution of inflammation and corneal edema. Intraocular pressure should also be checked frequently, as the toxic insult can damage the trabecular meshwork, cause inflammation (acute trabeculitis), and lead to increased IOP. Ophthalmologists should be aware that the IOP can initially be low due to a disruption in aqueous humor production, but with recovery of aqueous production, the IOP can increase rapidly, thus illustrating the need for close follow-up for several days after the initial insult. In some cases there can be permanent damage to the trabecular meshwork, leading to a glaucoma that is refractory to treatment. Patients should also be monitored for the formation of anterior synechiae, secondary to the inflammatory response, which can lead to a secondary glaucoma. Topical NSAIDs and systemic steroids have not been evaluated for use in TASS as of this writing; however, their use in TASS, especially severe cases, is recommended by some ophthalmologists. The reduction in inflammation associated with topical NSAIDs [2] makes their use logical in cases of severe TASS [12, 13].

4.2.2.5 Outcomes

The clinical outcomes for patients with TASS vary depending on the type, amount, and duration of the toxic insult. Patients with mild cases often recover fully, with the inflammation clearing rapidly and the cornea edema clearing over days to weeks with no long-term sequelae. Moderate cases can take weeks to months for the cornea edema to clear, with the possibility of some residual corneal edema and/or increased IOP. Severe cases often involve permanent damage to the eye, such as corneal edema that does not resolve, permanent iris damage resulting in a fixed, dilated pupil and thinned iris stroma, and significantly increased IOP secondary to trabecular meshwork damage and peripheral anterior synechiae that is refractory to medical treatment alone. Severe cases not uncommonly lead to endothelial or penetrating keratoplasty and/or glaucoma surgery [12, 13].

4.3 Subacute or Chronic Postoperative Intraocular Inflammation

TASS cases and patients with a virulent bacterial endophthalmitis will start experiencing typical symptoms and exhibiting typical signs hours (more likely TASS) to days (more likely endophthalmitis) after surgery. However, if the inflammation arises weeks to months or even years after surgery, other conditions should be considered. The differential for such a reaction is wide and includes mechanical damage and inflammation from an implanted IOL (uveitis-glaucoma-hyphema syndrome), an inflammatory reaction to retained lens protein or cortex, an inflammatory reaction to polymers used in IOL manufacturing, or a reaction to postoperative ointments that gain access to the anterior chamber. In addition, in any patient with a chronic, subacute postoperative inflammation, a low virulence bacterial or fungal infection should also be considered.

4.3.1 Uveitis-Glaucoma-Hyphema Syndrome

Uveitis-glaucoma-hyphema (UGH) syndrome is characterized by a mechanical rubbing or chaffing of the iris or angle structures by an intraocular lens implant. In the past this syndrome was associated with poorly designed or finished lenses, but improvements in IOL manufacturing and a predominance of posterior chamber IOL placement in the capsular bag has reduced the

incidence of UGH syndrome. The condition has been associated most often with anterior chamber lenses, but has also been seen with posterior chamber, sulcus-fixated, and iris-supported lenses. Symptoms can arise weeks to months and in some cases years after uneventful cataract extraction and intraocular lens placement. The pathology involves mechanical damage to the iris or angle tissue, a release of iris pigment into the anterior chamber, inflammation, and a collection of iris pigment, erythrocytes, and inflammatory markers in the trabecular meshwork resulting in a sudden rise in intraocular pressure. Over time, with multiple episodes of tissue trauma, the trabecular meshwork can be permanently damaged with resulting glaucoma [26].

A patient will present with blurry vision, redness, photophobia, and sometimes pain in addition to one or all of the typical exam findings of AC inflammation, microhyphema, and increased intraocular pressures. The uveitis can be treated topically with corticosteroids and may resolve if maximal damage has already been done, but recurrent episodes of tissue damage and inflammation is common. Removal or exchange of the offending IOL is the most definitive treatment, but does not always bring significant improvements in visual outcomes [26, 27].

4.3.2 Inflammation Secondary to Lens Protein

The normal eye appears to have an immunologic tolerance to a small amount of lens antigen, such that if a small amount of cortex remains after cataract surgery, it will not cause a reaction. However, if a moderate to large amount of lens protein or cortex is retained in the eye following surgery, an IgG immune-mediated granulomatous inflammation can occur. This inflammatory condition has been called by many names, including phacoantigenic uveitis, phacoanaphylactic uveitis, phacotoxic uveitis, phacoantigenic endophthalmitis, phacoanaphylactic endophthalmitis, and lens-induced granulomatous endophthalmitis. The pattern of inflammation on histology is that of a zonal granuloma. Often the center of the inflammatory response consists of a nidus of neutrophilic inflammation around the degenerating lens material followed by concentric layers of inflammatory cells. Present in the inner layers of the inflammation are multinucleated giant cells, with epithelioid cells, eosinophils, plasma cells, lymphocytes, and histiocytes containing phagocytized lens material seen in the intermediate and outer layers of cells [28]. Similar findings are also seen in cases of trauma during which the lens capsule is ruptured and lens protein is exposed to the anterior chamber.

The patient will often present with a red, painful eye, and anterior chamber inflammation with cells, flare, and keratic precipitates. The course of the disease may include a chronic cystoid macular edema. The patient may develop glaucoma from trabecular meshwork blockage and posterior synechiae formation, with late complications of cyclitic membrane formation, hypotony, and phthisis bulbi. Steroid treatment can bring a remission of symptoms if the amount of lens protein is small, but uveitis can recur upon cessation of treatment if all the lens material has not been resorbed. Treatment for more severe cases involves topical and systemic corticosteroids, with mydriatic and cycloplegic agents used as well. The definitive cure involves removing all lens protein, thus removing the source of the inflammatory reaction.

Involvement of the fellow eye, similar to sympathetic ophthalmia, has been observed, with the inflammation in the fellow eye following that of the first in time. In rare cases sensitization to lens protein during cataract surgery in one eye can lead to an early onset of inflammation when the capsule is ruptured (surgically or traumatically) in the fellow eye [28, 29].

4.3.3 Delayed-Onset TASS

Most TASS cases are acute, but there have been several instances of a sterile, postoperative inflammation that occurs further out from surgery than the typical TASS case. In these cases, the onset of inflammation is delayed for days to even several weeks and years postoperatively.

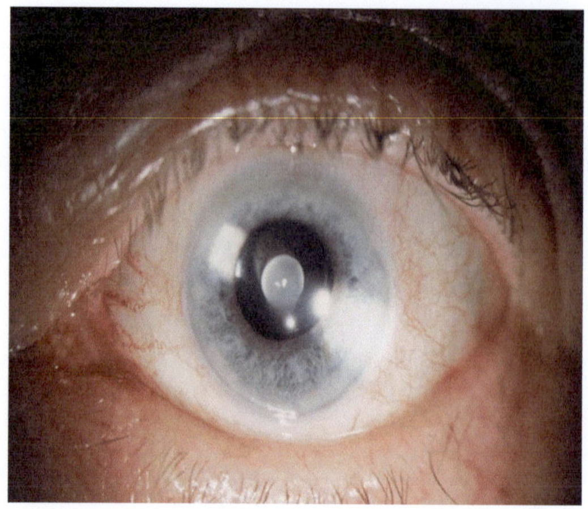

Fig. 4.6 Topical ointment in the anterior chamber (Reprinted from Mamalis et al. [12], copyright ©2006, with permission from Elsevier)

One etiology of this delayed-onset inflammatory response is postoperative ointment that has gained access to the anterior chamber. A report by Werner et al. surmised that if the application of ointment postoperatively is followed by tight patching, the risk of ointment moving into the anterior chamber is increased (Fig. 4.6) [25]. The response to the ointment appeared to be dose-dependent, with higher doses causing symptoms acutely and lower doses presenting after a delay in onset of inflammation. In addition, Jehan et al. described a series of 10 patients that experienced a delayed-onset (1–21 days postoperative) inflammatory reaction to a specific intraocular lens, the MemoryLens, which was felt to be secondary to a residual polishing compound used in the lens manufacturing [30]. Inflammatory reactions to lens material, rough edges, and substances used in lens manufacturing were more common in the 1970s–1980s, but have not been as prevalent in the past 10–20 years due to advances in the manufacturing process.

4.4 Infectious

While this chapter is primarily focused on noninfectious etiologies of postoperative inflammation, infectious etiologies form an important part of the differential diagnosis for subacute or chronic postoperative inflammation; thus, they will be mentioned briefly. In any patient with a delayed-onset, low-grade inflammation that is partially responsive to steroids or initially responsive but recurs with cessation of treatment, a fungal endophthalmitis or low-grade bacterial endophthalmitis should be considered. This type of endophthalmitis has been known by several terms over the years, including localized, chronic, indolent, and saccular endophthalmitis. The species most frequently associated with an infectious, delayed-onset inflammation following cataract surgery include *Propionibacterium acnes*, *Staphylococcus epidermidis*, *Candida parapsilosis*, and *Aspergilla* species [31, 32].

Patients with a low-grade, bacterial, or fungal endophthalmitis have a smoldering inflammation that can be unresponsive to corticosteroid treatment or initially responsive but recurring. The infection is characterized by bacteria or fungi that are sequestered in the capsular bag after the natural lens has been removed. The two most common causative agents are *Propionibacterium acnes* and coagulase-negative *Staphylococcus* (e.g., *Staph. epidermidis*), both of which are common skin and conjunctival flora. Classic findings upon examination include a white plaque that is seen within the capsule, representing a localized collection of the microbes, in the setting of decreased vision, conjunctival injection, inflammation with or without hypopyon, and keratic precipitates (Fig. 4.7) [33]. The localized collection of microbes has been found to be particularly difficult to eradicate without capsulectomy. While often localized, the collection of bacteria or fungi can also be spread around the bag 360°. Mild cases have seen resolution with corticosteroid drops and in some cases oral antibiotics [34], whereas moderate cases require surgical intervention. Fifty percent of patients who undergo pars plana vitrectomy, partial capsulotomy, and intravitreal injection of vancomycin have a recurrence of the inflammation, and the definitive treatment includes a vitrectomy with total capsulotomy [35, 36].

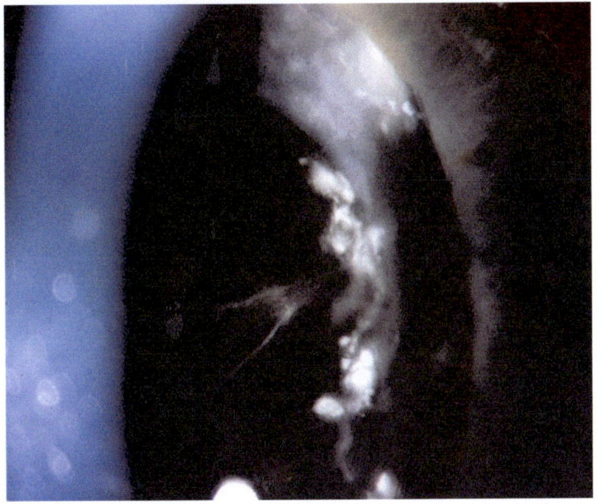

Fig. 4.7 *P. acnes* endophthalmitis – white exudative material on the posterior lens capsule

Conclusion

Inflammation following cataract surgery is a well-recognized aspect of cataract extraction, with cases ranging from mild and transient to severe and chronic. While many cases resolve with no lasting sequelae, more severe cases can lead to additional surgeries and long-term/permanent sequelae including corneal damage, glaucoma, cystoid macular edema, and chronic uveitis. Even though modern surgical techniques incite less inflammation than previous methods, perioperative NSAIDs and corticosteroids still play a beneficial role in reducing inflammation following cataract surgery. Cases of TASS should be differentiated from acute infectious endophthalmitis, treated appropriately, and a complete analysis of all operating room procedures and protocols, instrument cleaning and sterilization protocols, and medications and fluids used during surgery should be undertaken. Cases of subacute or chronic postoperative inflammation can be related to UGH syndrome, retained lens protein, delayed-onset TASS, or subacute infectious endophthalmitis. As cataract surgery with intraocular lens placement continues to evolve and include new techniques, products, instruments, and methodologies, new sources of inflammation may be encountered. Ophthalmologists must remain vigilant in identifying the sources of postoperative inflammation, be it recognized or new sources, and take all necessary and appropriate steps to reduce or eliminate their occurrence in future patients.

References

1. Meisler DM. Intraocular inflammation and extracapsular cataract surgery. AAO Focal Points. 1990; 7:1–10 (B).
2. Kim SJ, Flach AJ, Jampol LM. onsteroidal anti-inflammatory drugs in ophthalmology. Surv Ophthalmol. 2010;55(2):108–33 (B).
3. Decroos FC, Afshari NA. Perioperative antibiotics and anti-inflammatory agents in cataract surgery. Curr Opin Ophthalmol. 2008;19(1):22–6 (B).
4. Nelson RM, Cecconi O, Roberts WG, et al. Heparin oligosaccharides bind L- and P-selectin and inhibit acute inflammation. Blood. 1993;82:3253–8 (C).
5. Kohnen T, Dick B, Hessemer V, Koch DD, Jacobi KW. Effect of heparin in irrigating solution on inflammation following small incision cataract surgery. J Cataract Refract Surg. 1998;24(2):237–43 (C).
6. Kruger A, Amon M, Formanek CA, Schild G, Kolodjaschna J, Schauersberger J. Effect of heparin in the irrigation solution on postoperative inflammation and cellular reaction on the intraocular lens surface. J Cataract Refract Surg. 2002;28:87–92 (C).
7. Bayramlar H, Keskin UC. Heparin in the irrigation solution during cataract surgery. J Cataract Refract Surg. 2002;28(12):2070–1 (C).
8. Bayramlar H, Totan Y, Borazan M. Heparin in the intraocular irrigating solution in pediatric cataract surgery. J Cataract Refract Surg. 2004;30(10):2163–9 (C).
9. Rumelt S, Stolovich C, Segal ZI, Rehany U. Intraoperative enoxaparin minimizes inflammatory reaction after pediatric cataract surgery. Am J Ophthalmol. 2006;141(3):433–7 (C).
10. Monson MC, Mamalis N, Olson RJ. Toxic anterior segment inflammation following cataract surgery. J Cataract Refract Surg. 1992;18:184–9 (C).
11. Peck CM, Brubaker J, Clouser S, Danford C, Edelhauser HF, Mamalis N. Toxic anterior segment syndrome: common causes. J Cataract Refract Surg. 2010;36:1073–80 (B).
12. Mamalis N, Edelhauser HF, Dawson DG, Chew J, Leboyer RM, Werner L. Toxic anterior segment syndrome. J Cataract Refract Surg. 2006;32:324–33 (B).
13. Mamalis N. Toxic anterior segment syndrome. AAO Focal Points. 2009;10:1–13 (B).
14. Hellinger WC, Hasan SC, Bacalis LP, et al. Outbreak of toxic anterior segment syndrome following cataract surgery associated with impurities of autoclave steam moisture. Infect Control Hosp Epidemiol. 2006;27: 294–8 (C).
15. Parikh CH, Sippy BD, Martin DF, Edelhauser HF. Effects of enzymatic sterilization detergents on the corneal endothelium. Arch Ophthalmol. 2002; 120:165–72 (C).
16. Kriesler KR, Martin SS, Young CW, Anderson CW, Mamalis N. Postoperative inflammation following cataract extraction caused by bacterial contamination of the cleaning bath detergent. J Cataract Refract Surg. 1992;18:106–10 (C).
17. American Society of Cataract and Refractive Surgery, The American Society of Ophthalmic Registered Nurses. Recommended practices for cleaning and sterilizing intraocular surgical instruments. J Cataract Refract Surg. 2007;33:1095–100. Available at http:// www.ascrs.org/TASS/upload/TASS_guidelines.pdf. Accessed 31 Jan 2011 (D)
18. Hull DS, Chemotti MT, Edelhauser HF, et al. Effect of epinephrine on the corneal endothelium. Am J Ophthalmol. 1975;79:245–50 (C).
19. Liu H, Routley I, Teichmann K. Toxic endothelial cell destruction from intraocular benzalkonium chloride. J Cataract Refract Surg. 2001;27: 1746–50 (C).
20. Parikh CH, Edelhauser HF. Ocular surgical pharmacology: corneal endothelial safety and toxicity. Curr Opin Ophthalmol. 2003;14:178–85 (B).
21. Kadonosono K, Ito N, Yazama F, et al. Effect of intracameral anesthesia on the corneal endothelium. J Cataract Refract Surg. 1998;24:1377–81 (C).
22. Kutty PK, Forster TS, Wood-Koob C, Thayer N, Nelson RB, Berke SJ, Pontacolone L, Beardsley TL, Edelhauser HF, Arduino MJ, Mamalis N, Srinivasan A. Multistate outbreak of toxic anterior segment syndrome, 2005. J Cataract Refract Surg. 2008;34: 585–90 (B).
23. Gonnering R, Edelhauser HF, Van Horn DL, et al. The pH tolerance of rabbit and human corneal endothelium. Invest Ophthalmol Vis Sci. 1979;18:373–90 (B).
24. Edelhauser HF, Van Horn DL, Schultz RO, et al. Comparative toxicity of intraocular irrigating solutions on the corneal endothelium. Am J Ophthalmol. 1976;81:473–81 (B).
25. Werner L, Sher JH, Taylor JR, Mamalis N, Nash WA, Csordas JE, Green G, Maziarz EP, Liu XM. Toxic anterior segment syndrome and possible association with ointment in the anterior chamber following cataract surgery. J Cataract Refract Surg. 2006;32:227–35 (C).
26. Apple DJ, Hansen SO, Richards SC, et al. Anterior Chamber lenses. Part 1: Complications and pathology and a review of designs. J Cataract Refract Surg. 1987;13:157–74 (B).
27. Doren GS, Stern GA, Driebe WT. Indications for and results of intraocular lens explantation. J Cataract Refract Surg. 1992;18(1):79–85 (B).
28. Marak Jr GE. Phacoanaphylactic endophthalmitis. Survey Ophthalmol. 1991;36(5):325–39 (B).
29. Shetler DJ, Chevez-Barrios P, Dubovy S, Rosa RH, Nasreen S, Wilson MW, Pelton RW, Pe'er J. Ophthalmic Pathology and Intraocular tumors. In: Basic Clinical Science Course. 2009–10; 4:112–113. American Academy of Ophthalmology; 2009 (D).

30. Jehan FS, Mamalis N, Spencer TS, et al. Postoperative sterile endophthalmitis (TASS) associated with the MemoryLens. J Cataract Refract Surg. 2000;26:1773–7 (C).
31. Fox GM, Joondeph BC, Flynn Jr HW, et al. Delayed-onset pseudophakic endophthalmitis. Am J Ophthalmol. 1991;111:163–73 (C).
32. Al-Mezaine HS, Al-Assiri A, Al-Rajhi AA. Incidence, clinical features, causative organisms, and visual outcomes of delayed-onset pseudophakic endophthalmitis. Eur J Ophthalmol. 2009;19:804–11 (C).
33. Meisler DM, Mandelbaum S. Propionibacterium-associated endophthalmitis after extracapsular cataract extraction. Review of reported cases. Ophthalmology. 1989;96:54–61 (B).
34. Abreu JA, Cordovés L. Chronic or saccular endophthalmitis: diagnosis and management. J Cataract Refract Surg. 2001;27:650–1 (C).
35. Aldave AJ, Stein JD, Deramo VA, et al. Treatment strategies for postoperative Propionibacterium acnes endophthalmitis. Ophthalmology. 1999;106:2395–401 (B).
36. Clark WL, Kaiser PK, Flynn HW, et al. Treatment strategies and visual acuity outcomes in chronic postoperative Propionibacterium acnes endophthalmitis. Ophthalmology. 1999;106:1665–70 (B).

Corneal Inflammation Following Excimer Laser Surgery

5

Jaime Javaloy, Jorge L. Alió,
and Alfredo Vega Estrada

Contents

J. Javaloy, MD, PhD
Anterior Segment and Refractive Surgery, VISSUM
Alicante (Spain), Cabañal s/n. Pinar de Vistahermosa,
Alicante, Alicante 03016, Spain

Department of Ophthalmology,
Miguel Hernández University of Elche,
Alicante, Spain
e-mail: jjavaloy@coma.es

J.L. Alió, MD, PhD (⊠)
Department of Ophthalmology,
Miguel Hernandez University,
Vissum-Instituto Oftalmologico, Alicante, Spain

Vissum-Instituto Oftalmologico de Alicante, Vissum
Corporation, Spain, Avda de Denia s/n,
Edificio Vissum, Alicante 03016, Spain
e-mail: jlalio@vissum.com

A.V. Estrada, MD
Cornea, Cataract and Refractive Surgery,
Vissum Corporacion, Calle Cabañal s/n,
Alicante 03016, Spain
e-mail: alfredovega@vissum.com

5.1 PRK and Inflammation

Modelling corneal curvature by using excimer laser indeed implies tissular injury and consequently wound healing response. This phenomenon definitively affects the refractive outcome and can be responsible for visual impairment. Understanding inflammatory and healing reactions after photoablations appears essential for the safety and accuracy of the procedures.

After destroying keratocytes and the extracellular matrix, photorefractive procedures activate stromal corneal fibroblasts to produce cytokines and chemokines that may modulate wound healing [1]. Several chemokines are involved in the recruitment and activation of inflammatory cells in the corneal wound healing process [2, 3].

Analysis of extracellular matrix proteins and cytokines in tear fluid after PRK showed increased levels of tenascin, TNF-α, and several growth factors, suggesting that growth-modulating cytokines may be involved in healing processes [4–8].

5.1.1 Postoperative Inflammation and Corneal Wound Healing

The inflammatory response associated with the corneal healing process after excimer laser PRK is characterised predominantly by macrophage infiltration [9].

Macrophages play a central role in the innate immune response by engulfing, processing, and destroying foreign invaders. Macrophages also

U. Pleyer et al. (eds.), *Immune Modulation and Anti-Inflammatory Therapy in Ocular Disorders*,
DOI 10.1007/978-3-642-54350-0_5, © Springer-Verlag Berlin Heidelberg 2014

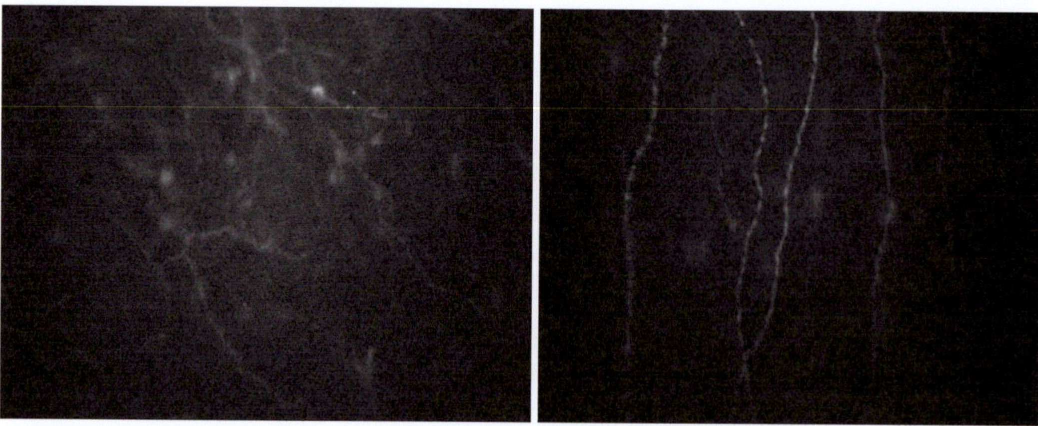

Fig. 5.1 Confocal microphotographs of a normal subepithelial plexus (*right*) and morphological abnormalities in the nerves after ablation (*left*)

play a crucial role in cell-mediated immune responses as antigen-presenting cells that initiate specific immune responses, as a source of various cytokines and growth factors, or as effector inflammatory cells to perform inflammatory, tumoricidal, or microbicidal activity. In addition, macrophages can secrete elastase and collagenase and ingest dead tissue or degenerated cells that are important for tissue repair and reorganisation [10, 11]. Therefore, it is not surprising that macrophages are present in the cornea following excimer laser PRK. However, during the laser procedure, there are no foreign antigens or infectious factors. Thus, the macrophage may be recruited to the ablation site as an effector cell to engulf cellular debris and assist reorganisation of the laser sculpted cornea.

Langerhans cells remained relatively stable after excimer laser PRK. This is consistent with the lack of antigen-presenting activity in the excimer laser-related corneal recovery process. Furthermore, the mechanism by which corticosteroids substantially reduced haze intensity could be related to its effect on macrophages [9].

5.1.1.1 Confocal Microscopy Findings

During PRK the corneal epithelium is physically or chemically debrided. After that, the Bowman's layer and part of the anterior stroma are ablated by excimer laser. A few hours later, re-epithelisation begins from the periphery, and the process is completed in 3–4 days [12, 13].

Nerve Fibre Repair

One week after surgery the first sprouts of subepithelial plexus and the stromal trunks appear, although some authors report these initial changes 1 or 2 months after procedures [14, 15].

Reinnervation starts from the periphery in the form of thin branches in such a way that the subepithelial plexus is formed 6–8 months later, always containing morphological abnormalities (Fig. 5.1). The nervous regeneration is relatively fast due to neurological inflammation and the direct interaction of the ablated fibres with the neurotrophic factors produced by the regenerating epithelium. Hypoesthesia during the 3 first months appears as a consequence of the initial loss of nerve fibres although some investigators find almost normal sensitivity 1 month after PRK [16].

Stromal Healing

The stromal repair is responsible for the transparency and refractive outcome.

An acellular layer is appreciable between 25 and 100 μm of depth immediately after PRK caused by apoptosis of the anterior keratocytes [17]. This cellular disappearance is followed by a progressive repopulation from the subjacent activated keratocytes which migrate to the ablated stroma during the first weeks after surgery. These cells transform into myofibroblasts and are associated with an increase in the extracellular matrix (ECM), being responsible for new collagen creation. It is assumed that the surgical-induced apoptosis and the keratocyte repopulation, activation, and transformation regulate both the normal wound healing and the formation of haze [18]. Different cytokines and matrix metalloproteinases related to inflammation and wound repair play an important role in the changes in the keratocyte population and in the production of ECM. Some of these cytokines seem to proceed from the tear [5, 7, 19, 20].

Usually, the healing response is more evident in the first 30–50 µm between 1 and 3 months after procedures, with the deeper area of the corneal stroma remaining unaltered. Even in cases with complete transparence of the cornea, some morphological alterations can be seen over 30 months after PRK. However, the intensity of these phenomena is less after the 6th month [12, 14].

An inadequate healing response with large amounts of activated keratocytes and an exaggerated production of ECM provoke the presence of haze.

Haze

Haze is described as a subepithelial opacity with variable degrees of intensity which alters the visual function, decreasing contrast sensitivity and visual acuity. The presence of activated keratocytes and the synthesis of types III and IV of new collagen which is anatomically structured in an abnormal way are clearly documented (Fig. 5.2). Before the use of mitomycin C (MMC), the appearance of some traces of haze was frequent, but only patients suffering pathological healing present clinically relevant haze [21]. Different authors have found that the intensity of haze is greater during the first 6 months after PRK and tending to decrease in the following 12–24 months [12]. Its development can be modified by using postoperative steroids and its appearance prevented with intraoperative topical application of MMC [12, 22]. Adequate control of the postoperative inflammatory response is essential for preventing the formation of haze.

Haze and Re-epithelisation

The corneal surface is normally fully covered by a thin layer of epithelium in 3–4 days. Many authors have pointed out the impact of the

Fig. 5.2 Activated anterior keratocytes and abnormal ECM in a patient with subclinical haze after PRK

relationship between the epithelium and the surface of the ablated stroma [12, 23]. When the re-epithelisation is delayed, the appearance of subepithelial haze is greater [13]. The impact of the interaction of the wound healing epithelium has been demonstrated after the observation that LASEK-treated eyes showed less keratocyte apoptosis, myofibroblast transformation, and upregulation in the synthesis of chondroitin sulphate than PRK-treated eyes [24].

Using confocal microscope (CM) and confocal microscopy through focusing (CMTF) analysis, several aspects related to the haze can be studied:

- *Depth*
  In most cases, the haze is located between 60 and 150 µm from the ocular surface. CMTF allows measurement of the thickness of this opaque layer, such manoeuvre being essential before performing phototherapeutical keratectomy (PTK).
- *Optical Density*
  In 1997, Möller-Pedersen et al. first used CM for measuring the degree of haze. The degree of opacity is estimated by calculating the peak of luminous reflectivity (WHO index) that can be observed after the CMTF analysis [14, 25–29].

CMTF analysis allows evaluation of the development of haze over time and appreciation of the efficacy of different medical or surgical strategies for treatment.

5.1.1.2 Pharmacological Approaches for Controlling Corneal Inflammation After PRK

In the usual management of postoperative inflammation, highly powerful topical steroids are used during the first week. Some authors recommend carrying on with nonabsorbable corticosteroids such as fluorometholone for modulating the inflammatory response and therefore the wound healing process in the midterm.

When combining topical steroids and nonsteroidal anti-inflammatory drugs (NSAIDs), there is an increased risk of suffering corneal melting and even ocular perforation [30]. As NSAIDs alone are not enough for controlling postoperative inflammation after PRK, its use appears as inefficient and potentially hazardous.

Newly designed substances are currently being tested in the laboratory to control the postoperative inflammation after PRK [31].

The outcome and stability of PRK can be improved by controlling keratocyte apoptosis. This can be achieved by inhibiting the transmission of the apoptosis signal from the damaged corneal epithelium to the keratocytes and so attenuating cell activation. Omega-6 essential fatty acids have been used to control the release of the mediators of the inflammation and to stimulate tear production [32].

5.1.1.3 Effect of MMC

The appearance of haze has been one of the complications that has limited the use of PRK or photoablative surface ablations for deep ablations to correct high refractive defects. It has been seen that the greater incidence of haze after PRK when compared to LASIK can be explained in part because PRK acts more on superficial stromal areas. At these levels, the density and the capability of the keratocytes to be activated are much greater. As seen before, these cells transform into myofibroblasts and can produce ECM and haze [17].

A study from our investigational team pointed out that the opacity index related to the wound healing process after photoablative surgery was greater in eyes operated by surface ablations (LASEK) and in LASIK after performing flaps thinner than 100 µm. This increase can be considered to be subclinical because it is hardly visible under biomicroscopic exam, but we have also demonstrated an impact on the contrast sensitivity [25]. Even considering that these facts have a limited impact on the visual outcome after LASIK, these findings have the same physiopathological basis explaining the genesis of haze after PRK, namely, the exaggerated activation of anterior keratocytes.

The topical intraoperative application of MMC has been used as cytostatic agent and to avoid excessive scarring in surgical procedures such as the treatment of CIN or the prophylaxis of bleb failure in filtering antiglaucomatous surgery. The appearance of secondary effects after the use of this drug has been controlled by a better knowledge of the dosage. Mitomycin C is an alkylating agent with cytotoxic and antiproliferative effects that reduces the myofibroblast repopulation after laser surface ablation and, therefore, reduces the risk of postoperative corneal haze [33].

Topical intraoperative MMC has been successfully used during surface photoablative procedures with the aim of reducing the incidence and intensity of haze [22, 34, 35]. MMC has proved to be efficient in preventing haze even in PRK to correct residual errors after penetrating keratoplasties [36, 37] or in radial keratotomy [38, 39]. The substance has been used prophylactically to avoid haze after primary surface ablation but also therapeutically to treat preexisting haze [33].

No relevant ocular or systemic adverse effects have been reported with such use of the drug. A delay in the epithelial healing has been observed in 3.5 % of the treated corneas, but such incidence does not increase the risk of suffering postoperative haze [40].

The substance has been used as well in some special circumstances during LASIK surgery [41–43].

The prophylactic effect seems to produce a reduction in the capability of activation of keratocytes and in the transformation into myofibroblasts [44], but it seems that in the long term the use of 0.02 % topical MMC has no significant side effects on corneal keratocytes regarding the density and morphology compared to standard PRK, as documented by in vivo corneal confocal microscopy [45].

However, experimental papers have evidenced some dosage-dependent endothelial damage after the application of different concentrations of

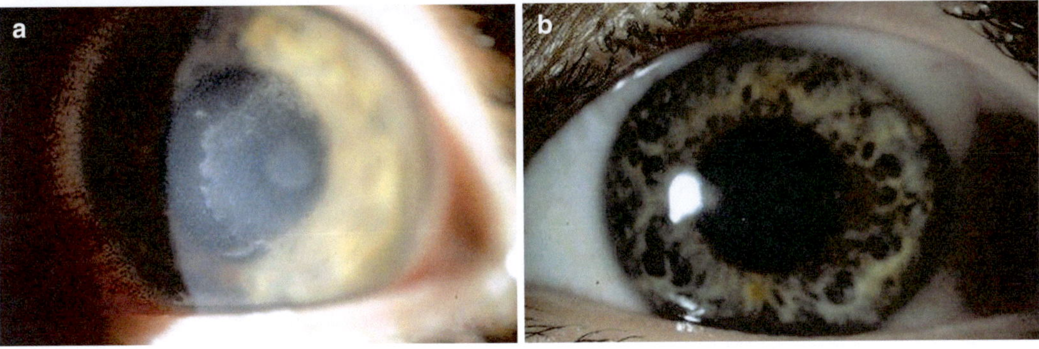

Fig. 5.3 Slit lamp pictures of (**a**) post-PRK infection and (**b**) same eye 10 days after treatment

MMC over the denudated corneal stroma once the epithelium had been mechanically removed. It has been pointed out as well that mitomycin C is detectable in the aqueous humour of the hen eye after topical application in PRK-treated eyes and in eyes with intact epithelium [46].

Some clinical studies have demonstrated as well that a significant reduction in the endothelial cell density (ECD) can be found after using 0.02 % MMC during PRK and that such effect is proportional to the time of exposure [47, 48]. In fact, if the drug application is no longer than 15 s, such toxic ECD reduction is not appreciated [49]. It seems that for moderate myopia and shallow depth, low dosing of MMC (0.002 %) appears to be as effective as the classic concentration of 0.02 % [50].

Furthermore, a case of clinically relevant haze after retreatment with photorefractive keratectomy with mitomycin C following laser in situ keratomileusis has been recently published [51], being suggested by the authors that in such cases, applications of over 15 s should be used.

But even taking into account these aspects, the use of 0.02 % MMC during surface ablations is routinely used in most refractive surgery units due to its unquestionable ability to prevent haze formation (grade of recommendation: B).

5.1.2 Corneal Infections After PRK: Prevalence, Diagnosis, and Treatment

Postoperative PRK infections (Fig. 5.3) are considered to be a rare occurrence. Such complications have been reported in the literature in 30 cases [52–59]. Higher concentrations of antibiotics in the ablated corneal surface, a non-anaerobic ambient at this level, or even the presence of bacteriostatic substances in the tear fluid can explain the lower incidence of such infections [60]. However, bacterial [58, 59, 61, 62], viral [63], fungal [56], and even Acanthamoeba keratitis [64] have been reported after PRK. Gram-positive bacteria is thought to be the most common cause of post-PRK infectious keratitis, and *Staphylococcus aureus*, *Staphylococcus epidermidis*, *Streptococcus pneumoniae*, and *Streptococcus viridans* are the most commonly cultured organisms [55].

Although microorganisms such as *S. aureus* induce acute fulminant keratitis after PRK, other uncommon microorganisms such as nontuberculous mycobacteria and *Nocardia* species may lead to late-onset infection [55, 65].

Possible sources of contamination in post-PRK keratitis are the patient's skin or conjunctival surfaces, surgical instruments, topical anaesthetic agents, and airborne particles [55].

Risk factors for post-PRK infections are corneal epithelial defects, use of extended-wear bandage soft contact lenses, and topical steroids [55, 66]. Contact lenses and use of corticosteroids after PRK may also be considered contributing factors. Application of MMC during PRK is another potential factor because of the predisposition to development of persistent corneal epithelial defects [67].

Considering the most frequent microorganisms which produce bacterial keratitis after surface ablations, taking specimens for culture and the prescription of an intensive empirical topical therapy with fortified first-generation cephalosporins and aminoglycosides or second-generation fluoroquinolones seem to be a reasonable approach for initial management.

5.2 Corneal Inflammation After LASIK

(a) Corneal healing after LASIK: confocal microscopy features
(b) Infections after LASIK: diagnosis and therapeutic approach
(c) Diffuse lamellar keratitis
(d) Central toxic keratopathy

Although the inflammatory and healing response is less after LASIK than after PRK, all refractive surgery procedures induce the activation of corneal cells and the release of several cytokines to modulate the corneal inflammatory and healing processes.

The cellular, molecular, and neural regulatory phenomena associated with postoperative inflammation and wound healing are likely to be involved in the adverse effects of LASIK such as flap melting, epithelial ingrowth, and regression. For these reasons, corticosteroid or nonsteroidal anti-inflammatory agents are always used to minimise inflammation in the postoperative period [1].

Stimulated keratocytes can produce several chemokines that might potentially initiate severe corneal inflammation, leading to corneal haze and other unsatisfactory sequelae [2, 68–71].

Keratocyte activation induced by LASIK has a short duration compared to that reported after photorefractive keratectomy (PRK). In a recent study, regardless of the method of flap formation, all corneas showed early transformed morphology of the keratocytes located below the flap [72].

LASIK and laser-assisted subepithelial keratectomy seem to be less traumatic than PRK because a lower amount of tear transforming growth factor (TGF-b) is released and expressed in the early postoperative days than in PRK, indicating that different techniques stimulate different corneal cell activation [73–75].

Several studies have focused on tear proteins such as cytokines, chemokines, and growth factors that are known to modulate wound healing, apoptosis, cell cycling, and migration on the ocular surface in physiological, postsurgical, and pathological conditions [1, 4–6, 8, 76, 77].

A recent paper has studied the changes in the levels of chemokines in the tears of eyes after LASIK surgery. Some of the interesting results from this article can be resumed as follows:[1]

- It has been found that *in nonstimulated tears before surgery* (a condition that can be considered equivalent to normal), IL-8 was the only cytokine consistently present in all patients, while the levels of Th1-type and Th2-type cytokines were low or below detection limits.

- It was observed *after surgeries* that:
  - Tear IL-12, although at low levels, was increased 1 h after operations probably as a result of corneal dendritic cell stimulation.
  - Eotaxin, a chemokine involved in the recruitment of eosinophils, monocytes, and mast cells, was increased in tears 24 h following surgeries. Eotaxin has been shown to be produced by keratocytes and conjunctival fibroblasts, but not by corneal and epithelial cells. In the in vitro model, eotaxin was detectable at baseline and 24 h after treatment, when corneal fibroblasts were growing during the healing process.
  - MCP-1 and IL-8 were significantly increased 24 h after laser treatment, confirming that stimulated corneal fibroblasts produce these factors after injury. Interleukin-8, produced by keratocytes and neutrophils, was shown to contribute to the development of diffuse lamellar keratitis in an animal model. It is possible that overexpression of these chemokines is responsible for noninfective LASIK complications.
  - The symptom score after surgery was correlated only with IL-6 tear levels, indicating that this cytokine is directly involved in the development of postsurgical inflammation and in the wound healing process.

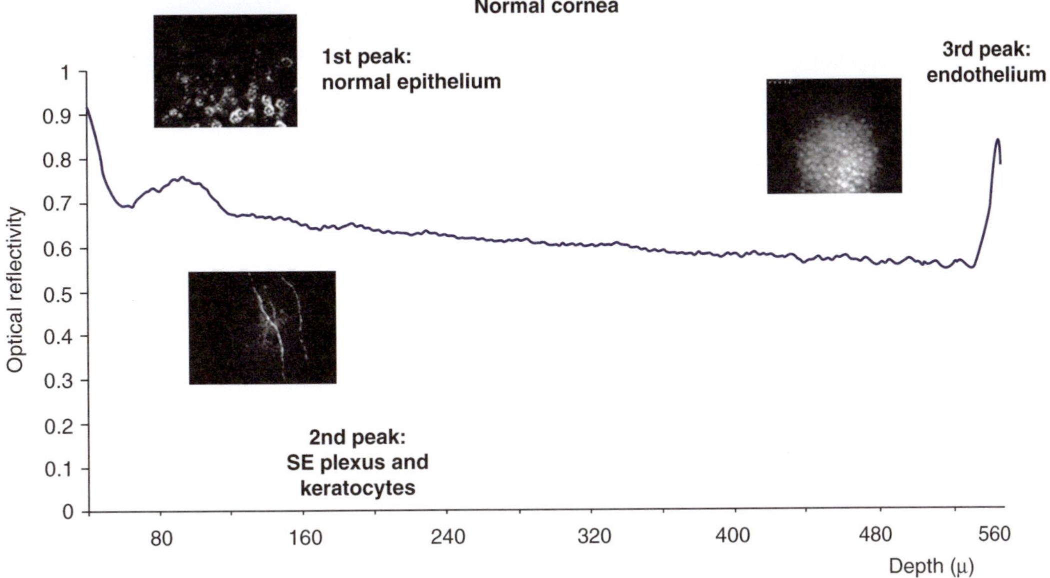

Fig. 5.4 CMTF graph in a normal cornea. The confocal microscope software creates a bidimensional graph, whose *horizontal axis* represents the corneal thickness in microns, being indicated the optical reflectivity in the *vertical* one

5.2.1 Corneal Healing After LASIK: Confocal Microscopy Features

Although the wound healing process is similar for surface ablations and for LASIK, the differences in the surgical techniques clearly determine the inflammatory response and the intensity, location, and wound repair events.

Significant inflammatory cell infiltration was noted in both PRK and LASIK but appeared to be greater in PRK [17].

Some other differences include the absence in the interaction between stroma and regenerating epithelium or the absence with cytokines and biological active substances which are present in the fluid tear. As the subepithelial nerve plexus is not ablated, less pain and neurogenic inflammation but a more delayed recovery of corneal sensitivity are differential features between LASIK and PRK.

On the other hand, in LASIK surgeries a deeper ablation level (which respects the most anterior keratocytes) produces less intense keratocyte activation and the usual absence of clinically detectable haze.

Finally, the presence of a new virtual space – the surgical interface – generates specific situations regarding the collection of liquid or particles, the spreading of inflammatory cells, or the inoculation and proliferation of microorganisms during the postoperative period.

In the same way as in the surface ablations, confocal microscopy appears as a useful tool for helping to understand the tissular phenomena which occur after LASIK.

CMTF analysis provides precise records of the cornea and flap thickness [16, 25–28]. The depth of ablation and flap thickness have been related to different degrees of luminous reflectivity in the CMTF profiles. So, thinner flaps require photoablations to be performed over more superficial keratocytes. As the capability of these cells to be activated and transformed into myofibroblasts is greater, a larger peak of reflectivity can be appreciated after performing thin flaps even when clinical haze is not detectable at the slit lamp [25, 26, 28, 78, 79].

So, using CM it is possible to evaluate the surgical interface, the stromal bed, the nervous regeneration, the corneal and flap thickness, and, finally, the luminous reflectivity which implies an indirect way for evaluating the corneal transparency (Fig. 5.4) [68].

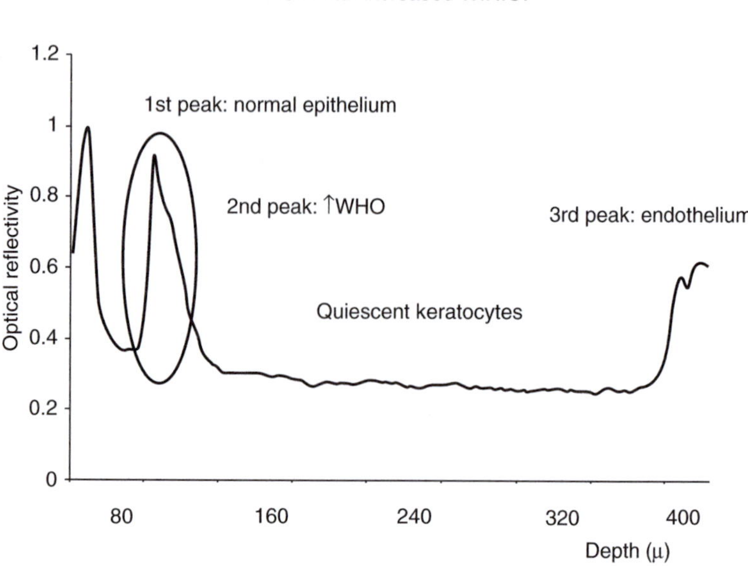

Fig. 5.5 CMTF graph in a cornea operated with LASIK and suffering a subclinical degree of haze. The peak which is inside of the ellipse represents the increased optical reflectivity generated by the mild opacity which is produced by the activation of anterior keratocytes and abnormal ECM

5.2.1.1 Flap and Stromal Thickness

The remaining stromal bed and the flap thickness are important parameters to be taken into account when planning retreatment of a LASIK-operated eye. The possibility of intraoperative incidences when lifting an ultrathin flap or the need to respect between 250 and 300 μm of corneal stroma makes an accurate estimation of the thickness of these structures obligatory. The accuracy of CMTF analysis for performing precise pachymetries of the natural or artificial sublayers of the operated corneas has been pointed out in several studies [27, 28, 80, 81].

It has been previously suggested that the flap thickness can have some influence on the corneal transparency. It is well known that the keratocyte population which is present in the most anterior part of the stroma is more able to suffer activation, apoptosis, and transformation into myofibroblasts and to produce ECM and haze (Fig. 5.5) [25, 78, 79]. The presence of significant amounts of cytokines and inflammatory mediators in the most anterior part of the stroma has been reported [17].

However, not in all eyes which have been operated by LASIK with thin flaps is possible to see the increase in reflectivity. That implies that an individual susceptibility should exist to explain the different healing responses [26].

5.2.1.2 Analysis of the Stromal Changes

A significant decrease in the density of the anterior keratocytes is clearly seen from early stages after LASIK. The cellular disappearance is greater in the most superficial areas (overall in the posterior flap and anterior retroablation layer, the regions adjacent to the lamellar cut) and has been related to apoptosis, the loss of communication between the keratocytes, the presence of inflammatory cells, and the denervation. Keratocytes that die in the anterior stroma following the lamellar cut after LASIK are replenished in 2–4 days by proliferation and migration. The replenishing cells are activated myofibroblastic keratocytes that produce collagen, hyaluronic acid, growth factors modulating epithelial healing, and other components of the wound healing response [78, 82–85].

On the other hand, some studies have found that the cellular density remains altered for over 12 months after LASIK and even decreases over the time. The impact of these observations in the biomechanical stability of the corneas in the long term is not yet clarified [86].

5.2.1.3 Nerve Regeneration

Although the first regenerating sprouts can be appreciated in the wound in the first week after LASIK, the density of the nerves is clearly low

Fig. 5.6 Confocal microscopy of the LASIK interface. Particles are visible as small hyperreflective (*white*) dots

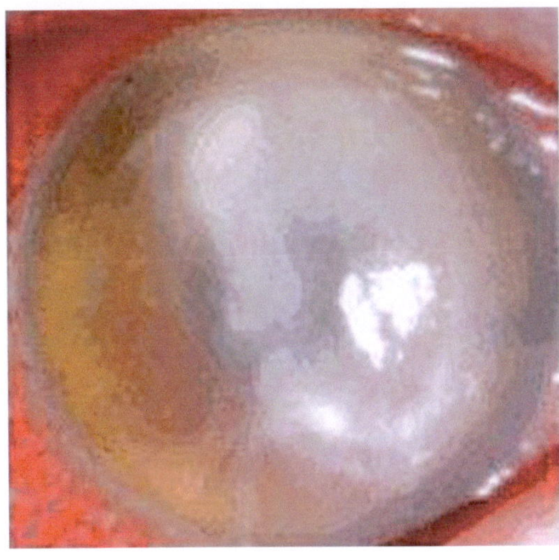

Fig. 5.7 Corneal abscess in a bacterial keratitis post-LASIK

until 6–8 months after the surgeries, and the pattern is, even at this time, abnormal [87, 88]. It is well known that the nerve regeneration and the recovery of the corneal sensitivity are slower after LASIK than after surface ablations [26, 87, 88].

5.2.1.4 The Interface

The morphological specific changes that can be observed with CM involve 15–50 μm of thickness. Apart from the mentioned changes in the keratocyte density, it is possible to see inflammatory cells and necrotic spindle-shaped debris if diffuse lamellar keratitis occurs, microfolds in the Bowman's layer in 96 % of cases, and hyperreflective particles in 100 % of cases (Fig. 5.6) [26, 79, 88].

The nature of these foreign particles seems to be varied, metallic, plastic, or organic, but does not have a relevant clinical impact in the visual function of the patient and does not originate special inflammatory responses in normal conditions [16, 25, 26, 78, 79, 88, 89].

5.2.2 Infections After LASIK: Diagnosis and Therapeutic Approach

Infectious keratitis is a potentially devastating complication following LASIK which has become increasingly recognised as a sight-threatening problem (Figs. 5.7 and 5.8).

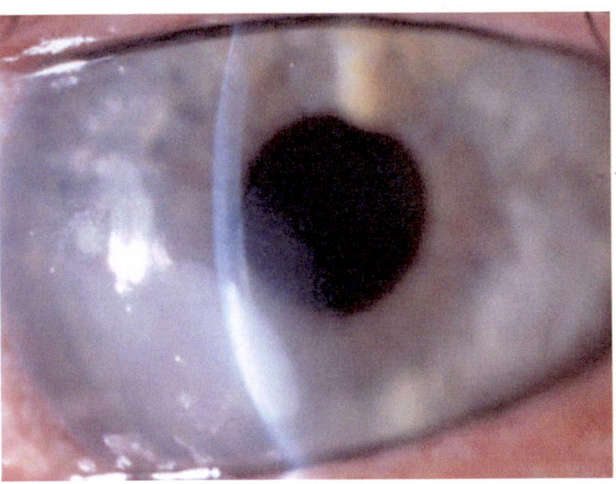

Fig. 5.8 Biomicroscopic aspect of a post-LASIK infectious keratitis at the moment of the diagnosis

The incidence of infectious keratitis following LASIK is difficult to estimate and can vary widely depending on the source of the information.

5.2.2.1 Incidence

- A recent case series of LASIK-associated infections encountered at a single institution reports an estimated incidence of between 1:1,000 and 1:5,000 [90].
- Chang et al. state that the incidence of infection after LASIK can vary widely (0–1.5 %) [91].

5.2.2.2 Aetiology

The organisms encountered in infectious keratitis following LASIK can be unusual, difficult to predict, and will often not respond to empirical therapy with older-generation topical fluoroquinolone antibiotic agents.

- In a survey of ASCRS, the incidence reported by LASIK surgeons who had experienced an infectious keratitis was 1 in 2,919. The most common organisms cultured were atypical mycobacteria (28 %) and staphylococci (20 %) [92].
- A review of the published reports of LASIK-associated microbial keratitis in the peer-reviewed literature reveals over 100 cases with a striking preponderance of atypical mycobacterial (47 %) and staphylococcal (19 %) species [91].

It has been communicated that in early-onset infectious keratitis (under 10 days), common bacterial pathogens are Gram-positive staphylococcal and streptococcal species.

The organisms seen in late-onset infectious keratitis (over 10 days) are usually opportunistic such as fungi, *Nocardia*, and atypical mycobacteria [91, 93].

The Centers for Disease Control and Prevention (CDCP) concluded that LASIK-associated keratitis from atypical mycobacteria may be more common than previously thought and also suggested that LASIK could be a risk factor for the development of atypical mycobacterial keratitis which can occur in clusters [90].

5.2.2.3 Management

It seems to be advisable to lift the flap and take corneal scrapings for appropriate stains and cultures if any suspicious infiltrates appear following LASIK. The results of these stains and cultures can be helpful in guiding antimicrobial therapy. A high degree of suspicion coupled with a rapid diagnosis and appropriate therapy can result in eradication of the infection and visual recovery. It is recommendable for any focal infiltrate following LASIK to be considered infectious, and we discourage the practice of empirical antibiotic treatment without culturing [93].

5.2.2.4 Diagnosis [93]

It is highly recommendable to lift the flap to take cultures, as many of the organisms responsible for infectious keratitis following LASIK will often not respond to empirical therapy.

- The following media should be used for cultures:
  - Blood agar–chocolate agar: for aerobic bacteria
  - Thioglycolate broth for facultative anaerobic bacteria
  - Sabouraud's agar for fungi
  - Lowenstein–Jensen or Middlebrook 7H-9 agar for atypical mycobacteria (especially if the keratitis develops 10 days or more after the surgery)
- It is also recommendable to perform stains such as Gram stain, Gomori methenamine silver stain, and Ziehl–Neelsen stain on unusual pathogens such as nocardia, atypical mycobacteria, and fungi.
- If the disease remains uncontrolled with negative cultures, a PCR or corneal biopsy can be performed.

5.2.2.5 Treatment [93] (Grade of Recommendation: C)

While the results of the microbiological study are being processed, it will be necessary to start empirical treatment. Depending on the presentation, the following can be recommended:

1. Early-onset keratitis (under 10 days):
   (a) The interface can be irrigated with a solution of fortified vancomycin 50 mg/ml during the flap lifting after the cultures.
   (b) Quinolones of fourth generation (gatifloxacin 0.3 % or moxifloxacin 0.5 %) given in a loading dose every 5 minutes for 3 doses and later every 30 minutes associated to.
   (c) Fortified cefazolin 50 mg/mL every 30 minutes. If the patient works in a hospital, an MRSA infection is, so in these patients, the substitution of fortified vancomycin 50 mg/ml for cefazolin every 30 min can be advisable to provide more effective therapy against MRSA.
   (d) Oral doxycycline 100 mg twice a day to inhibit collagenase production.
   (e) Discontinuation of corticosteroids.

2. Late-onset keratitis (less than 10 days):
   (a) Amikacin 35 mg/ml every 30 min
   (b) Alternating with a fourth-generation fluoroquinolone (gatifloxacin 0.3 % or moxifloxacin 0.5 %) every 30 min
   (c) Oral doxycycline 100 mg twice a day
   (d) Discontinuation of corticosteroids

5.2.2.6 Differential Diagnosis [68]

DLK infectious keratitis following LASIK often presents inflammation in the corneal interface, which can mimic diffuse lamellar keratitis. Some clinical keys to differentiate both diseases are as follows:

- Presentation: DLK usually appears during the 3–4 days following the surgery. The appearance of an interface inflammation over 1 week after LASIK should be presumed to be of an infectious origin.
- Appearance: Diffuse lamellar keratitis is characterised by a diffuse appearance, while infectious keratitis has a focal area of infiltration surrounded by diffuse inflammation or even focal inflammation limited to the area of the infiltrate. The eye usually presents more redness in the case of bacterial keratitis.
- Response to steroids: DLK tends to respond well to intensive steroidal therapy. However, the inflammation associated to LASIK-associated infections usually persists despite topical corticosteroids, and the underlying infections can potentially worsen with corticosteroid tapering.

5.2.2.7 Prophylaxis

- Careful preoperative treatment of any infectious lid disease with hot compresses and an antibiotic ointment applied on the lids and lacrimal apparatus.
- Correct sterilisation techniques.
- Several epidemics of atypical mycobacteria have been associated to the use of nonsterile water to clean instruments or the use of ice during LASIK [94, 95].
- Use of sterile drapes, gowns, gloves, and masks by the treating physician and assisting technician.
- Povidone–iodine solution (Betadine 10 %) lid preparation before surgery.

- All fluids applied to the eye before, during, and after LASIK should be sterile.

5.2.3 Diffuse Lamellar Keratitis

Diffuse lamellar keratitis is a multietiologic syndrome characterised by an inflammatory reaction confined to the interface of eyes operated by LASIK surgery which appears during the first week after surgery [96–99].

In 1998, Smith and Maloney published 13 cases belonging to 12 patients who presented diffuse multifocal infiltrates between the 2nd and 6th day after LASIK limited to the interface without anterior or posterior extension and accompanied by pain, photophobia, red eye, and tearing. All cases disappeared without sequels after being treated with antibiotics or fluorometholone [99].

Several terms have been used for this entity: "Sahara's Sands Syndrome (SSS)" due to the granulated and undulated pattern, "PostLASIK Interface's Keratitis (PLIK)", "Non-specific and Diffuse Interstitial Keratitis (NSDIK)", and "Diffuse Intralamellar Keratitis (DIK)". However, DLK is the most frequently used term when referring to this disease [97, 98].

Since the first cases of this condition were described, it has been recognised that the syndrome can occur either in isolated cases or in epidemic outbreaks [97]. Cluster DLK has been defined as a variable concentration of diffuse lamellar keratitis cases over time. Johnson et al. proposed a classification system considering a single case described in a surgical session as sporadic and when more than one case is detected as cluster [96, 100]. The incidence of sporadic DLK can range between 0.58 and 3.54 % reaching 50 % in clusters [28, 68, 101–124].

In this chapter, we will overview this topic considering the physiopathology, treatment, and prophylactic measures of DLK and our experience when managing this entity.

5.2.3.1 Aetiology

A great variety of causes have been proposed as causing DLK, but differences in the prognosis exist when comparing clusters to sporadic cases. Central scars involving central cornea with irregular astigmatism, hyperopic shift, and loss of BCVA are more frequent after epidemic cases [96]. Usually, epidemics have been described as related to sterilisation problems, the cleaning of instruments or environmental aspects such as ventilation air circuits in the theatres or toxic substances touching the eye during surgeries [28, 96, 99, 103, 106–108, 112, 115, 120, 124–126]. Epithelial defects, bleeding, trauma, and surface or intraocular inflammation have been described as potential causes of sporadic-, early-, or even late-onset DLK after LASIK [68, 96, 97, 105, 110, 111, 113, 114, 116, 119, 121, 123, 127].

Lipopolysaccharide Endotoxin of Gram-Negative Bacteria

The implication of LPS endotoxin in the genesis of the disease has been proposed as the most likely condition able to provoke epidemics of DLK by Holland et al. [125] and has been clinically and experimentally tested in many studies [100, 107, 108, 121, 125, 126, 128–130]. Gram-negative bacteria and endotoxins are frequently present in water supplies, and although the bacteria are killed in a sterilisation machine, the endotoxins remain and can therefore be transferred by LASIK instruments onto the flap interface [130]. Until today, in the majority of short cycle autoclaves, the water reservoir cannot be removed for complete cleaning and sterilisation. A new model of these sterilisation machines (Statim 7000®) allows the extraction of the water reservoir.

Other Agents

Metallic particles were initially related to the origin of the syndrome, but later studies did not confirm any inflammatory reaction around these kinds of particles when inserted at the interface of operated rabbits. On the other hand, the authors of this paper suggest a more possible implication of plastic particles [131].

The presence of remains of detergents such as Palmolive ultra 100 %, Klenzyme 100 %, or sterilising substances as glutaraldehyde on the instruments or lubricant oils on the microkeratome blade have also been proposed [96, 97, 124, 132].

Associated Conditions

A greater risk of DLK has been described for atopic patient, even under antihistaminic treatment [102].

Meibomian secretions and exotoxins of *S. aureus* present in patients suffering chronic blepharitis have been associated to DLK, due to the ability of these toxins to promote lymphocyte T activation and inflammatory response. For such reasons, strict cleaning of the edge of the lids is recommended before surgery [133, 134].

Epithelial Defects

A strong association between DLK and intraoperatory epithelial defect has been reported, with increases in the risk of suffering the disease of between 13 and 24 times compared to eyes with undamaged epithelium [96, 119, 127].

Others

Our investigational team first described the association between the presentation of DLK and high levels of energy when using femtosecond laser for creating flaps during LASIK [28, 135]. This condition is now rare due to the use of the low energetic parameters of the 30 and 60 KHz femtolasers currently marketed. In a large series of DLK outbreaks, our investigational team found that several factors can act simultaneously to generate an epidemic and that a dramatic reduction in the incidence to normal levels can be achieved after applying a progressive strategy acting at all levels of the surgical procedure even when the exact cause of the outbreak could not be determined [136].

5.2.3.2 Classification

- Linebarger et al. (1999) proposed a classification taking into account the severity and location of the lamellar interface inflammation [98].

Stage 1: Presence of white granular infiltrates at the periphery of the flap outside the visual axis. The incidence is 1/25–50 cases.

Stage 2 (Fig. 5.9): Visual axis is affected. The incidence is 1/200 cases.

Stage 3 (Fig. 5.10): The pattern of white cell infiltration appears condensed in the visual axis, and this is often associated to a decrease

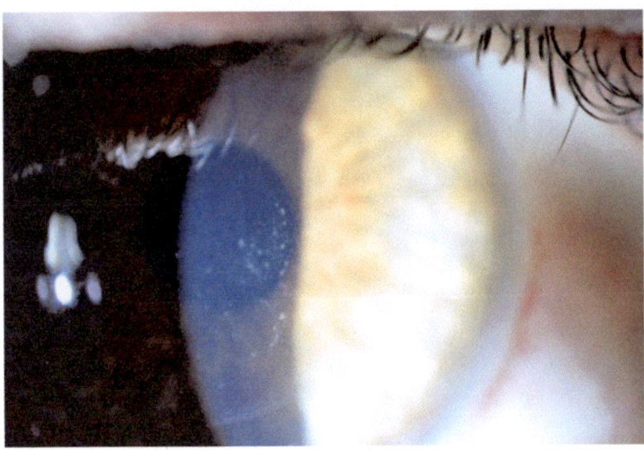

Fig. 5.9 Stage 2 DLK at the moment of the diagnosis

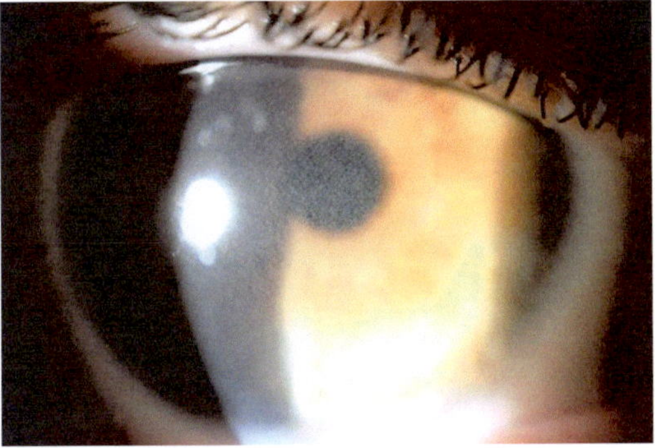

Fig. 5.10 Slit lamp aspect of a DLK stage 3

in the visual acuity of less than 2 lines. The incidence is 1/500 cases.

Stage 4 (Fig. 5.11): Severe lamellar keratitis with stromal melting due to the enzymatic digestion caused by the collagenases produced by white cells. This results in stromal volume loss and hyperopic shift. The incidence is approximately 1/5,000 cases.

• Jonson and coauthors proposed a new classification (2000) based on the extent of centripetal migration of inflammatory cells and if the occurrence is sporadic or in cluster [96].

Type I is designated as scarce affectation of the centre and subdivided into:

IA sporadic

IB Cluster

An association between epithelial defects and DLK seems to exist especially in the type IA.

Type II involves the visual axis and is subdivided into:

IIA sporadic

IIB Cluster

The occurrence of clusters is an important factor when managing DLK. Type IIB is associated to a greater risk of visual loss and is strongly related to endotoxins [96].

• Bühren and coauthors proposed a four-stage classification based on confocal microscopy in relation to the findings under the slit lamp; with this technology we can study the resulting inflammatory activity [17].

DLK stage	Slit lamp features	Confocal microscopic features
1	Infiltrate in the periphery, sparing the centre	Granulocytes and monocytes in the anterior stroma and at the flap interface
2	Infiltrate involves the centre	Granulocytes and monocytes in the anterior stroma and at the interface, involvement of the central cornea, spindle-shaped structures mostly in dense infiltrates
3	Infiltrate more condensed at the corneal centre	Accumulation of decayed inflammatory cells in the flap interface, spindle-shaped structures
4	Folds, stromal opacity	No inflammatory cells detectable, microfolds and activated keratocytes at the interface

5.2.3.3 Visual Outcome

The impact of DLK on the visual function varies with the severity, therapeutic approach, and the concurrence of an epidemic. So, while DLK 1 and 2 rarely affect the refractive or visual outcome of LASIK, DLK 3 and 4 can induce hyperopic shift, irregular astigmatism, and loss of best corrected visual acuity.

Recent studies of our investigational team on the impact of an outbreak of DLK on the refraction, visual abilities, and corneal aberrations of a group of over 200 affected cases concluded that this is scarce if with early diagnosis and an adequate treatment [137]. These findings are consistent to those of other authors regarding clusters or sporadic DLK [100, 112].

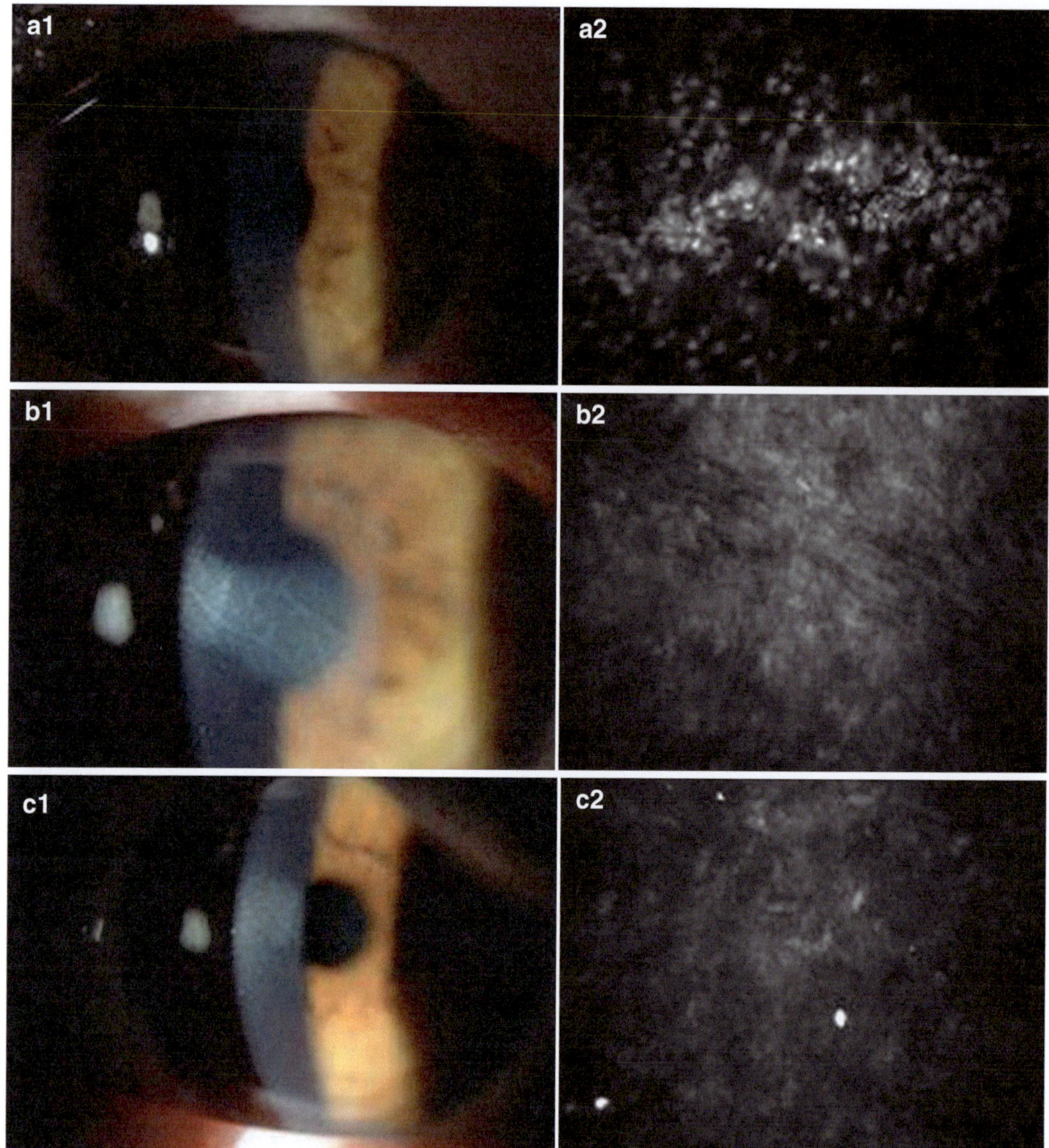

Fig. 5.11 Full slit lamp and confocal microscopy evolution in a DLK four case belonging to our series. *Left side column* of pictures (**a**1, **b**1, and **c**1) shows the biomicroscopic aspect at 24 h, first month, and third month, respectively. *Right images* (**a**2, **b**2, and **c**2) correspond to confocal microscopy exams done in the same day than the photographs were taken

5.2.3.4 Differential Diagnosis [68]

- Epithelial Ingrowth
  Epithelial cells appear at the interface without inflammatory signs as a few scattered fine translucent cells. The cells are more transparent and fewer than would be present in diffuse lamellar keratitis. In addition, a smaller area is affected.
- Microbial Keratitis

Acute microbial keratitis presents decreased visual acuity, pain, and inflammation (redness). Microbial keratitis does not respect the boundaries of the flap interface. A single or dominant focus extending anteriorly into the flap and posteriorly into the stroma is present. Conjunctival/ciliary injection, epithelial defects over the infiltrate, and inflammatory cells in the anterior chamber are also present. DLK can be distinguished from microbial infiltrates by clinical presentation and close follow-up.

- Nonmicrobial Interface Opacities
  Nonmicrobial interface opacities are common in the first postoperative weeks and are related to tear film debris or foreign particles from the microkeratome, blade, sponge, or airborne. Interface debris can also be caused by the powder on the gloves, meibomian secretions, or blood from cut pannus. Usually, it is not difficult to recognise these interface opacities. The foreign bodies are usually well tolerated, although they may sometimes be a nidus for infection or inflammation. If inflammation is present, flap repositioning and foreign body removal can be considered.

5.2.3.5 Treatment (Grade of Recommendation: D)

Linebarger recommended the intensive application of topical steroids (methylprednisolone acetate 1 % hourly during the day and dexamethasone ointment at bedtime) for stages 1 and 2. The patients should be seen 48 h later for evaluation and tapering treatment.

For stage 3, early flap lifting and careful irrigation of the interface were indicated for removing white cells and to avoid stromal melting. Cultures can be taken if differential diagnosis with microbial keratitis is considered. After flap lifting, the same routine of topical steroids must be applied [98, 126]. Hoffman [106] standardised additional systemic treatment (oral prednisone 40–80 mg each day) for the initial management of stage 3.

Although initially a similar protocol was described for stage 4, it was soon seen that flap lifting could increase the possibility of stromal volume loss, and so, worsening the visual prognosis by hyperopic shift and irregular astigmatism. In the same way, if CTK is suspected, the application of high doses of topical steroids can be contraindicated given its noninflammatory nature [138–140]. So, some authors recommend waiting until the eye heals itself and the hyperopic shift is resolved rather than subject the patient to any of the aforementioned invasive procedures [98, 138, 139].

Regarding prophylactic treatments, it has been reported that the prophylactic use of hourly postoperative prednisolone acetate and dexamethasone sodium during a DLK epidemic resulted in a significant decrease in the rate of DLK [141]. However such preventive effect has not been proved with hourly fluorometholone on a patient's fellow eye if the first eye developed sporadic (non-epidemic) DLK [142].

5.2.4 Central Toxic Necrosis (CTK)

There is some discussion about whether DLK 4 stage is an independent entity which should be called central toxic keratopathy as the pathogenesis of the tissue damage has been proposed as different to DLK [139, 143] or could be considered as a spectrum of disorders forming part of a single syndrome [144].

It has been proposed that CTK could differ from DLK 4 in the absence of inflammation and in an affectation of flap stroma without interface infiltration. Affected eyes present central stromal opacification within 1 week of laser refractive surgery, resulting in stromal thinning and a hyperopic shift in most eyes. The opacity clears without treatment, and the remaining refractive error can be corrected with later enhancement surgery without recurrence of the opacity. The syndrome can also occur after photorefractive keratectomy (PRK).

References

1. Leonardi A, Tavolato M, Curnow SJ, Fregona IA, Violato D, Alio JL. Cytokine and chemokine levels in tears and in corneal fibroblast cultures before and after excimer laser treatment. J Cataract Refract Surg. 2009;35(2):240–7.
2. Wilson SE, Mohan RR, Mohan RR, Ambrosio Jr R, Hong J, Lee J. The corneal wound healing response: cytokine-mediated interaction of the epithelium, stroma, and inflammatory cells. Prog Retin Eye Res. 2001;20(5):625–37.
3. Fini ME. Keratocyte and fibroblast phenotypes in the repairing cornea. Prog Retin Eye Res. 1999;18(4):529–51.

4. Tervo T, Vesaluoma M, Bennett GL, Schwall R, Helena M, Liang Q, et al. Tear hepatocyte growth factor (HGF) availability increases markedly after excimer laser surface ablation. Exp Eye Res. 1997;64(4):501–4.

5. Vesaluoma M, Teppo AM, Gronhagen-Riska C, Tervo T. Platelet-derived growth factor-BB (PDGF-BB) in tear fluid: a potential modulator of corneal wound healing following photorefractive keratectomy. Curr Eye Res. 1997;16(8):825–31.

6. Vesaluoma M, Tervo T. Tear fluid changes after photorefractive keratectomy. Adv Exp Med Biol. 1998;438:515–21.

7. Vesaluoma MH, Tervo TT. Tenascin and cytokines in tear fluid after photorefractive keratectomy. J Refract Surg. 1998;14(4):447–54.

8. Tuominen IS, Tervo TM, Teppo AM, Valle TU, Gronhagen-Riska C, Vesaluoma MH. Human tear fluid PDGF-BB, TNF-alpha and TGF-beta1 vs corneal haze and regeneration of corneal epithelium and subbasal nerve plexus after PRK. Exp Eye Res. 2001;72(6):631–41.

9. O'Brien TP, Li Q, Ashraf MF, Matteson DM, Stark WJ, Chan CC. Inflammatory response in the early stages of wound healing after excimer laser keratectomy. Arch Ophthalmol. 1998;116(11):1470–4.

10. Nathan CF. Secretory products of macrophages. J Clin Invest. 1987;79(2):319–26.

11. Werb Z, Gordon S. Secretion of a specific collagenase by stimulated macrophages. J Exp Med. 1975;142(2):346–60.

12. Fagerholm P. Wound healing after photorefractive keratectomy. J Cataract Refract Surg. 2000;26(3):432–47.

13. Kourenkov VV, Mytiagina ON, Kasparov AA, Pavluk AG. Stimulating re-epithelialization after photorefractive keratectomy. J Refract Surg. 1999;15(2 Suppl):S234–7.

14. Linna T, Tervo T. Real-time confocal microscopic observations on human corneal nerves and wound healing after excimer laser photorefractive keratectomy. Curr Eye Res. 1997;16(7):640–9.

15. Kaufman SC, Kaufman HE. How has confocal microscopy helped us in refractive surgery? Curr Opin Ophthalmol. 2006;17(4):380–8.

16. Tervo T, Moilanen J. In vivo confocal microscopy for evaluation of wound healing following corneal refractive surgery. Prog Retin Eye Res. 2003;22(3):339–58.

17. Wilson SE. Analysis of the keratocyte apoptosis, keratocyte proliferation, and myofibroblast transformation responses after photorefractive keratectomy and laser in situ keratomileusis. Trans Am Ophthalmol Soc. 2002;100:411–33.

18. Moller-Pedersen T, Cavanagh HD, Petroll WM, Jester JV. Corneal haze development after PRK is regulated by volume of stromal tissue removal. Cornea. 1998;17(6):627–39.

19. Vesaluoma M, Ylatupa S, Mertaniemi P, Tervo K, Partanen P, Tervo T. Increased release of tenascin in tear fluid after photorefractive keratectomy. Graefes Arch Clin Exp Ophthalmol. 1995;233(8):479–83.

20. Vesaluoma M, Teppo AM, Gronhagen-Riska C, Tervo T. Increased release of tumour necrosis factor-alpha in human tear fluid after excimer laser induced corneal wound. Br J Ophthalmol. 1997;81(2):145–9.

21. Durrie DS, Lesher MP, Cavanaugh TB. Classification of variable clinical response after photorefractive keratectomy for myopia. J Refract Surg. 1995;11(5):341–7.

22. Shalaby A, Kaye GB, Gimbel HV. Mitomycin C in photorefractive keratectomy. J Refract Surg. 2009;25(1 Suppl):S93–7 (Level of evidence: 2-).

23. Moller-Pedersen T, Li HF, Petroll WM, Cavanagh HD, Jester JV. Confocal microscopic characterization of wound repair after photorefractive keratectomy. Invest Ophthalmol Vis Sci. 1998;39(3):487–501.

24. Esquenazi S, He J, Bazan NG, Bazan HE. Comparison of corneal wound-healing response in photorefractive keratectomy and laser-assisted subepithelial keratectomy. J Cataract Refract Surg. 2005;31(8):1632–9.

25. Javaloy EJ, Vidal MT, Quinto A, De Rojas V, Alio JL. Quality assessment model of 3 different microkeratomes through confocal microscopy. J Cataract Refract Surg. 2004;30(6):1300–9.

26. Javaloy J, Vidal MT, Ruiz-Moreno JM, Alio JL. Confocal microscopy of the cornea in photorefractive surgery. Arch Soc Esp Oftalmol. 2005;80(9):497–509.

27. Javaloy J, Vidal MT, Ruiz-Moreno JM, Alio JL. Confocal microscopy of disposable and nondisposable heads for the Moria M2 microkeratome. J Refract Surg. 2006;22(1):28–33.

28. Javaloy J, Vidal MT, Abdelrahman AM, Artola A, Alio JL. Confocal microscopy comparison of intralase femtosecond laser and Moria M2 microkeratome in LASIK. J Refract Surg. 2007;23(2):178–87.

29. Möller-Pedersen T, Li HF, Petroll WM, Cavanagh HD, Jester JV. Confocal microscopic characterization of wound repair after photorefractive keratectomy. Invest Ophthalmol Vis Sci. 1998;39(3):487–501.

30. Mian SI, Gupta A, Pineda R. Corneal ulceration and perforation with ketorolac tromethamine (Acular) use after PRK. Cornea. 2006;25(2):232–4 (Level of evidence: 3).

31. Esquenazi S, He J, Li N, Bazan NG, Esquenazi I, Bazan HE. A novel platelet activating factor receptor antagonist reduces cell infiltration and expression of inflammatory mediators in mice exposed to desiccating conditions after PRK. Clin Dev Immunol. 2009;2009:138513 (Level of evidence: 2++).

32. Querques G, Russo V, Barone A, Iaculli C, Delle NN. [Efficacy of omega-6 essential fatty acid treatment before and after photorefractive keratectomy]. J Fr Ophtalmol. 2008;31(3):282–6 (Level of evidence: 2-).

33. Teus MA, de Benito-Llopis L, Alio JL. Mitomycin C in corneal refractive surgery. Surv Ophthalmol. 2009;54(4):487–502 (Level of evidence: 2++).

34. Solomon R, Donnenfeld ED, Perry HD. Photorefractive keratectomy with mitomycin C for the management of a LASIK flap complication following a penetrating keratoplasty. Cornea. 2004;23(4):403–5 (Level of evidence: 3).

35. Xu H, Liu S, Xia X, Huang P, Wang P, Wu X. Mitomycin C reduces haze formation in rabbits after excimer laser photorefractive keratectomy. J Refract Surg. 2001;17(3):342–9 (Level of evidence: 2+).

36. Forseto AS, Marques JC, Nose W. Photorefractive keratectomy with mitomycin C after penetrating and lamellar keratoplasty. Cornea. 2010;29(10):1103–8 (Level of evidence: 2-).

37. Leccisotti A. Photorefractive keratectomy with mitomycin C after deep anterior lamellar keratoplasty for keratoconus. Cornea. 2008;27(4):417–20 (Level of evidence: 2-).

38. Ghanem RC, Ghanem EA, Kara-Jose N. Safety of photorefractive keratectomy with mitomycin-C for the treatment of hyperopia after radial keratotomy. Arq Bras Oftalmol. 2010;73(2):165–70 (Level of evidence: 2-).

39. Koch DD, Maloney R, Hardten DR, Dell S, Sweeney AD, Wang L. Wavefront-guided photorefractive keratectomy in eyes with prior radial keratotomy: a multicenter study. Ophthalmology. 2009;116(9):1688–96 (Level of evidence: 2-).

40. Kremer I, Ehrenberg M, Levinger S. Delayed epithelial healing following photorefractive keratectomy with mitomycin C treatment. Acta Ophthalmol. 2010;90(3):271–6 (Level of evidence: 2-).

41. Kymionis GD, Portaliou DM, Karavitaki AE, Krasia MS, Kontadakis GA, Stratos A, et al. LASIK flap buttonhole treated immediately by PRK with mitomycin C. J Refract Surg. 2010;26(3):225–8 (Level of evidence: 3).

42. Lane HA, Swale JA, Majmudar PA. Prophylactic use of mitomycin-C in the management of a buttonholed LASIK flap. J Cataract Refract Surg. 2003;29(2):390–2 (Level of evidence: 3).

43. Utz VM, Krueger RR. Management of irregular astigmatism following rotationally disoriented free cap after LASIK. J Refract Surg. 2008;24(4):383–91 (Level of evidence: 3).

44. Kim TI, Pak JH, Lee SY, Tchah H. Mitomycin C-induced reduction of keratocytes and fibroblasts after photorefractive keratectomy. Invest Ophthalmol Vis Sci. 2004;45(9):2978–84 (Level of evidence: 2+).

45. Midena E, Gambato C, Miotto S, Cortese M, Salvi R, Ghirlando A. Long-term effects on corneal keratocytes of mitomycin C during photorefractive keratectomy: a randomized contralateral eye confocal microscopy study. J Refract Surg. 2007;23(9 Suppl):S1011–4 (Level of evidence: 2+).

46. Torres RM, Merayo-Lloves J, Daya SM, Blanco-Mezquita JT, Espinosa M, Nozal MJ, et al. Presence of mitomycin-C in the anterior chamber after photorefractive keratectomy. J Cataract Refract Surg. 2006;32(1):67–71 (Level of evidence: 2++).

47. Morales AJ, Zadok D, Mora-Retana R, Martinez-Gama E, Robledo NE, Chayet AS. Intraoperative mitomycin and corneal endothelium after photorefractive keratectomy. Am J Ophthalmol. 2006;142(3):400–4 (Level of evidence: 2+).

48. Nassiri N, Farahangiz S, Rahnavardi M, Rahmani L, Nassiri N. Corneal endothelial cell injury induced by mitomycin-C in photorefractive keratectomy: nonrandomized controlled trial. J Cataract Refract Surg. 2008;34(6):902–8 (Level of evidence: 2+).

49. Diakonis VF, Pallikaris A, Kymionis GD, Markomanolakis MM. Alterations in endothelial cell density after photorefractive keratectomy with adjuvant mitomycin. Am J Ophthalmol. 2007;144(1):99–103 (Level of evidence: 2+).

50. Thornton I, Xu M, Krueger RR. Comparison of standard (0.02 %) and low dose (0.002 %) mitomycin C in the prevention of corneal haze following surface ablation for myopia. J Refract Surg. 2008;24(1):S68–76 (Level of evidence: 2-).

51. Liu A, Manche EE. Visually significant haze after retreatment with photorefractive keratectomy with mitomycin-C following laser in situ keratomileusis. J Cataract Refract Surg. 2010;36(9):1599–601 (Level of evidence: 3).

52. Amayem A, Ali AT, Waring III GO, Ibrahim O. Bacterial keratitis after photorefractive keratectomy. J Refract Surg. 1996;12(5):642–4.

53. Bertschinger DR, Hashemi K, Hafezi F, Majo F. Infections after PRK could have a happy ending: a series of three cases. Klin Monbl Augenheilkd. 2010;227(4):315–8.

54. Brancato R, Carones F, Venturi E, Cavallero A, Gesu G. Mycobacterium chelonae keratitis after excimer laser photorefractive keratectomy. Arch Ophthalmol. 1997;115(10):1316–8.

55. Donnenfeld ED, O'Brien TP, Solomon R, Perry HD, Speaker MG, Wittpenn J. Infectious keratitis after photorefractive keratectomy. Ophthalmology. 2003; 110(4):743–7.

56. Dunphy D, Andrews D, Seamone C, Ramsey M. Fungal keratitis following excimer laser photorefractive keratectomy. Can J Ophthalmol. 1999;34(5):286–9.

57. Faschinger CW. Phototherapeutic keratectomy of a corneal scar due to presumed infection after photorefractive keratectomy. J Cataract Refract Surg. 2000;26(2):296–300.

58. Heidemann DG, Clune M, Dunn SP, Chow CY. Infectious keratitis after photorefractive keratectomy in a comanaged setting. J Cataract Refract Surg. 2000;26(1):140–1.

59. Kouyoumdjian GA, Forstot SL, Durairaj VD, Damiano RE. Infectious keratitis after laser refractive surgery. Ophthalmology. 2001;108(7):1266–8.

60. Aho VV, Holopainen JM, Tervo T, Moilanen JA, Nevalainen T, Saari KM. Group IIA phospholipase A(2) content in tears of patients having photorefractive keratectomy. J Cataract Refract Surg. 2003;29(11):2163–7.

61. Wee WR, Kim JY, Choi YS, Lee JH. Bacterial keratitis after photoreactive keratectomy in a young, healthy man. J Cataract Refract Surg. 1997;23(6):954–6.

62. Wroblewski KJ, Pasternak JF, Bower KS, Schallhorn SC, Hubickey WJ, Harrison CE, et al. Infectious keratitis after photorefractive keratectomy in the United States army and navy. Ophthalmology. 2006;113(4):520–5.

63. Wulff K, Fechner PU. Herpes simplex keratitis after photorefractive keratectomy. J Refract Surg. 1997; 13(7):613.

64. Kaldawy RM, Sutphin JE, Wagoner MD. Acanthamoeba keratitis after photorefractive keratectomy. J Cataract Refract Surg. 2002;28(2):364–8.

65. Chandra NS, Torres MF, Winthrop KL, Bruckner DA, Heidemann DG, Calvet HM, et al. Cluster of Mycobacterium chelonae keratitis cases following laser in-situ keratomileusis. Am J Ophthalmol. 2001;132(6):819–30.

66. Schein OD, Buehler PO, Stamler JF, Verdier DD, Katz J. The impact of overnight wear on the risk of contact lens-associated ulcerative keratitis. Arch Ophthalmol. 1994;112(2):186–90.

67. Javadi MA, Kanavi MR, Zarei S, Mirbabaei F, Jamali H, Shoja M, et al. Outbreak of Nocardia keratitis after photorefractive keratectomy: clinical, microbiological, histopathological, and confocal scan study. J Cataract Refract Surg. 2009;35(2):393–8.

68. Alio JL, Perez-Santonja JJ, Tervo T, Tabbara KF, Vesaluoma M, Smith RJ, et al. Postoperative inflammation, microbial complications, and wound healing following laser in situ keratomileusis. J Refract Surg. 2000;16(5):523–38.

69. Tran MT, Tellaetxe-Isusi M, Elner V, Strieter RM, Lausch RN, Oakes JE. Proinflammatory cytokines induce RANTES and MCP-1 synthesis in human corneal keratocytes but not in corneal epithelial cells. Beta-chemokine synthesis in corneal cells. Invest Ophthalmol Vis Sci. 1996;37(6):987–96.

70. Hong JW, Liu JJ, Lee JS, Mohan RR, Mohan RR, Woods DJ, et al. Proinflammatory chemokine induction in keratocytes and inflammatory cell infiltration into the cornea. Invest Ophthalmol Vis Sci. 2001; 42(12):2795–803.

71. McInnis KA, Britain A, Lausch RN, Oakes JE. Synthesis of alpha-chemokines IP-10, I-TAC, and MIG are differentially regulated in human corneal keratocytes. Invest Ophthalmol Vis Sci. 2005;46(5): 1668–74.

72. Sonigo B, Chong SD, Ancel JM, Auclin F, Bokobza Y, Baudouin C. In vivo confocal microscopy evaluation of corneal changes induced after LASIK using the IntraLase femtosecond laser technique. J Fr Ophtalmol. 2005;28(5):463–72.

73. Kaji Y, Soya K, Amano S, Oshika T, Yamashita H. Relation between corneal haze and transforming growth factor-beta1 after photorefractive keratectomy and laser in situ keratomileusis. J Cataract Refract Surg. 2001;27(11):1840–6.

74. Lee JB, Choe CM, Kim HS, Seo KY, Seong GJ, Kim EK. Comparison of TGF-beta1 in tears following laser subepithelial keratomileusis and photorefractive keratectomy. J Refract Surg. 2002;18(2):130–4.

75. Long Q, Chu R, Zhou X, Dai J, Chen C, Rao SK, et al. Correlation between TGF-beta1 in tears and corneal haze following LASEK and epi-LASIK. J Refract Surg. 2006;22(7):708–12.

76. Nakamura Y, Sotozono C, Kinoshita S. Inflammatory cytokines in normal human tears. Curr Eye Res. 1998;17(6):673–6.

77. Tuominen I, Vesaluoma M, Teppo AM, Gronhagen-Riska C, Tervo T. Soluble Fas and Fas ligand in human tear fluid after photorefractive keratectomy. Br J Ophthalmol. 1999;83(12):1360–3.

78. Pisella PJ, Auzerie O, Bokobza Y, Debbasch C, Baudouin C. Evaluation of corneal stromal changes in vivo after laser in situ keratomileusis with confocal microscopy. Ophthalmology. 2001;108(10):1744–50.

79. Vesaluoma M, Perez-Santonja J, Petroll WM, Linna T, Alio J, Tervo T. Corneal stromal changes induced by myopic LASIK. Invest Ophthalmol Vis Sci. 2000;41(2):369–76.

80. Javaloy J, Vidal MT, Villada JR, Artola A, Alio JL. Comparison of four corneal pachymetry techniques in corneal refractive surgery. J Refract Surg. 2004;20(1): 29–34.

81. Li HF, Petroll WM, Moller-Pedersen T, Maurer JK, Cavanagh HD, Jester JV. Epithelial and corneal thickness measurements by in vivo confocal microscopy through focusing (CMTF). Curr Eye Res. 1997;16(3): 214–21.

82. Wilson SE. Everett Kinsey Lecture. Keratocyte apoptosis in refractive surgery. CLAO J. 1998;24(3): 181–5.

83. Helena MC, Baerveldt F, Kim WJ, Wilson SE. Keratocyte apoptosis after corneal surgery. Invest Ophthalmol Vis Sci. 1998;39(2):276–83.

84. Wilson SE, Kim WJ. Keratocyte apoptosis: implications on corneal wound healing, tissue organization, and disease. Invest Ophthalmol Vis Sci. 1998;39(2):220–6.

85. Ivarsen A, Laurberg T, Moller-Pedersen T. Role of keratocyte loss on corneal wound repair after LASIK. Invest Ophthalmol Vis Sci. 2004;45(10):3499–506.

86. Mitooka K, Ramirez M, Maguire LJ, Erie JC, Patel SV, McLaren JW, et al. Keratocyte density of central human cornea after laser in situ keratomileusis. Am J Ophthalmol. 2002;133(3):307–14.

87. Kauffmann T, Bodanowitz S, Hesse L, Kroll P. Corneal reinnervation after photorefractive keratectomy and laser in situ keratomileusis: an in vivo study with a confocal videomicroscope. Ger J Ophthalmol. 1996;5(6):508–12.

88. Linna TU, Vesaluoma MH, Perez-Santonja JJ, Petroll WM, Alio JL, Tervo TM. Effect of myopic LASIK on corneal sensitivity and morphology of subbasal nerves. Invest Ophthalmol Vis Sci. 2000;41(2):393–7.

89. Ivarsen A, Thogersen J, Keiding SR, Hjortdal JO, Moller-Pedersen T. Plastic particles at the LASIK interface. Ophthalmology. 2004;111(1):18–23.

90. Karp CL, Tuli SS, Yoo SH, Vroman DT, Alfonso EC, Huang AH, et al. Infectious keratitis after LASIK. Ophthalmology. 2003;110(3):503–10.

91. Chang MA, Jain S, Azar DT. Infections following laser in situ keratomileusis: an integration of the published literature. Surv Ophthalmol. 2004;49(3):269–80.

92. Solomon R, Donnenfeld ED, Azar DT, Holland EJ, Palmon FR, Pflugfelder SC, et al. Infectious keratitis after laser in situ keratomileusis: results of an ASCRS survey. J Cataract Refract Surg. 2003;29(10):2001–6.

93. Donnenfeld ED, Kim T, Holland EJ, Azar DT, Palmon FR, Rubenstein JB, et al. ASCRS White Paper: management of infectious keratitis following laser in situ keratomileusis. J Cataract Refract Surg. 2005;31(10): 2008–11 (Level of evidence: 2+).

94. Fulcher SF, Fader RC, Rosa Jr RH, Holmes GP. Delayed-onset mycobacterial keratitis after LASIK. Cornea. 2002;21(6):546–54.

95. Winthrop KL, Steinberg EB, Holmes G, Kainer MA, Werner SB, Winquist A, et al. Epidemic and sporadic cases of nontuberculous mycobacterial keratitis associated with laser in situ keratomileusis. Am J Ophthalmol. 2003;135(2):223–4.

96. Johnson JD, Harissi-Dagher M, Pineda R, Yoo S, Azar DT. Diffuse lamellar keratitis: incidence, associations, outcomes, and a new classification system. J Cataract Refract Surg. 2001;27(10):1560–6.

97. Linebarger EJ, Hardten DR, Lindstrom RL. Diffuse lamellar keratitis: diagnosis and management. J Cataract Refract Surg. 2000;26(7):1072–7.

98. Linebarger EJ, Hardten DR, Lindstrom RL. Diffuse lamellar keratitis: identification and management. Int Ophthalmol Clin. 2000;40(3):77–86 (Level of evidence: 3).

99. Smith RJ, Maloney RK. Diffuse lamellar keratitis. A new syndrome in lamellar refractive surgery. Ophthalmology. 1998;105(9):1721–6.

100. Stulting RD, Randleman JB, Couser JM, Thompson KP. The epidemiology of diffuse lamellar keratitis. Cornea. 2004;23(7):680–8.

101. Aldave AJ, Hollander DA, Abbott RL. Late-onset traumatic flap dislocation and diffuse lamellar inflammation after laser in situ keratomileusis. Cornea. 2002;21(6):604–7.

102. Boorstein SM, Henk HJ, Elner VM. Atopy: a patient-specific risk factor for diffuse lamellar keratitis. Ophthalmology. 2003;110(1):131–7.

103. Castoro CJ. Causes of diffuse lamellar keratitis. Ophthalmology. 2003;110(5):873.

104. Gris O, Guell JL, Wolley-Dod C, Adan A. Diffuse lamellar keratitis and corneal edema associated with viral keratoconjunctivitis 2 years after laser in situ keratomileusis. J Cataract Refract Surg. 2004;30(6):1366–70.

105. Harrison DA, Periman LM. Diffuse lamellar keratitis associated with recurrent corneal erosions after laser in situ keratomileusis. J Refract Surg. 2001;17(4):463–5.

106. Hoffman RS, Fine IH, Packer M. Incidence and outcomes of lasik with diffuse lamellar keratitis treated with topical and oral corticosteroids. J Cataract Refract Surg. 2003;29(3):451–6 (Level of evidence: 2-).

107. Holland SP. Update in cornea and external disease: solving the mystery of "sands of the Sahara" syndrome (diffuse lamellar keratitis). Can J Ophthalmol. 1999;34(4):193–4.

108. Holland SP, Peters NT, Iskander NG. More to the mysterious tale: the search for the cause of 100+ cases of diffuse lamellar keratitis. J Refract Surg. 2004;20(1):85–6.

109. Javaloy J, Barrera C, Munoz G, Perez-Santonja JJ, Vidal MT, Alio JL. Spontaneous bilateral, recurrent, late-onset diffuse lamellar keratitis after LASIK in a patient with Cogan's syndrome. J Refract Surg. 2008;24(5):548–50.

110. Jin GJ, Lyle WA, Merkley KH. Late-onset idiopathic diffuse lamellar keratitis after laser in situ keratomileusis. J Cataract Refract Surg. 2005;31(2):435–7.

111. Keszei VA. Diffuse lamellar keratitis associated with iritis 10 months after laser in situ keratomileusis. J Cataract Refract Surg. 2001;27(7):1126–7.

112. Lazaro C, Perea J, Arias A. Surgical-glove-related diffuse lamellar keratitis after laser in situ keratomileusis: long-term outcomes. J Cataract Refract Surg. 2006;32(10):1702–9.

113. Mirshahi A, Buhren J, Kohnen T. Clinical course of severe central epithelial defects in laser in situ keratomileusis. J Cataract Refract Surg. 2004;30(8):1636–41.

114. Mulhern MG, Naor J, Rootman DS. The role of epithelial defects in intralamellar inflammation after laser in situ keratomileusis. Can J Ophthalmol. 2002;37(7):409–15.

115. Nakano EM, Nakano K, Oliveira MC, Portellinha W, Simonelli R, Alvarenga LS. Cleaning solutions as a cause of diffuse lamellar keratitis. J Refract Surg. 2002;18(3 Suppl):S361–3.

116. Perez-Santonja JJ, Galal A, Cardona C, Artola A, Ruiz-Moreno JM, Alio JL. Severe corneal epithelial sloughing during laser in situ keratomileusis as a presenting sign for silent epithelial basement membrane dystrophy. J Cataract Refract Surg. 2005;31(10):1932–7.

117. Samuel MA, Kaufman SC, Ahee JA, Wee C, Bogorad D. Diffuse lamellar keratitis associated with carboxymethylcellulose sodium 1 % after laser in situ keratomileusis. J Cataract Refract Surg. 2002;28(8):1409–11.

118. Schwartz GS, Park DH, Schloff S, Lane SS. Traumatic flap displacement and subsequent diffuse lamellar keratitis after laser in situ keratomileusis. J Cataract Refract Surg. 2001;27(5):781–3.

119. Shah MN, Misra M, Wihelmus KR, Koch DD. Diffuse lamellar keratitis associated with epithelial defects after laser in situ keratomileusis. J Cataract Refract Surg. 2000;26(9):1312–8.

120. Shen YC, Wang CY, Fong SC, Tsai HY, Lee YF. Diffuse lamellar keratitis induced by toxic chemicals after laser in situ keratomileusis. J Cataract Refract Surg. 2006;32(7):1146–50.

121. Thammano P, Rana AN, Talamo JH. Diffuse lamellar keratitis after laser in situ keratomileusis with the Moria LSK-One and Carriazo-Barraquer microkeratomes. J Cataract Refract Surg. 2003;29(10):1962–8.

122. Weisenthal RW. Diffuse lamellar keratitis induced by trauma 6 months after laser in situ keratomileusis. J Refract Surg. 2000;16(6):749–51.

123. Wilson SE, Ambrosio Jr R. Sporadic diffuse lamellar keratitis (DLK) after LASIK. Cornea. 2002;21(6):560–3.

124. Yuhan KR, Nguyen L, Wachler BS. Role of instrument cleaning and maintenance in the development of diffuse lamellar keratitis. Ophthalmology. 2002;109(2):400–3.

125. Holland SP, Mathias RG, Morck DW, Chiu J, Slade SG. Diffuse lamellar keratitis related to endotoxins released from sterilizer reservoir biofilms. Ophthalmology. 2000;107(7):1227–33.
126. Villarrubia A, Palacin E, del Gomez RM, Martinez P. Description, etiology, and prevention of an outbreak of diffuse lamellar keratitis after LASIK. J Refract Surg. 2007;23(5):482–6 (Level of evidence: 2+).
127. Sachdev N, McGhee CN, Craig JP, Weed KH, McGhee JJ. Epithelial defect, diffuse lamellar keratitis, and epithelial ingrowth following post-LASIK epithelial toxicity. J Cataract Refract Surg. 2002;28(8):1463–6.
128. de Rojas Silva MV, Abraldes MJ, Diez-Feijoo E, Yanez PM, Javaloy J, Sanchez-Salorio M. Confocal microscopy and histopathological examination of diffuse lamellar keratitis in an experimental animal model. J Refract Surg. 2007;23(3):299–304.
129. Levinger S, Landau D, Kremer I, Merin S, Aizenman I, Hirsch A, et al. Wiping microkeratome blades with sterile 100 % alcohol to prevent diffuse lamellar keratitis after laser in situ keratomileusis. J Cataract Refract Surg. 2003;29(10):1947–9.
130. Peters NT, Iskander NG, Anderson Penno EE, Woods DE, Moore RA, Gimbel HV. Diffuse lamellar keratitis: isolation of endotoxin and demonstration of the inflammatory potential in a rabbit laser in situ keratomileusis model. J Cataract Refract Surg. 2001;27(6):917–23.
131. Bissen-Miyajima H, Minami K, Miyake-Kashima M, Taira Y, Nakamura M. Observation of the corneal flap interface with metal particles in a rabbit model. J Cataract Refract Surg. 2005;31(7):1409–13.
132. Holzer MP, Solomon KD, Vroman DT, Vargas LG, Sandoval HP, Kasper TJ, et al. Diffuse lamellar keratitis: evaluation of etiology, histopathologic findings, and clinical implications in an experimental animal model. J Cataract Refract Surg. 2003;29(3):542–9.
133. Fogla R, Rao SK, Padmanabhan P. Diffuse lamellar keratitis: are meibomian secretions responsible? J Cataract Refract Surg. 2001;27(4):493–5.
134. Holzer MP, Solomon KD, Sandoval HP, Auffarth GU. Diagnosis and treatment of mycobacterial keratitis following LASIK. Case report and review of the literature. Ophthalmologe. 2003;100(7):550–3.
135. Javaloy J, Artola A, Vidal MT, Munoz G, de Rojas V, Alio JL. Severe diffuse lamellar keratitis after femtosecond lamellar keratectomy. Br J Ophthalmol. 2007;91(5):699.
136. Javaloy J, Alio JL, Rodríguez A, González A, Perez-Santonja JJ. Epidemiological analysis of an outbreak of DLK. J Refract Surg. 2011;27(11):796–803.
137. Javaloy J, Alió JL, El Kady B, Muñoz G, Barraquer RI, Maldonado MJ. Refractive outcomes and quality of vision related to an epidemic outbreak of diffuse lamellar keratitis. J Refract Surg. 2011;27(11):804–10.
138. Moshirfar M, Welling JD, Feiz V, Holz H, Clinch TE. Infectious and noninfectious keratitis after laser in situ keratomileusis Occurrence, management, and visual outcomes. J Cataract Refract Surg. 2007;33(3):474–83 (Level of evidence: 2-).
139. Sonmez B, Maloney RK. Central toxic keratopathy: description of a syndrome in laser refractive surgery. Am J Ophthalmol. 2007;143(3):420–7 (Level of evidence: 3).
140. Moshirfar M, Kurz C, Ghajarnia M. Contact lens-induced keratitis resembling central toxic keratopathy syndrome. Cornea. 2009;28(9):1077–80 (Level of evidence:3).
141. Cosar CB, Sener AB, Sen N, Coskunseven E. The efficacy of hourly prophylactic steroids in diffuse lamellar keratitis epidemic. Ophthalmologica. 2004;218(5):318–22 (Level of evidence: 2-).
142. McLeod SD, Tham VM, Phan ST, Hwang DG, Rizen M, Abbott RL. Bilateral diffuse lamellar keratitis following bilateral simultaneous versus sequential laser in situ keratomileusis. Br J Ophthalmol. 2003;87(9):1086–7 (Level of evidence: 2-).
143. Hainline BC, Price MO, Choi DM, Price Jr FW. Central flap necrosis after LASIK with microkeratome and femtosecond laser created flaps. J Refract Surg. 2007;23(3):233–42.
144. Parolini B, Marcon G, Panozzo GA. Central necrotic lamellar inflammation after laser in situ keratomileusis. J Refract Surg. 2001;17(2):110–2.

6

Prevention and Treatment of Transplant Rejection in Keratoplasty

Uwe Pleyer and Anna-Karina Brigitte Maier

Contents

U. Pleyer, MD (✉)
Department of Ophthalmology, Charité,
Augustenburger Platz 1, Berlin 13353, Germany
e-mail: uwe.pleyer@charite.de

A.-K.B. Maier, MD
Department of Opthalmology, Charité –
Universitätsmedizin Berlin,
Augustenburger Platz 1, Berlin 13353, Germany
e-mail: anna-karina.maier@charite.de

6.1 Introduction

6.1.1 Definition/Background of Corneal Transplantation

With more than 100.000 procedures a year, keratoplasty is the most frequent transplantation procedure in humans. Technical advances in microsurgery have moved forward to transplant isolated layers of the cornea. However, immune-mediated rejection remains a key problem. Continued preventive and therapeutic efforts are therefore required to improve the prognosis after keratoplasty.

Reports on the incidence of graft rejection after penetrating keratoplasty vary between 5 and 40 % (Table 6.1) [3, 6, 12, 21, 60, 67, 73, 90, 105, 111, 113–115]. Whereas the short-term survival (1-year follow-up) of penetrating corneal transplants is excellent, the long-term prognosis (10-year follow-up) is even inferior to solid organ transplantation and estimated to be approximately 50 % [3, 6, 102, 114]. In particular, the issue of "chronic rejection" and continuous endothelial cell loss is still under debate. Continued preventive and therapeutic efforts are therefore

U. Pleyer et al. (eds.), *Immune Modulation and Anti-Inflammatory Therapy in Ocular Disorders*,
DOI 10.1007/978-3-642-54350-0_6, © Springer-Verlag Berlin Heidelberg 2014

Table 6.1 Immune reaction after penetrating keratoplasty

Author	Number	Incidence (%)	Irreversible (%)
Völker-Dieben et al. [113]	290	28	n.m.
Alldredge and Krachmer [3]	156	29	5
Arentsen [6]	869	n.m.	5
Severin [90]	226	43	13
Pleyer et al. [67]	740	4–37[a]	3–28[a]
Williams et al. [115]	7,741	n.m.	32–33
Reinhard et al. [73]	646	18	n.m.
Patel et al. [60]	394	23	7
Birnbaum et al. [12]	417	n.m.	28–40
Varssano et al. [111]	126	37	30
Tan et al. [105]	901	n.m.	29
Williams et al. [114]	14,622	n.m.	34

n.m. Not mentioned
[a]Dependent from risk factors

required to improve the long-term prognosis after penetrating keratoplasty.

6.1.2 Aetiology of Corneal Graft Rejection

6.1.2.1 Immunological Features of Cornea

The eye has unique features which makes it quite different from other organs in respect to its immunobiology. Accordingly, some principles involved in general transplantation immunology usually cannot be applied directly in corneal transplantation. Experimental models have provided many details on the immunobiology of corneal grafts [65].

6.1.2.2 Corneal Immunogenicity

The cornea has been thought to lack of immunogenicity because of its low antigen expression. HLA class I antigens are expressed particularly in the corneal epithelium and, much less densely, in the stroma and endothelium. HLA class II antigens have been found only scattered in the corneal epithelium, particularly at the limbus region and in the corneal stroma [61]. However, the expression can change under certain conditions. An enhanced expression of HLA class I and II antigens could be detected during allograft rejection and even induced by the surgical process itself [61]. In contrast, extending storage [5] or low-dose UVB radiation [18] decreased HLA class II antigens (DR) expression in human corneas. Moreover, studies using rodent models of keratoplasty have shown that, in some strain combinations, allografts carrying minor histocompatibility (H) alloantigens are more likely to be rejected than those bearing MHC alloantigens [33, 87, 99]. Since in humans these antigens are less well characterised, this issue remains open for future clinical approaches.

A brief summary of immunological events is presented in Figs. 6.1 and 6.2.

6.1.3 Technical Factors

6.1.3.1 Role of Trephination Technique in Penetrating Keratoplasty

The role of different trephination techniques and instruments, e.g. mechanical vs. laser-guided systems on graft rejection, remains uncertain. Very few studies have focused attention on this issue. In a prospective study using excimer laser guided vs. mechanical trephination, no difference in the rejection rate was observed in normal-risk recipients followed up to 40 months [89 (EBM: 1+, A)].

6.1.3.2 Lamellar Transplantation Techniques Versus Penetrating Keratoplasty

Recent years have seen the evolution of several lamellar transplantation techniques. Fast optical and visual rehabilitation and less invasive surgical procedures are encouraging. In general, endothelial graft rejection seems to occur much less often after endothelial keratoplasty (EK) [2 (**EBM: 2+, C**), [8 (EBM: 1+, B), [32 (EBM: 2++, B)]. It certainly can also be considered that the risk for epithelial and stromal rejection should be lower in EK recipients. Also the absence of graft sutures in these patients may reduce the risk of rejection

a Immune privilege

- Blood–ocular barrier
- Absence of blood and lymphatic vessels
- Immunosuppressive factors
- Immature APCs
- Presence of regulatory T cells
- Low expression of MHC class I
- Lack of MHC class II molecules
- FasL expression

High risk factors

- Inflammation
- Neovascularization
- Lymphangiogenesis
- Pre–sensitization (previous rejection)
- Large or eccentric grafts
- Infection
- Viral replication (Herpes simplex virus)

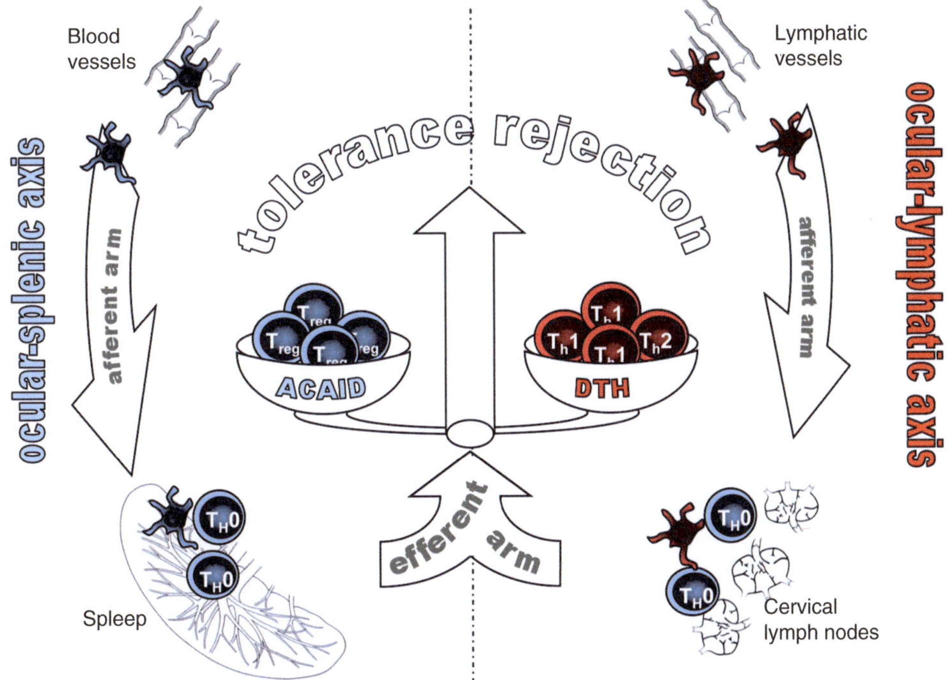

Fig. 6.1 (**a**) Local factors contributing to immune privilege ligand (*left*), and risk factors leading to ablation of corneal privilege (*right*). Abbreviations: *α-MSH* α-melanocyte stimulating hormone, *APCs* antigen-presenting cells, *FasL* Fas ligand, *IL* interleukin, *TGF-β* transforming growth factor-β, *TNF-α* tumour necrosis factor-α, *T_reg* regulatory T cells, *VIP* vasoactive intestinal peptide. (**b**) Systemic factors that contribute to the immune privilege

Antigen presentation pathways

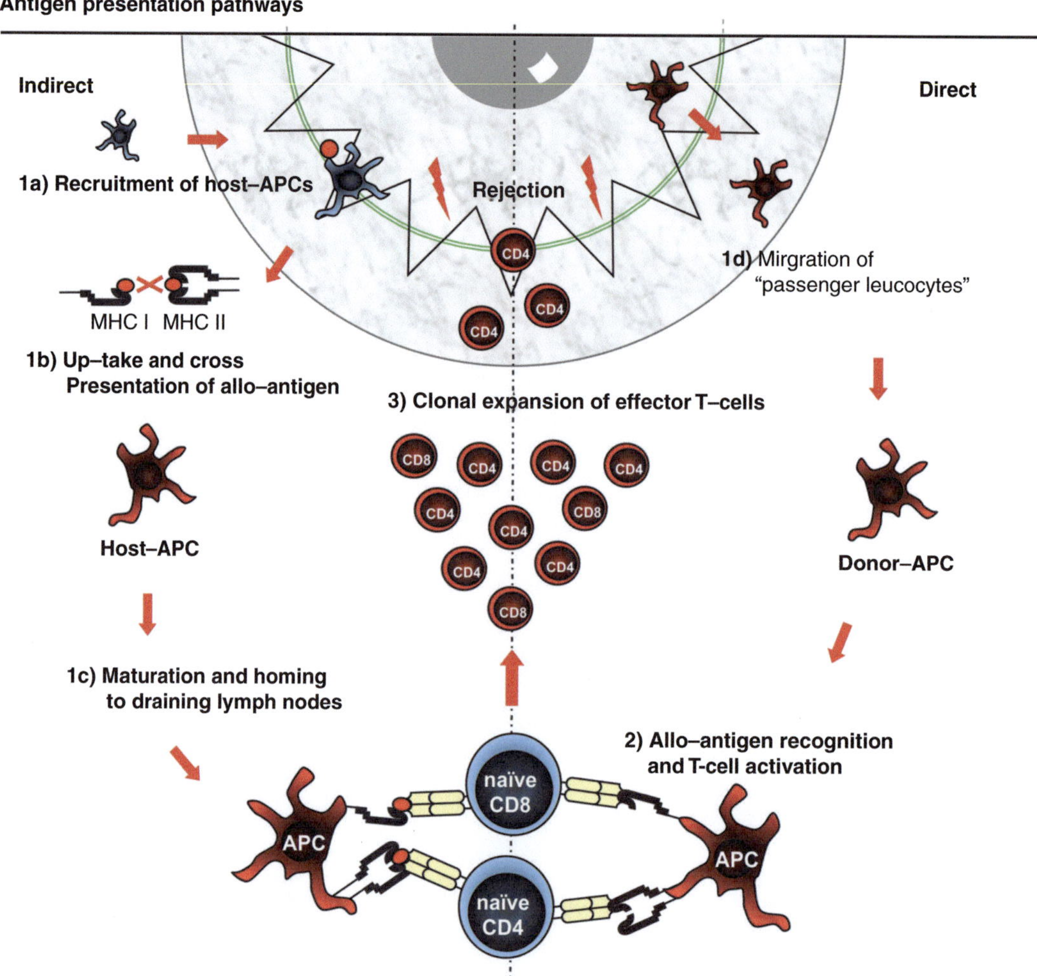

Fig. 6.2 Indirect (*left*) and direct (*right*) antigen presentation. (*1*) Recipient antigen-presenting cells (*APCs*) migrate from the limbus centripetally into the corneal graft. There they either internalise and process alloantigens (*1a*) or acquire shed donor MHC molecules (*1b*). Mature recipient APCs migrate to draining lymph nodes (*2*) and present alloantigens indirectly or semidirectly, respectively. (*1c*) Donor APCs migrate out of the allograft and prime directly T cells in the draining lymph nodes. (*3*) Alloantigen-specific T cells recognise either presented corneal antigens or allogenic epitopes on the MHC molecules

since these may trigger an immune response related to wound dehiscence and infectious keratitis [80, 114]. In addition, a meta-analysis supports the conclusion that endothelial keratoplasty is superior to PK for preservation of corneal endothelial cells [76 (**EBM: 1+A**)]. This may allow to reduce postoperative immune modulation and simplify long-term management of EK eyes compared with PK eyes [76 (**EBM: 1+A**)]. Interestingly, if corneal transplant rejection occurs, it may be less severe after EK than after PK.

It has to be noticed, however, that the reduced rejection rate in EK patients could be simply a product of a relatively prolonged postoperative topical steroid cover. Most patients received topical steroids even 2 years post-op [2 (**EBM: 2+, C**)].

Core Messages
- Even when the short-term survival (1-year follow-up) of penetrating corneal transplants is excellent, the long-term prognosis is inferior to solid organ transplantation and estimated to be approximately 50 % (EBM: 2+).

- Technical factors, such as different trephination techniques and instruments, are unlikely to cause consequences for corneal graft rejection. Mechanical vs. laser-guided systems did not demonstrate any long-term difference (EBM: 1+ A).
- Recent data support the conclusion that endothelial keratoplasty is superior to penetrating corneal transplants with a lower endothelial rejection rate (EBM: 1+ B) and better preservation of corneal endothelial cells (EBM: 1+ A).
- The prolonged use of topical corticosteroid treatment following endothelial keratoplasty may have contributed to this favourable outcome and has to be further elucidated.

6.2　Clinical Signs and Symptoms

6.2.1　Clinical Presentation of Graft Rejection: Signs

As a consequence of HLA antigen distribution in all cellular layers, corneal allograft rejection can occur in each of the three main layers independently or simultaneously. Corneal graft rejection most commonly occurs during the first year after surgery. Fortunately, most episodes of graft rejection do not cause irreversible graft failure if recognised early and treated adequately.

6.2.1.1 Epithelial Rejection

Epithelial rejection is considered relatively unimportant, as the donor epithelium can be replaced by recipient epithelium derived from the limbus without further consequences. It occurs within 1–13 months postoperatively, at a rate of 1–10 %, as after this time the donor epithelium is replaced by host epithelium. Clinical manifestation of epithelial rejection includes the appearance of an elevated epithelial rejection line that consists of damaged donor epithelial cells. It usually starts from the periphery, stains with fluorescein and migrates towards the centre of the graft like the Khodadoust line (Fig. 6.3).

6.2.1.2 Subepithelial Rejection

Subepithelial rejection presents as subepithelial infiltrates of 0.2–0.5 mm in diameter located in the anterior stroma (Fig. 6.4) [3]. They occur within 2–24 months after keratoplasty and resemble infiltrates similar to that in adenoviral keratitis. This is the second most common form of corneal graft rejection with a reported incidence of 2–15 % [66]. Subepithelial graft rejection leaves no sequelae if treated, but it may precede the more severe endothelial rejection [66].

6.2.1.3 Stromal Rejection

Stromal rejection is relatively rare (1–2 %) [66]. It is characterised by peripheral stromal infiltrates and haze in a previously clear graft. Stromal rejection usually occurs simultaneously with endothelial rejection.

6.2.1.4 Endothelial Rejection

Endothelial rejection is the most common form of graft rejection with reported rates of 8–37 % [66]. In terms of corneal function, this type of rejection is of greatest interest. Human endothelial cells do not replicate, and thus, donor cell loss is irreversible. During endothelial rejection, it is possible to visualise linear or multifocal deposits of leucocytes adhering to the endothelium associated with segmental corneal oedema. An endothelial rejection line (i.e. Khodadoust line) starts in the periphery of the graft, usually in the vicinity of stromal vessels, and moves towards to the centre of the graft (Fig. 6.3c). Hence, although intensive treatment with topical steroids reverses the acute inflammation in most patients, the goal is to reverse the rejection episode as early as possible to minimise endothelial cell loss.

6.2.2　Clinical Presentation of Endothelial Graft Rejection: Symptoms

- Decrease of visual acuity
- Redness
- (Pain)
- Irritation
- Photophobia

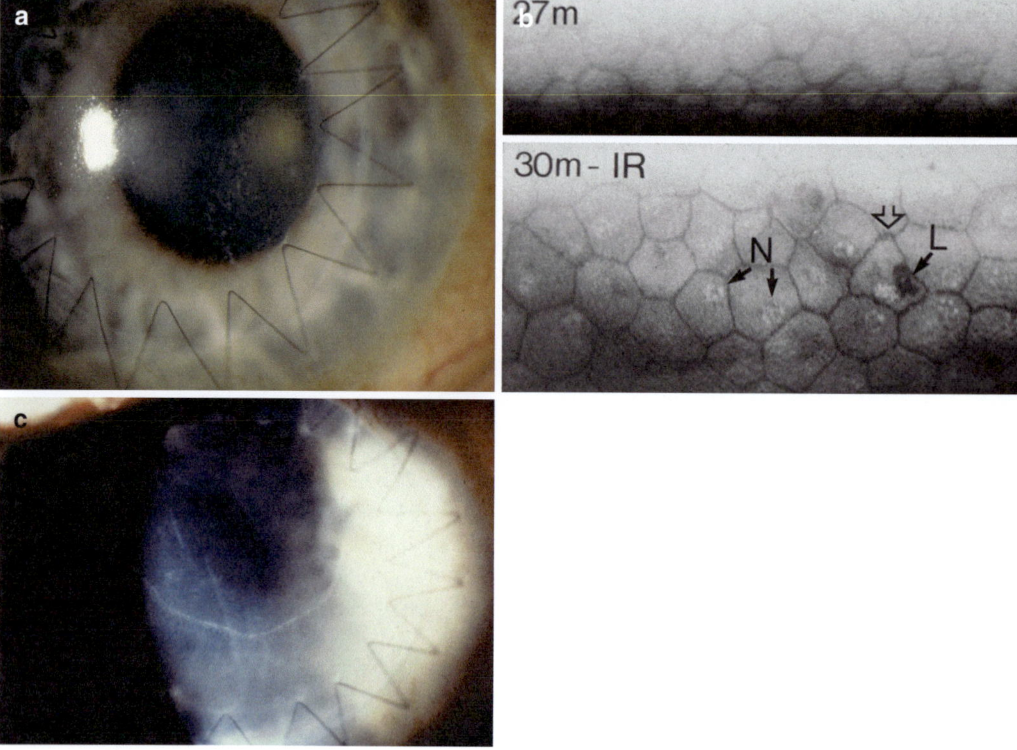

Fig. 6.3 Corneal graft rejection. Since all layers of the tissue are able to express MHC antigens, rejection may occur at the epithelial (**a**) and endothelial level (**b+c**). (**b**) Illustrates endothelial cell loss as seen by specular microscopy with adherent neutrophil granulocyte (*N*) and lymphocyte (*L*). (**c**) Demonstrates Khodadoust rejection line

Depending on the severity of graft rejection and postoperative time interval, patients may be asymptomatic.

Clinical presentation	Differential diagnosis
Endothelial rejection	Corneal oedema from endothelial insufficiency
	Late graft failure
	Recurrent herpetic keratitis
	Epithelial downgrowth
	Remaining endothelial precipitates
	Endothelial decompensation due to secondary glaucoma

6.2.3 Differential Diagnosis of Graft Rejection (Table 6.2)

Table 6.2 Differential diagnosis of graft rejection

Clinical presentation	Differential diagnosis
Epithelial rejection	Recurrent or acquired herpetic keratitis
	Epitheliopathy (dry eye syndrome)
	Ocular surface alteration (e.g. following chemical burn, atopic keratoconjunctivitis)
	Stem cell damage
Subepithelial rejection	Macular corneal dystrophy
	Adenoviral keratoconjunctivitis

Core Messages
- Corneal allograft rejection can occur in each of the three main layers independently or simultaneously (EBM: 2+).
- Acute corneal graft rejection occurs most commonly during the first year after surgery (EBM: 1+).
- A wide spectrum of differential diagnoses of different types of rejection has to be considered.

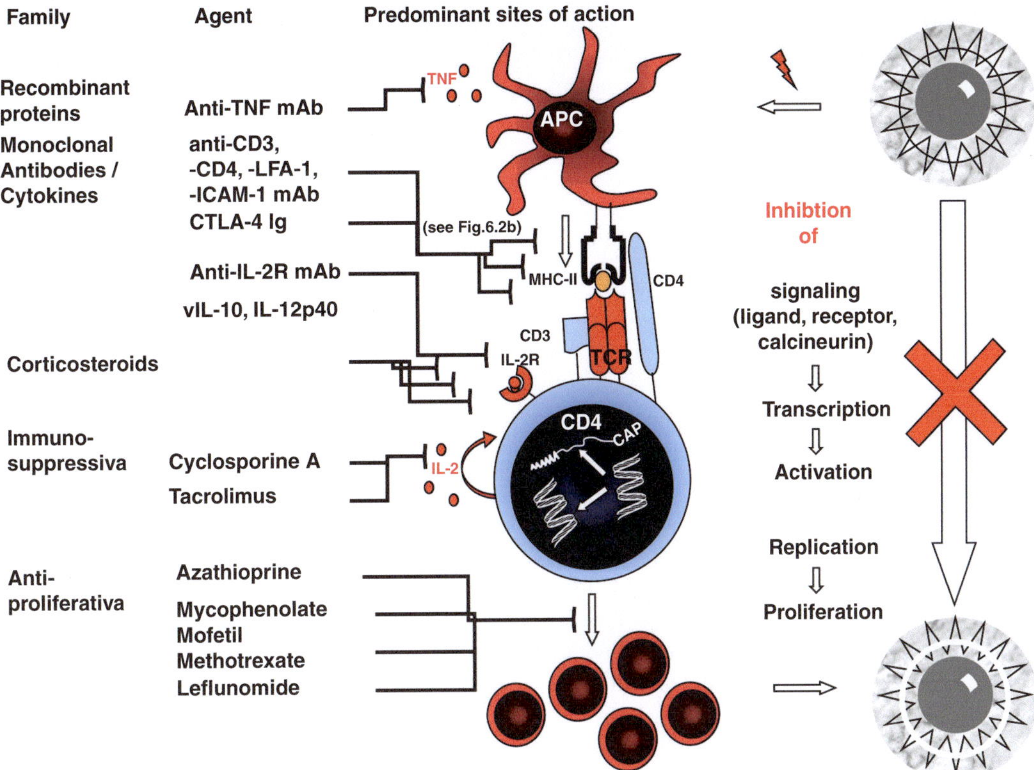

Fig. 6.4 Immunomodulatory agents in keratoplasty. This figure schematically shows the sites of action of currently clinically used compounds (corticosteroids, immune modulatory and antiproliferative agents) and of recombinant proteins as potential future therapeutics

6.3 Prevention of Corneal Graft Rejection in Penetrating Keratoplasty

6.3.1 Strategies to Prevent Allograft Rejection

Several options are used to reduce the risk of corneal allograft rejection. Most are derived from other areas in transplantation medicine.

Two major strategies are used to improve corneal graft survival:

- Decrease of the recipient's sensibility by reduction of antigen difference between the donor and recipient (histocompatibility complex (HLA) matching)
- Reduction of the recipient's afferent or efferent immune response by pharmacological modulation

6.3.2 Use of HLA-Matched Donor Tissue to Prevent Corneal Graft Rejection

Based on the immune biology of the cornea, rational arguments can be easily generated in favour to HLA matching in keratoplasty. However, in clinical practice, HLA matching is still widely neglected, even when growing evidence shows a benefit in corneal transplantation. Whereas mainly in Europe several studies support a significant benefit for HLA-A, HLA-B and HLA-DR matching, this is not generally accepted elsewhere [31, 86, 112]. Interestingly, the prospective randomised "CCTS study" demonstrated no effect for neither class I nor class II matching even when that same study demonstrated an increased risk of graft rejection in patients with lymphocytotoxic antibodies to HLA class I and

II antigens [1]. However, the validity of this study has been discussed because of high error rates in the matching procedures and a concomitant high dose of topical corticosteroids [37]. More conflicting results derived from other well-designed studies that came to the conclusion that HLA matching may even have a negative outcome on graft survival [19, 110]. The fact that certain HLA mismatches differ in immunogenicity and may have an impact on graft survival has been known for some time in kidney transplantation and in keratoplasty, but just recently got adequate attention. For HLA class I/II loci, the structural basis of this phenomenon has been established [7, 46, 57, 110]. Therefore, in order to select the optimal donor for this category of patients, it will be important to take advantage of the differential immunogenicity and thus differential importance of mismatched HLA antigens. Indeed, it has been possible to define "acceptable or permissible mismatches" with a low immunogenicity, which are associated with a favourable graft survival, vs. "taboo mismatches" with a high immunogenicity and a poor graft survival [17]. It can be expected that further experience in this direction will allow new strategies for future HLA matching, which will not only suit a rare number of patients with frequent haplotypes but also provide an acceptable waiting time for great percentage of most other patients. Recently, a computer-based approach, "HLA Matchmaker", a molecularly based algorithm for histocompatibility algorithm, has been introduced which respects this problem. It can identify immunologically acceptable mismatches and reduces the time on the waiting list substantially [16] (Table 6.3).

Still some limitations of HLA matching in keratoplasty remain. These include:

- Adequate "logistics"
- Additional costs for HLA typing and distribution
- Monitoring and quality control of typing procedures
- The uncertain role of factors such as minor histocompatibility antigens

Core Messages

- HLA matching reduces graft rejections in normal-risk as well as in high-risk keratoplasty (EBM: 2).
- Most patients can be served with an HLA compatible graft within well below a year, even in a monocentre setup (EBM: 3).
- The HLA-A1/H-Y minor antigen equals immunogenicity of HLA mismatches: allocating male HLA-A1 positive donors for female recipients should be avoided (EBM: 3).
- Long-term graft survival can probably be improved upon routinely matching major and selected minor histocompatibility antigens.

6.3.3 Use of Immune Modulatory Agents to Prevent Corneal Graft Rejection

No generally accepted "guidelines" on the use of anti-inflammatory and immune modulating agents to prevent corneal graft rejection are available. Several surveys of corneal transplant societies indicate that a broad pattern of clinical practices exists [10, 83].

6.3.3.1 Use of Immune Modulatory Agents in "Normal-Risk" Recipients

Whereas most studies deal with the prevention of allograft rejection in "high-risk" patients, only few studies focused on postoperative care in "normal-risk" recipients. Commonly, topical postoperative treatment with corticosteroids is considered as sufficient.

Topical Corticosteroids

Topical corticosteroids are used as standard treatment for the prevention of corneal allograft rejection for over 40 years [17]. Main advantages

Table 6.3 Clinical studies on HLA matching

Autors	Mono-/multi-center	(n)	Median (years)	Prognosis	Determined antigens			Criteria	Method of HLA-typing	Results/comments
					HLA class 1	HLA class 2	Others			
Beekhuis et al. (2003)	Mono	303	4	High-risk	A, B			Immune rejection	Control-sero	Retrospective study; significant positive effect of HLA-A and B matching (irreversible rejection); HLA split matching is superior as followed for 3–12 years
Reinhard et al. (2003)	Mono	398	3	Normal-risk	A, B	DR		Irreversible rejection; graft failure	Control-sero (HLA class 1) DNA (HLA class 2)	Retrospective study; HLA matching (HLA-A, B, DR) reduces immune rejection and improves long term survival
Khaireddin et al. [46]	Mono	459	3	Normal- and high-risk	A, B	DR		Immune rejection	Control-sero	Retrospective study; HLA matching (HLA-A, B, DR) reduces immune rejection and improves long term survival significantly for high- and normal-risk grafts; no significant benefit for split matching
Bartels et al. (2001)	Mono	64	3	Normal- and high-risk	A, B	DR		Immune rejection	DNA (retrospective)	Case-control study; significant benefit of HLA-A and HLA-DR matching in high-risk grafts
Völker-Dieben et al. [112]	Mono	1,681	5	Normal- and high-risk	A, B	DR		Immune rejection irrev. IR	Control-sero	Significant benefit of HLA-A and HLA-B matching in high- and normal-risk grafts
Roy et al. (1997)	Mono	693	3	Normal- and high-risk	A, B		Lewis-antigens	Immune rejection	n.d.	Significant benefit of HLA-A and HLA-B and Lewis-antigens in normal-risk grafts

include immediate and potent anti-inflammatory effects, favourable pharmacological properties and low price. Steroids rapidly permeate the cellular membrane and act intracellularly through glucocorticoid-responsive elements that regulate the expression of more than 200 different genes [72].

Biological effects include downregulation of interleukin (IL)-1, IL-3, IL-6 and IL-8 which are secreted predominantly by antigen-presenting cells. In addition, reduction of IL-1 and IL-6 leads to inhibition of IL-2 secretion and subsequent T cell inhibition. Important for the postoperative use of corticosteroids in corneal grafts is their broad spectrum of antiphlogistic properties. They reduce the permeability of vascular endothelium (blood-aqueous barrier, blood-retina barrier) and inhibit migration of monocytes. Experimental data demonstrate a dose-dependent inhibitory effect on cytokine production. Already very low doses (10–100 nM) inhibit resting cells, while far higher doses are necessary to block also activated cells.

The pharmacological preparation of topically used corticosteroids is important for the intraocular effects of the drug. Prednisolone acetate penetrates the cornea very well even with an intact epithelium, whereas the topical application of prednisolone phosphate leads to intraocular availability only when the epithelium is abraded. The effects of different corticosteroids on the migration of leucocytes in the cornea vary widely [50]. It is important to emphasise that the biological effect of local steroid therapy is mainly anti-inflammatory. Although local steroids are commonly applied for postoperative treatment after keratoplasty, there are different opinions about dosage and duration of treatment. There are no controlled clinical studies from which a "gold standard" could be derived. In normal-risk patients, topical application of 1 % prednisolone acetate q.i.d. has been suggested for the first 2–4 weeks, reduced to 1 drop/day after 3 months and then continued up to the 12th postoperative month. Nguyen et al. demonstrated in a prospective, randomised interventional trial that long-term treatment (continued steroids once daily for 12 months) significantly reduced ($p=0.001$) graft rejections as compared to 6 months short term (stop topical steroid treatment) [59 (EBM: 1+, B)].

6.3.3.2 Topical Calcineurin Inhibitors (Cyclosporine A, Tacrolimus)

Since long-term treatment with corticosteroids is likely to cause adverse effects, the use of topical calcineurin inhibitors (CsA, tacrolimus) has been investigated. Perry et al. [62] suggested that topical CsA (0.5 %) may substitute local steroids in secondary glaucoma responders; however, the rejection rate in CsA-treated patients increased. Another calcineurin inhibitor tacrolimus (FK506) was used as topical immune modulatory eye drop (0.06 %) in a 3-year prospective trial. Even when the use of topical eye drops resulted in a lower number of graft rejections as compared to topical prednisolone acetate 1 % eye drops, there was no statistical significant difference. Unfortunately, eight patients in the FK 506 group concluded the study early due to local side effects. An optimised galenic formulation of tacrolimus might be a therapeutic option to prevent graft rejection [77 (EBM: 1+, B)].

Undesired Effects of Topical Immune Modulatory Treatment

Well-known undesired side effects of local corticosteroids are altered wound healing, increased risk for infection, reactivation of herpes virus keratitis, secondary glaucoma and cataract formation [92]. Whether topical steroid therapy alters re-epithelialisation of the cornea is not proven [101]. However, prolonged wound healing after keratoplasty can be expected due to fibroblast inhibition and reduced collagen synthesis. The increase in intraocular pressure due to steroid response is a well-known side effect in up to 30 % of patients. This is of particular importance in keratoplasty recipients, since corneal graft endothelial cells are susceptible to pressure rise. Often incorrect pressure measurements after keratoplasty are another challenge in these patients. Several new agents are in focus of clinical studies to prove whether the rate of IOP increase can be reduced by application of less pressure-altering steroids. The use of loteprednol has been recommended since the likelihood of IOP increase

Table 6.4 Major agents used for systemic immune modulation in keratoplasty

Generic	Effect	Initial dosage	Maximum dosage	Time to be effective	Major undesired effects	Control parameters
Cyclosporine A	Calcineurin inhibitor	3–5 mg/kg/day	10 mg/kg/day	2–6 weeks	Nephrotoxicity	CsA blood level
					Hypertension	Creatinine
					Tremor	RR control
					Hirsutismus	Serum electrolytes
					Gingival hyperplasia	
Mycophenolate mofetil	Purine synthesis	2 × 500 mg/day	2 × 1.5 g/day	2–12 weeks	Diarrhoea	Complete blood count
					Gastrointestinal irritation	Liver enzymes
					Infection	
					Neutropenia	
Tacrolimus	Calcineurin inhibitor	0.15–0.3 mg/kg/day	0.30 mg/kg/day	2–8 weeks	Nephrotoxicity	Complete blood count
					Infection	Creatinine

seems less likely. Currently, a new class of agents labelled as selective receptor agonists (SEGRA) [68] might be promising. Cataract formation has been observed after a cumulative dose of 740 drops of 0.1 % dexamethasone [51] (Table 6.4).

Systemic Corticosteroid Treatment in Normal-Risk Patients

Systemic treatment with corticosteroids has not only antiphlogistic but also immunosuppressive effects. Suggestions for dosage and duration of systemic treatment vary as much as for topical treatment [107]. For the perioperative period, some authors suggest 100–250 mg/day prednisolone intravenously. Prolonged monotherapy with systemic corticosteroids should be avoided because of the high potential of side effects. In a randomised prospective study, there was no benefit for normal-risk patients that received systemic fluocortolone for a 3-week period in addition to topical prednisolone acetate [54]. It is of clinical importance that the inhibition of cytokine synthesis by corticosteroids is quickly reversible and the effect on T cells and antigen-presenting cells diminishes rapidly. Sudden termination of corticosteroid therapy can provoke rebound effects resulting in immediate adverse effects. Marked T cell proliferation after corticosteroid termination could be detected possibly because of upregulation of T cell receptors. These findings indicate that steroid therapy should be terminated by tapering of the drug. Systemic steroid therapy provokes all the side effects of local therapy and may lead additionally to severe metabolic alterations.

Core Messages

- Based on current evidence, topical corticosteroids remain the gold standard to prevent graft rejection in normal-risk recipients. Prolonged "low-dose (1/day prednisolone 1 %) treatment" for 12 months was superior to a 6-month application and should be considered in penetrating keratoplasty patients (EBM: 1+ B).
- Long-term corticosteroid treatment bears the risk of secondary IOP elevation and subsequent chronic endothelial cell alteration. Switching to, e.g. loteprednol etabonate from prednisolone acetate should be considered in known steroid responders, since it was successful in reducing IOP and did not increase the risk of allograft rejection (EBM: 2+).
- Topical calcineurin inhibitors, including CsA and tacrolimus, did not demonstrate a significant benefit to reduce

graft rejection in any controlled study (EBM: 1+ B).

- Systemic corticosteroid treatment did not demonstrate an additional benefit to topical application for normal-risk patients. Since systemic side effects are more likely to occur, additional systemic treatment is not recommended (EBM: 1+B).

6.3.3.3 Use of Immunomodulatory Agents in "High-Risk" Recipients

It is commonly agreed that a certain subpopulation of patients exist that can be classified as "high-risk" individuals. Subsequently, these patients are handled differently regarding postoperative immunomodulatory prophylaxis.

Well-known risk factors for corneal graft rejection include:

- More than 2/4 vascularisation of the recipient's cornea
- Preoperative inflammation of the anterior segment
- Keratoplasty à chaud
- Anterior synechiae
- Large graft (>7.7 mm diameter)
- Grafts near the limbus
- Multiple grafts

Identification and proper handling of these patients is essential to provide an optimal result. Pharmacotherapy for prophylaxis and treatment of corneal graft rejection is warranted in these "high-risk" patients. Even when recipients will often get HLA-matched corneas, immune modulatory agents are applied in addition.

Topical Corticosteroids in High-Risk Patients

Because of their rapid and broad anti-inflammatory effect, topical corticosteroids are also a "standard" in high-risk patients. Frequency and duration of treatment are adapted to the individual clinical situation of the patient. For "high-risk" patients, recommendations vary for prednisolone acetate drops from b.i.d. to up to 24 times per day [10, 83]. But even a high-dose local corticosteroid therapy (>5× daily) cannot avoid graft rejection, and undesired side effects may instead dominate. Therefore, alternative/additional therapeutic options are necessary.

Topical Calcineurin Inhibitors (Cyclosporine A, Tacrolimus)

Cyclosporine A

Inhibition of calcineurin in the intracellular signalling pathway interferes with DNA transcription and thus leads to a decreased function of immune cells. Calcineurin inhibitors are potent immunosuppressive drugs acting predominantly through inhibition of T cell activation. As a lipophilic compound, CsA can pass the cellular membrane by diffusion and binds to specific receptors called cyclophilins. Cyclophilins have enzymatic activity and contribute to intracellular protein benching [94]. Target molecules of the CsA-cyclophilin complex are proteins that regulate the gene transcription in the nucleus (NF-AT, AP-3, NF-B), which are involved in the transcription of IL-2 genes [103]. In different tissues, various types of cyclophilins exist indicating that the effect on IL-2 regulation might vary in different tissues. Until now, cyclophilins A, B, C and S have been characterised. It could be shown that cyclophilin A is highly expressed in the corneal epithelium but only weakly in the endothelium and in the uvea [64]. The regulation pathway of CsA activity is not completely revealed, but the main effect is the inhibition of cytokine synthesis, especially of IL-2 but also IL-4 and tumour necrosis factor. CsA acts dose dependently on the afferent and efferent arc of the immune response. The MHC_{50} of CsA is 10–20 ng/ml for IL-2 production and 20–50 ng/ml for the proliferation of cytotoxic lymphocytes.

Topical Cyclosporine A in High-Risk Recipients

A number of experimental and clinical studies dealt with topically applied CsA, but pharmacological properties limit its clinical benefit. As a lipophilic compound, CsA penetrates easily the corneal epithelium, but intraocular levels remain very low. Improved solvent preparations like cyclodextrin, azone, collagen lenses and liposomes led to higher intraocular concentrations. Subsequent experimental studies using these preparations demonstrated a significant therapeutic effect [48, 55, 57]. In an experimental study of Lee et al., episcleral CsA implants were safe and effective at delivering therapeutic CsA levels to the cornea and able to prevent corneal allograft rejection [49].

However, human studies using topical CsA demonstrated little benefit. In a retrospective clinical study, a positive effect of topically applied CsA (2 %) on graft survival in high-risk but not low-risk patients could be seen [39]. However, subsequent prospective, randomised multicenter studies could not demonstrate a benefit of topical CsA eye drops using either 2 or 0.05 % in preventing graft rejection as compared to topical corticosteroids [41, 97, 108 (EBM: 1+, B)]. Perry et al. [62] suggested that topical CsA (0.5 %) may substitute local steroids in secondary glaucoma responders. However, an increased rejection rate in CsA-treated patients was observed. More recently, an episcleral CsA implant was investigated in a prospective, randomised study and compared to standard prednisolone treatment. Again, no significant benefit could be seen in using this potential alternative to corticosteroids. On the contrary, Shi et al. reported about a CsA drug-delivery system in the anterior chamber. It seems to be effective for the prophylaxis of immune rejection after high-risk keratoplasty without toxicity to the cornea and the iris of patients [95 (EBM: 3, D)].

Topical Tacrolimus in High-Risk Recipients

Like CsA, FK506 is a lipophilic compound with similar limitation following local application, but intraocular drug levels are higher than with CsA [63]. A clinical study demonstrated that topical FK506 was at least as effective in preventing graft rejection as topical steroids in a prospective pilot study. However, local discomfort limited further use [74].

Core Messages
- Current evidence indicates that topical corticosteroids remain the gold standard to prevent graft rejection in high-risk recipients. Prolonged "low-dose (1/day prednisolone 1 %) treatment" for 12 months should be considered in penetrating keratoplasty patients (EBM: 1+).
- Topical CsA did not demonstrate a significant benefit to reduce graft rejection in any prospective, randomised controlled study. It remains inconclusive whether this is related to their particular (unfavourable) pharmacological properties or its spectrum of immune modulatory activity (EBM: 1+, B).
- Topical FK506 was at least as effective in preventing graft rejection as topical steroids in a prospective pilot study. However, local discomfort remains a limiting factor, and currently no commercial product is available (EBM: 1+, B).

Systemic Cyclosporine A in High-Risk Recipients

In general, systemic application of CsA is more effective to reduce the risk of graft rejection in penetrating keratoplasty. There are a number of controlled and uncontrolled clinical studies that support the use of CsA in high-risk patients [34, 35, 102]. A prospective study showed that combined systemic CsA treatment with topical dexamethasone was superior to topical corticosteroid treatment alone [34 (EBM: 1+, B)]. However, different opinions exist on the duration of CsA application. Though a positive effect of a short-term therapy (3 months) was reported in one study [56], there are later results showing a better efficacy with 1 year of CsA treatment. The limited benefit of a short-term (3 months) CsA treatment was confirmed by others. In addition, some studies could not confirm a benefit of CsA at all [40, 69, 85, 96]. A prospective, randomised study could not demonstrate an efficacy of systemic cyclosporine A (mean follow-up of 42.7 months) [96, (EBM: 1+, B)]. Potential side effects of CsA include nephrotoxicity, increase in arterial blood pressure and hepatotoxic effects. Therefore, serum creatinine, liver enzymes and arterial blood pressure need to be monitored. Taken together, CsA is the most frequently used immunomodulatory agent for preventive treatment in high-risk keratoplasty patients [69].

Systemic Tacrolimus in High-Risk Recipients

The acting mechanism is similar to CsA, but, e.g. inhibition of lymphocyte proliferation is 10- to 100-fold stronger compared to CsA [20]. In two noncomparative case series, tacrolimus was effective in the prevention of rejection in patients with high-risk corneal and limbal grafts [98, 116 (EBM: 3, C)]. However, a high rate of undesired side effects and a narrow therapeutic index have limited the clinical use in other fields of transplantation medicine. Predominantly reported side effects are nephrotoxicity and neurotoxicity [91].

Systemic Mycophenolate Mofetil in High-Risk Recipients

Mycophenolate mofetil (MMF) has been introduced some 30 years ago. When its immunomodulatory effects were revealed, it was approved for use in kidney and heart transplantation. After oral intake, MMF is transformed into MPA, the biologically active compound acting as a selective inhibitor of lymphocyte proliferation. A significant preventive effect was demonstrated in a prospective, randomised, multicenter study [14]. MMF given $2 \times 1,000$ mg/day improved the rejection-free graft survival following high-risk keratoplasty significantly ($p = 0.044$) [14 (EBM: 1+, B)]. In a small randomised study [75], MMF was equally effective as CsA in high-risk keratoplasty patients. A recent survey of German keratoplasty centres revealed good acceptance of this agent in high-risk recipients [10]. Side effects of MMF include gastrointestinal symptoms, increase in serum levels of liver enzymes, anaemia as well as increase in respiratory and urogenital tract infections. Interestingly, MMF provides a synergistic antiviral effect with acyclovir treatment that supports corneal graft survival in patients with HSV-associated keratitis [53].

Systemic Rapamycin (Sirolimus) in High-Risk Recipients

A number of experimental studies dealt with topical and systemic applied rapamycin, a well-known agent in renal transplantation for 15 years [27, 42, 93, 100]. A first prospective study on the use of rapamycin after penetrating high-risk keratoplasty demonstrated a comparable efficacy of rapamycin and MMF in preventing immune reactions. However, a broad spectrum of side effects limit the use of rapamycin [15 (EBM: 1+, B)]. Chatel et al. presented a prospective interventional case series. Six patients were treated with oral MMF in combination with sirolimus for 1 year and afterwards with sirolimus only for additional 2 years. The combination seemed to be effective in extending corneal transplant survival in most but not all high-risk patients and generally was well tolerated [22 (EBM: 3, D)].

> **Core Messages**
>
> - Based on current evidence, systemically applied immune modulatory agents such as calcineurin inhibitors (CsA, tacrolimus) and mycophenolate mofetil provide a significant benefit to reduce graft rejection in high-risk patients (EBM: 1+B; EBM: 3).
> - Long-term treatment using CsA (12 months vs. 3 months) was superior in high-risk recipients, but has its limitation by adverse effects in individual cases (EBM: 1+B).
> - Mycophenolate mofetil was equally effective as CsA in high-risk keratoplasty patients and was better tolerated in several studies. Additional advantage may result from MMF treatment in HED recipients due to its synergistic effect with antiviral medication (EBM: 1+B).
> - Systemic rapamycin (sirolimus) might be a promising agent in high-risk recipients as indicated by small case series (EBM: 3D).

6.3.4 Special Situations and Conditions

6.3.4.1 Recurrence of Herpetic Eye Disease (HED) Following Penetrating Keratoplasty

Herpetic eye disease (HED) remains a major indication for keratoplasty [44]. Graft failure in herpetic keratitis is most commonly attributed to either HED recurrences or allograft rejection [23, 29]. The reported survival rate of postherpetic corneal transplants varies from 54 to 86 % at 5 years [9, 23, 29] and is significantly worse as compared to normal-risk patients.

One of the major problems following penetrating keratoplasty for HSV keratitis is recurrent disease in the transplant and secondly corneal graft rejection following or concurrent with herpetic eye disease (HED). Corneal nerve disruption from surgical trauma after keratoplasty causes early reactivation of latent HSV-1 and its shedding in the tear film [11, 58]. In addition, topical corticosteroids enhance herpetic infections. Most episodes of HED occur within the first year following PK, with a reported rate of up to 25 % [43]. Recurrent HED is usually thought to be caused by reactivation of the initial infecting viral strain in the trigeminal ganglion. However, superinfection with a new strain is also possible [80].

Prevention of Reactivation in HED Recipients

Long-term antiviral therapy has proven to reduce the risk of recurrent HED and associated graft rejection. Oral acyclovir 400 mg twice daily demonstrated a significant reduction of HSV recurrences and a better graft prognosis [81, 104, 109]. Since most episodes of HSK occur within the first year following penetrating keratoplasty, it appears reasonable to maintain preventive treatment for at least 1 year postoperatively. In a retrospective study [104], no recurrences were reported in patients receiving oral acyclovir within the first year, as compared to 21 % in untreated patients. Furthermore, a prospective placebo-controlled multicenter trial demonstrated a significant reduction of recurrent HED while for 1 year on acyclovir (9 % vs. 27 %) [109].

Corneal Graft Rejection in HED Recipients

The incidence of immunological graft rejections in patients with underlying HED is higher than in normal-risk grafts [28, 30, 45]. HSV-1 DNA has been detected more frequently in the corneas of patients undergoing repeat corneal transplantation and has been suggested as a possible risk factor for graft failure [4, 44]. Herpes simplex virus has also been found as a rare cause of primary graft failure, probably due to transfer from the donor tissue to the host [24].

In the absence of pathognomonic signs such as a donor endothelial rejection line, a dendritic or geographic ulcer bridging the donor-recipient interface, graft rejection and viral recurrence can be difficult to distinguish clinically. Further analysis based on virus detection, e.g. in the aqueous humour by polymerase chain reaction (PCR) or antibody synthesis, can be very useful [43].

Prevention of Graft Rejection in HED Recipients

Not only reactivation of HED but also the rejection rate could be reduced by treatment with oral acyclovir. Therefore, combined treatment using antiviral medication plus an immune modulatory agent is the logic consequence. Garcia et al. reported a rejection-free survival of 69.4 % after 3 years in patients, receiving prophylactic oral acyclovir (400 mg twice a day), vs. 42.9 % in patients without treatment ($P=0.006$) [30 (EBM: 3, C)]. Reis et al. analysed the effect of MMF 1 g twice daily combined with acyclovir 5×200 mg/day in patients following penetrating keratoplasty with HED. In this uncontrolled study, the immune reaction rate was low with just 13.3 % during a 12-month follow-up [78 (EBM: 3, C)].

6.3.4.2 Risk to Acquire HED After Penetrating Keratoplasty

Interestingly, the incidence of newly acquired HSV keratitis after penetrating keratoplasty is 14-fold higher increased [79]. Molecular biological studies of human ganglia have found evidence of HSV infection in as many as 94 % specimens in humans older than 60 years of age. Therefore, even without a history of HSV keratitis, a patient may be at risk for HSV corneal disease after PKP [82]. Although the trigeminal ganglion is the primary site for harbouring latent HSV-1 in terms of eye disease, there is considerable evidence that HSV-1 may remain within the cornea, for a long period, in either a latent or low-grade infection [43].

Potential Side Effects of Antiviral Long-Term Treatment

Acyclovir is an acyclic nucleoside analogue of guanosine that inhibits HSV replication in the host cells. In terms of dosage, acyclovir 400 mg five times per day provides therapeutic levels in the aqueous, while 400 mg b.i.d. is considered as prophylactically effective. Low-dose oral acyclovir therapy is generally well tolerated, and evaluation of renal function is not recommended routinely. However, acyclovir should be avoided in patients with known renal disease, and people at risk for kidney problem should be cleared before using this drug.

> **Core Messages**
> - Graft failure in herpetic keratitis is most commonly attributed to HED recurrences and allograft rejection (EBM: 2+).
> - Based on current evidence, long-term (12 months) prophylaxis using low-dose antiviral treatment (e.g. 400 mg acyclovir twice daily) significantly reduced recurrent HED (EBM: 1+).
> - The incidence of immunological graft rejections in patients with underlying HED is more than 10 times higher than in normal-risk grafts and often associated with reactivated HED (EBM: 2+).
> - The rejection rate could be significantly reduced by additional long-term antiviral treatment (EBM: 3, C).
> - Combined antiviral prevention and immunomodulatory treatment should be therefore considered in HED patients. Mycophenolate mofetil might be a particular interesting agent since it demonstrated an additional supportive effect (EBM: 3, C).

6.4 Management and Treatment of Corneal Graft Rejection

Despite all progress made in preventive measures, corneal graft rejection still occurs. Thus, early recognition and effective treatment of graft rejection remains critical for the success of corneal transplantation. The treatment of corneal graft rejection varies according to its clinical presentation.

6.4.1 Epithelial and SEI Rejection

Epithelial and SEI rejection is usually treated on an outpatient basis with frequent topical steroids, such as prednisolone acetate 1 % every 2 h.

6.4.2 Endothelial Rejection

Endothelial rejection needs probably a more aggressive treatment strategy. A questionnaire, designed to evaluate the practice patterns for corneal graft rejection, demonstrated that up to 42 % experts preferred to admit these patients and to treat them with topical prednisolone 1 % every hour [47 (EBM: 4, D)]. It is mainly agreed upon that additional treatment to topical steroids is supportive as either systemic or periocular steroids [47].

Whether subconjunctival or systemic steroid treatment is superior to each other is less clear.

Costa et al. presented a case control study that analysed the reversion rate in patients with an initial episode of corneal endothelial rejection. A single subconjunctival injection of 20 mg triamcinolone showed a significant better outcome ($p=0.025$) as compared to a single intravenous injection of 500 mg methylprednisolone when combined with topical 1 % prednisolone [25 (EBM: 2+, C)]. In contrast, Hudde et al. compared in a prospective, randomised trial the use of a single intravenous pulse of methylprednisolone 500 mg with a single subconjunctival betamethasone 2 mg injection in addition to local corticosteroid treatment. No statistically significant difference was found between the two groups with regard to reversal of the graft rejection episode [38 (EBM: 1+, B)]. In a retrospective case-control study, 67 patients were treated with 1 % topical prednisolone acetate and pulsed intravenous methylprednisolone 500 mg vs.14 patients receiving topical treatment only [26 (EBM: 3, D)]. There was a statistically significant association ($p<0.05$) to greater success with pulsed steroids. Analysing different systemic steroids therapies, Hill et al. showed that prednisolone acetate 1 % drops and single i.v. pulse of 500 mg methylprednisolone ($n=24$), vs. topical therapy plus oral 60–80 mg prednisolone demonstrated a significant better outcome using pulse therapy ($p<0.05$) [36 (EBM: 1+, B)].

The use of oral steroids remained a constant treatment element for graft rejection in a Castroviejo Society survey. Also respondents of a Bowman Club survey reported significantly higher use of oral steroids for routine management of high-risk graft and definite graft rejection [71, 118 (EBM: 4, D)].

Interestingly, a single-centre study demonstrated a significant better response to reverse rejection after treatment with i.v. dexamethasone as compared to i.v. methylprednisolone, when used in addition to topical steroids ($p=0.018$) [106]. In addition, a case report demonstrated that a single intracameral injection of triamcinolone acetonide may be an option to treat endothelial graft rejection when other steroid therapies have failed [52 (EBM: 3, D)]. Another case-control study reported about an effect in reducing the time to improvement of endothelial graft rejection after intravitreal injection of triamcinolone [117 (EBM: 2+, C)].

6.4.2.1 Additional Topical CsA Treatment in Endothelial Graft Rejection

Other options such as topical CsA 0.05 % were less effective. Poon et al. demonstrated that as an adjunct use to topical steroids, it does not improve the outcome of graft rejection [70, 71 (EBM: 2+, C)].

> **Core Messages**
> - Epithelial and SEI rejection can be effectively treated with frequent topical steroids, such as prednisolone acetate 1 % every 2 h (EBM: 3+).
> - Reversal of endothelial graft rejection is more difficult to obtain. Corticosteroids used as either subconjunctival injection or systemic therapy demonstrated a significant benefit when used in addition to topical treatment (EBM: 1+, B).
> - Based on current evidence, the use of 500 mg intravenous methylprednisolone in addition to 1 % topical prednisolone acetate is superior in reverting corneal allograft rejection when compared to isolated use of 1 % topical prednisolone (EBM: 3, D).
> - Pulse therapy, using i.v. 500 mg methylprednisolone, was superior to oral systemic steroid application (EBM: 1+, B).
> - Intracameral injection of triamcinolone acetonide might be an additional option to treat endothelial graft rejection when other steroid therapies have failed (EBM: 3, D).

6.5 New Developments and Future Perspectives in Immune Modulation

6.5.1 New Developments in Immune Modulation

The pathophysiologic basis of modern immune pharmacology is focused on T cell modulation and the interaction with antigen-presenting cells. Identification of pathophysiologic pathways such as costimulatory signals, T cell receptor antagonists and cytokine signalling have also resulted in a more tailored immune modulation. These approaches are already used in other fields of transplantation, but are not approved so far in human keratoplasty.

6.5.2 Monoclonal Antibodies and Other "Biologicals" to Prevent Corneal Graft Rejection

First clinical studies dealt with basiliximab, a monoclonal antibody with a high specific binding affinity to the IL-2 receptor of activated T cells. A first prospective pilot study on the use of basiliximab after penetrating high-risk keratoplasty demonstrated that using this antibody immediately following surgery and four days postoperatively has a lower efficacy in preventing immune reactions after risk keratoplasty than CsA [13 (EBM: 1+, B)]. However, the side effect profile of basiliximab was more favourable than that of CsA. Additionally, Schmitz et al. showed a potential promising effect of the combination of basiliximab perioperatively and cyclosporine postoperatively [88 (EBM: 3, D)].

6.5.3 Future Perspectives in Immune Modulation

New approaches to reduce the risk of allograft rejection may focus on topical rather than systemic therapies. New targets of "biologicals", agents that selectively interfere with key pathways, may include costimulatory molecules, antiapoptotic strategies and antiangiogenic and anti-lymphangiogenic factors. In addition, gene therapeutic approaches may be of particular interest [84]. Corneal grafts can be preserved for prolonged periods of time and allow modifying allografts ex vivo prior to transplantation. It is very likely that modulation of different pathways simultaneously may be necessary to improve clinical allograft survival.

References

1. The collaborative corneal transplantation studies (CCTS). Effectiveness of histocompatibility matching in high-risk corneal transplantation. The Collaborative Corneal Transplantation Studies Research Group. Arch Ophthalmol 1992;110:1392–403.
2. Allan BD, Terry MA, Price Jr FW, Price MO, Griffin NB, Claesson M. Corneal transplant rejection rate and severity after endothelial keratoplasty. Cornea. 2007;26(9):1039–42.
3. Alldredge OC, Krachmer JH. Clinical types of corneal transplant rejection. Their manifestations, frequency, preoperative correlates, and treatment. Arch Ophthalmol. 1981;99:599–604.
4. Al-Yousuf N, Mavrikakis I, Mavrikakis E, Daya SM. Penetrating keratoplasty: indications over a 10 year period. Br J Ophthalmol. 2004;88(8):998–1001.
5. Ardjomand N, Berghold A, Reich ME. Loss of corneal Langerhans cells during storage in organ culture medium, Optisol and McCarey-Kaufman medium. Eye. 1998;12:134–8.
6. Arentsen JJ. Corneal transplant allograft reaction: possible predisposing factors. Trans Am Ophthalmol Soc. 1983;81:361–402.
7. Baggesen K, Lamm LU, Ehlers N. Significant effect of high-resolution HLA-DRB1 matching in high-risk corneal transplantation. Transplantation. 1996;62: 1273–7.
8. Bahar I, Kaiserman I, McAllum P, Slomovic A, Rootman D. Comparison of posterior lamellar keratoplasty techniques to penetrating keratoplasty. Ophthalmology. 2008;115(9):1525–33.
9. Beckingsale P, Mavrikakis I, Al-Yousuf N, Mavrikakis E, Daya SM. Penetrating keratoplasty: outcomes from a corneal unit compared to national data. Br J Ophthalmol. 2006;90(6):728–31.
10. Bertelmann E, Reinhard T, Pleyer U. Current practice of immune prophylaxis and therapy in perforating keratoplasty. A survey of members of the Cornea Section of the German Ophthalmological Society. Ophthalmologe. 2003;100:1031–5.
11. Beyer CF, Hill JM, Reidy JJ, et al. Corneal nerve disruption reactivates virus in rabbits latently infected with HSV-1. Invest Ophthalmol Vis Sci. 1990; 31:925–32.
12. Birnbaum F, Bohringer D, Sokolovska Y, Sundmacher R, Reinhard T. Immunosuppression with cyclosporine A and mycophenolate mofetil after penetrating high-risk keratoplasty: a retrospective study. Transplantation. 2005;79:964–8.
13. Birnbaum F, Jehle T, Schwartzkopff J, Sokolovska Y, Böhringer D, Reis A, Reinhard T. Basiliximab following penetrating risk-keratoplasty-a prospective randomized pilot study. Klein Monbl Augenheilkd. 2008;225(1):62–5.
14. Birnbaum F, Mayweg S, Reis A, Böhringer D, Seitz B, Engelmann K, Messmer EM, Reinhard T. Mycophenolate mofetil (MMF) following penetrating high-risk keratoplasty: long-term results of a prospective, randomised, multicentre study. Eye (Lond). 2009;23(11):2063–70.
15. Birnbaum F, Reis A, Böhringer D, Skokolowska Y, Mayer K, Voiculescu A, Oellerich M, Sundmacher R, Reinhard T. An open prospective pilot study on the use of rapamycin after penetrating high-risk keratoplasty. Transplantation. 2006;81(5):767–72 (EBM 1+, B).
16. Bohringer D, Reinhard T, Bohringer S, Enczmann J, Godehard E, Sundmacher R. Predicting time on the

waiting list for HLA matched corneal grafts. Tissue Antigens. 2002;59:407–11.

17. Bohringer D, Reinhard T, Duquesnoy RJ, Bohringer S, Enczmann J, Lange P, Claas F, Sundmacher R. Beneficial effect of matching at the HLA-A and -B amino-acid triplet level on rejection-free clear graft survival in penetrating keratoplasty. Transplantation. 2004;77:417–21.

18. Borderie VM, Kantelip BM, Genin PO, Masse M, Laroche L, Delbosc BY. Modulation of HLA-DR and CD1a expression on human cornea with low-dose UVB irradiation. Curr Eye Res. 1996;15:669–79.

19. Bradley BA, Vail A, Gore SM, Rogers CA, Armitage WJ, Nicholls S, Easty DL. Negative effect of HLA-DR matching on corneal transplant rejection. Transplant Proc. 1995;27:1392–4.

20. Bram RJ, Hung DT, Martin PK, Schreiber SL, Crabtree GR. Identification of the immunophilins capable of mediating inhibition of signal transduction by cyclosporin A and FK506: roles of calcineurin binding and cellular location. Mol Cell Biol. 1993;13:4760–9.

21. Casey TA, Gibbs D. Complications in corneal grafting. Trans Ophthalmol Soc UK. 1972;92:517–30.

22. Chatel MA, Larkin DF. Sirolimus and mycophenolate as combination prophylaxis in corneal transplant recipients at high rejection risk. Am J Ophthalmol. 2010;150(2):179–84.

23. Cobo LM, Coster DJ, Rice NS, Jones BR. Prognosis and management of corneal transplantation for herpetic keratitis. Arch Ophthalmol. 1980;98:1755–9.

24. Cockerham GC, Bijwaard K, Sheng ZM, Hidayat AA, Font RL, McLean IW. Primary graft failure: a clinicopathologic and molecular analysis. Ophthalmology. 2000;107(11):2083–90; Discussion 2090–1.

25. Costa DC, de Castro RS, Kara-Jose N. Case-control study of subconjunctival triamcinolone acetonide injection vs intravenous methylprednisolone pulse in the treatment of endothelial corneal allograft rejection. Eye (Lond). 2009;23(3):708–14.

26. Castro DC, Castro RS, Camargo MS, Kara-José N. Corneal allograft rejection: topical treatment vs. pulsed intravenous methylprednisolone - ten years' result. Arq Bras Oftalmol. 2008;71(1):57–61.

27. Dong Y, Huang YF, Wang LQ, Chen B. Experimental study on the effects of rapamycin in prevention of rat corneal allograft rejection. Zhonghua Yan Ke Za Zhi. 2005;41(10):930–5.

28. Epstein RJ, Seedor JA, Dreizen NG, et al. Penetrating keratoplasty for herpes simplex keratitis and keratoconus. Allograft rejection and survival. Ophthalmology. 1987;94(8):935–44.

29. Ficker LA, Kirkness CM, Rice NS, Steele AD. The changing management and improved prognosis for corneal grafting in herpes simplex keratitis. Ophthalmology. 1989;96:1587–96.

30. Garcia DD, Farjo Q, Musch DC, et al. Effect of prophylactic oral acyclovir after penetrating keratoplasty for herpes simplex keratitis. Cornea. 2007; 26(8):930–4.

31. Gore SM, Vail A, Bradley BA, Rogers CA, Easty DL, Armitage WJ. HLA-DR matching in corneal transplantation. Systematic review of published evidence. Corneal Transplant Follow-up Study Collaborators. Transplantation. 1995;60:1033–9.

32. Guilbert E, Bullet J, Sandali O, Basli E, Laroche L, Borderie VM. Long-term rejection incidence and reversibility after penetrating and lamellar keratoplasty. Am J Ophthalmol. 2013;155:560–9.

33. Haskova Z, Sproule TJ, Roopenian DC, Ksander AB. An immunodominant minor histocompatibility alloantigen that initiates corneal allograft rejection. Transplantation. 2003;75:1368–74.

34. Hill JC. Systemic cyclosporine in high-risk keratoplasty. Short- versus long-term therapy. Ophthalmology. 1994;101:128–33.

35. Hill JC. Systemic cyclosporine in high-risk keratoplasty: long-term results. Eye. 1995;9:422–8.

36. Hill JC, Maske R, Watson P. Corticosteroids in corneal graft rejection. Oral versus single pulse therapy. Ophthalmology. 1991;98:329–33.

37. Hopkins KA, Maguire MG, Fink NE, Bias WB. Reproducibility of HLA-A, B, and DR typing using peripheral blood samples: results of retyping in the collaborative corneal transplantation studies. Collaborative Corneal Transplantation Studies Group (corrected). Hum Immunol. 1992;33:122–8.

38. Hudde T, Minassian DC, Larkin DF. Randomised controlled trial of corticosteroid regimens in endothelial corneal allograft rejection. Br J Ophthalmol. 1999;83:1348–52.

39. Inoue K, Amano S, Kimura C, Sato T, Fujita N, Kagaya F, Kaji Y, Oshika T, Tsuru T, Araie M. Long-term effects of topical cyclosporine A treatment after penetrating keratoplasty. Jpn J Ophthalmol. 2000; 44:302–5.

40. Inoue K, Kimura C, Amano S, Sato T, Fujita N, Kagaya F, Kaji Y, Tsuru T, Araie M. Long-term outcome of systemic cyclosporine treatment following penetrating keratoplasty. Jpn J Ophthalmol. 2001; 45:378–82.

41. Javadi MA, Feizi S, Karbasian A, Rastegarpour A. Efficacy of topical ciclosporin A for treatment and prevention of graft rejection in corneal grafts with previous rejection episodes. Br J Ophthalmol. 2010; 94(11):1464–7.

42. Jiang W, Sun HM, Li XR, Yuan XB, Wang YQ, Zhang SX, Tian EJ, Yuan JQ. Combined rapamycin eye drop in nanometer vector and poly (lactic acid) wafers of cyclosporine A effectively prevents high-risk corneal allograft rejection in rabbits. Zhonghua Yan Ke Za Zhi. 2009;45(6):550–5.

43. Kaye S, Choudhary A. Herpes simplex keratitis. Prog Retin Eye Res. 2006;25(4):355–80.

44. Kaye SB, Baker K, Bonshek R, Maseruka H, Grinfeld E, Tullo A, Easty DL, Hart CA. Human herpes viruses in the cornea. Br J Ophthalmol. 2000;84: 563–71.

45. Kersten A, Sundmacher R, Reinhard T. Postoperative complications of penetrating keratoplasty in herpes

infected eyes. Differential diagnosis, therapy and prognostic significance. Ophthalmologe. 1997;94(12): 889–96.

46. Khaireddin R, Wachtlin J, Hopfenmuller W, Hoffmann F. HLA-A, HLA-B and HLA-DR matching reduces the rate of corneal allograft rejection. Graefes Arch Clin Exp Ophthalmol. 2003;241:1020–8.

47. Koay PY, Lee WH, Figueiredo FC. Opinions on risk factors and management of corneal graft rejection in the United Kingdom. Cornea. 2005;24:292–6.

48. Lallemand F, Felt-Baeyens O, Besseghir K, Behar-Cohen F, Gurny R. Cyclosporine A delivery to the eye: a pharmaceutical challenge. Eur J Pharm Biopharm. 2003;56:307–18.

49. Lee SS, Kim H, Wang NS, Bungay PM, Gilger BC, Yuan P, Kim J, Csaky KG, Robinson MR. A pharmacokinetic and safety evaluation of an episcleral cyclosporine implant for potential use in high-risk keratoplasty rejection. Invest Ophthalmol Vis Sci. 2007;48(5):2023–9.

50. Leibowitz HM, Kupferman A. Kinetics of topically administered prednisolone acetate. Optimal concentration for treatment of inflammatory keratitis. Arch Ophthalmol. 1976;94:1387–9.

51. Mackay IR, Bignell JL, Smith PH, Crawford BA. Prevention of corneal-graft failure with the immunosuppressive drug azathioprine. Lancet. 1967;2: 479–82.

52. Maris Jr PJ, Correnti AJ, Donnenfeld ED. Intracameral triamcinolone acetonide as treatment for endothelial allograft rejection after penetrating keratoplasty. Cornea. 2008;27(7):847–50.

53. Mayer K, Reinhard T, Reis A, Voiculescu A, Sundmacher R. Synergistic antiherpetic effect of acyclovir and mycophenolate mofetil following keratoplasty in patients with herpetic eye disease: first results of a randomised pilot study. Graefes Arch Clin Exp Ophthalmol. 2003;241:1051–4.

54. Mayweg S, Reinhard T, Spelsberg H, Reis A, Godehardt E, Sundmacher R. Ranking of systemic steroids after normal-risk keratoplasty. Results of a randomized prospective study. Ophthalmologe. 2005; 102:497–501.

55. Milani JK, Pleyer U, Dukes A, Chou HJ, Lutz S, Ruckert D, Schmidt KH, Mondino BJ. Prolongation of corneal allograft survival with liposome-encapsulated cyclosporine in the rat eye. Ophthalmology. 1993;100:890–6.

56. Miller K, Huber C, Niederwieser D, Gottinger W. Successful engraftment of high-risk corneal allografts with short-term immunosuppression with cyclosporine. Transplantation. 1988;45:651–3.

57. Munkhbat B, Hagihara M, Sato T, Tsuchida F, Sato K, Shimazaki J, Tsubota K, Tsuji K. Association between HLA-DPB1 matching and 1-year rejection-free graft survival in high-risk corneal transplantation. Transplantation. 1997;63:1011–6.

58. Nicholls SM, Shimeld C, Easty DL, Hill TJ. Recurrent herpes simplex after corneal transplantation in rats. Invest Ophthalmol Vis Sci. 1996;37:425–35.

59. Nyugen NX, Seitz B, Martus P, Langenbucher A, Cursiefen C. Long-term topical steroid treatment improves graft survival following normal-risk penetrating keratoplasty. Am J Ophthalmol. 2007; 144(2):318–9.

60. Patel SV, Hodge DO, Bourne WM. Corneal endothelium and postoperative outcomes 15 years after penetrating keratoplasty. Trans Am Ophthalmol Soc. 2004;102:57–65.

61. Pepose JS, Gardner KM, Nestor MS, Foos RY, Pettit TH. Detection of HLA class I and II antigens in rejected human corneal allografts. Ophthalmology. 1985;92:1480–4.

62. Perry HD, Donnenfeld ED, Acheampong A, Kanellopoulos AJ, Sforza PD, D'Aversa G, Wallerstein A, Stern M. Topical Cyclosporine A in the management of postkeratoplasty glaucoma and corticosteroid-induced ocular hypertension (CIOH) and the penetration of topical 0.5 % cyclosporine A into the cornea and anterior chamber. CLAO J. 1998;24:159–65.

63. Pleyer U, Lutz S, Jusko WJ, Nguyen KD, Narawane M, Ruckert D, Mondino BJ, Lee VH, Nguyen K. Ocular absorption of topically applied FK506 from liposomal and oil formulations in the rabbit eye. Invest Ophthalmol Vis Sci. 1993;34:2737–42.

64. Pleyer U, Raphael B, Kosmidis P, Ryffel B, Thiel HJ. Verteilung von Cyclophilin in okularen Geweben. Ophthalmologe. 1993;90:118.

65. Pleyer U, Schlickeiser S. The taming of the shrew? The immunology of corneal transplantation. Acta Ophthalmol. 2009;87(5):488–97.

66. Pleyer U, Steuhl KP, Weidle EG, Lisch W, Thiel HJ. Corneal graft rejection: incidence, manifestation, and interaction of clinical subtypes. Transplant Proc. 1992;24:2034–7.

67. Pleyer U, Weidle EG, Lisch W, Steuhl KP, Möhrle C, Richter U, Zierhut M, Selbmann HK. Clinical types of immunologic transplant reactions following perforating keratoplasty. Fortschr Ophthalmol. 1990;87(1): 14–9.

68. Pleyer U, Yang J, Knapp S, Schacke H, Schmees N, Orlic N, Otasevic L, De Ruijter M, Ritter T, Keipert S. Effects of a selective glucocorticoid receptor agonist on experimental keratoplasty. Graefes Arch Clin Exp Ophthalmol. 2005;243:450–5.

69. Poon AC, Forbes JE, Dart JK, Subramaniam S, Bunce C, Madison P, Ficker LA, Tuft SJ, Gartry DS, Buckley RJ. Systemic cyclosporin A in high-risk penetrating keratoplasties: a case-control study. Br J Ophthalmol. 2001;85:1464–9.

70. Poon A, Constantinou M, Lamoureux E, Taylor HR. Topical Cyclosporin A in the treatment of acute graft rejection: a randomized controlled trial. Clin Experiment Ophthalmol. 2008;36(5):415–21.

71. Randleman JB, Stulting D. Prevention and treatment of corneal graft rejection: current practice patterns. Cornea. 2006;25:286–90.

72. Refojo D, Liberman AC, Holsboer F, Arzt E. Transcription factor-mediated molecular mechanisms

involved in the functional cross-talk between cytokines and glucocorticoids. Immunol Cell Biol. 2001; 79:385–94.

73. Reinhard T, Hutmacher M, Sundmacher R. Acute and chronic immune reactions after penetrating keratoplasty with normal immune risk. Klin Monatsbl Augenheilkd. 1997;210:139–43.

74. Reinhard T, Mayweg S, Reis A, Sundmacher R. Topical FK506 as immunoprophylaxis after allogeneic penetrating normal-risk keratoplasty: a randomized clinical pilot study. Transpl Int. 2005;18:193–7.

75. Reinhard T, Reis A, Bohringer D, Malinowski M, Voiculescu A, Heering P, Godehardt E, Sunmacher R. Systemic mycophenolate mofetil in comparison with systemic cyclosporin A in high-risk keratoplasty patients: 3 years' results of a randomized prospective clinical trial. Graefes Arch Clin Exp Ophthalmol. 2001;239:367–72.

76. Reinhart WJ, Musch DC, Jacobs DS, Lee WB, Kaufman SC, Shtein RM. Deep anterior lamellar keratoplasty as an alternative to penetrating keratoplasty a report by the american academy of ophthalmology. Ophthalmology. 2011;118(1):209–18.

77. Reis A, Mayweg S, Birnbaum F, Reinhard T. Long-term results of FK 506 eye drops following corneal transplantation. Klin Monbl Augenheilkd. 2008;225(1):57–61.

78. Reisr A, Reinhard T, Voiculescu A, et al. Highly active antiviral and immunosuppressive combination therapy with acyclovir and mycophenolate mofetil following keratoplasty in patients with herpetic eye disease. Klin Monbl Augenheilkd. 2001;218(3):183–6.

79. Remeijer L, Doornenbal P, Geerards AJ, Rijneveld WA, Beekhuis WH. Newly acquired herpes simplex virus keratitis after penetrating keratoplasty. Ophthalmology. 1997;104:648–52.

80. Remeijer L, Maertzdorf J, Buitenwerf J, Osterhaus AD, Verjans GM. Corneal herpes simplex virus type 1 superinfection in patients with recrudescent herpetic keratitis. Invest Ophthalmol Vis Sci. 2002;43:358–63.

81. Rezende RA, Bisol T, Hammersmith K, Hofling-Lima AL, Webster GF, Freitas JF, Rapuano CJ, Laibson PR, Cohen EJ. Epithelial herpetic simplex keratitis recurrence and graft survival after corneal transplantation in patients with and without atopy. Am J Ophthalmol. 2007;143(4):623–8.

82. Rezende RA, Uchoa UB, Raber IM, Rapuano CJ, Laibson PR, Cohen EJ. New onset of herpes simplex virus epithelial keratitis after penetrating keratoplasty. Am J Ophthalmol. 2004;137(3):415–9.

83. Rinne JR, Stulting RD. Current practices in the prevention and treatment of corneal graft rejection. Cornea. 1992;11:326–8.

84. Ritter T, Pleyer U. Novel gene therapeutic strategies for the induction for the induction of tolerance in cornea transplantation. Expert Rev Clin Immunol. 2009;5(6):749–64.

85. Rumelt S, Bersudsky V, Blum-Hareuveni T, Rehany U. Systemic cyclosporin A in high failure risk, repeated corneal transplantation. Br J Ophthalmol. 2002;86:988–92.

86. Sanfilippo F, MacQueen JM, Vaughn WK, Foulks GN. Reduced graft rejection with good HLA-A and B matching in high-risk corneal transplantation. N Engl J Med. 1986;315:29–35.

87. Sano Y, Ksander BR, Streilein JW. Minor H, rather than MHC, alloantigens offer the greater barrier to successful orthotopic corneal transplantation in mice. Transpl Immunol. 1996;4:53–6.

88. Schmitz K, Hitzer S, Behrens-Baumann W. Immune suppression by combination therapy with basiliximab and cyclosporin in high-risk keratoplasty. A pilot study. Ophthalmologe. 2002;99:38–45.

89. Seitz B, Langenbucher A, Diamantis A, Cursiefen C, Küchle M, Naumann GO. Immunological graft reactions after penetrating keratoplasty - a prospective randomized trial comparing corneal excimer laser and motor trephination. Klin Monbl Augenheilkd. 2001;218(11):710–9.

90. Severin M. Immune reactions following keratoplasty. Klin Monatsbl Augenheilkd. 1986;188:200–8.

91. Shapiro R, Fung JJ, Jain AB, Parks P, Todo S, Starzl TE. The side effects of FK 506 in humans. Transplant Proc. 1990;22:35–6.

92. Sherif Z, Pleyer U. Corticosteroids in ophthalmology: past-present-future. Ophthalmologica. 2002; 216:305–15.

93. Shi W, Gao H, Xie L, Wang S. Sustained intraocular rapamycin delivery effectively prevents high-risk corneal allograft rejection and neovascularization in rabbits. Invest Ophthalmol Vis Sci. 2006;47(8):3339–44.

94. Sigal NH, Dumont FJ. Cyclosporin A, FK-506, and rapamycin: pharmacologic probes of lymphocyte signal transduction. Annu Rev Immunol. 1992; 10:519–60.

95. Shi W, Chen M, Xie L, Liu M, Gao H, Wang T, Wu X, Zhao J. A novel cyclosporine a drug-delivery system for prevention of human corneal rejection after high-risk keratoplasty: a clinical study. Ophthalmology. 2013;120:695–702.

96. Shimazaki J, Den S, Omoto M, Satake Y, Shimmura S, Tsubota K. Prospective, randomized study of the efficacy of systemic cyclosporine in high-risk corneal transplantation. Am J Ophthalmol. 2011; 152:33–9.

97. Sinha R, Jhanji V, Verma K, Sharma N, Biswas NR, Vajpayee RB. Efficacy of topical cyclosporine A 2 % in prevention of graft rejection in high-risk keratoplasty: a randomized controlled trial. Graefes Arch Clin Exp Ophthalmol. 2010;248(8):1167–72.

98. Sloper CM, Powell RJ, Dua HS. Tacrolimus (FK506) in the management of high-risk corneal and limbal grafts. Ophthalmology. 2001;108:1838–44.

99. Sonoda Y, Streilein JW. Orthotopic corneal transplantation in mice–evidence that the immunogenetic rules of rejection do not apply. Transplantation. 1992;54:694–704.

100. Stanojlovic S, Schlickeiser S, Appelt C, Vogt K, Schmitt-Knosalla I, Haase S, Ritter T, Sawitzki B, Pleyer U. Influence of combined treatment of low dose rapamycin and cyclosporin A on corneal

allograft survival. Graefes Arch Clin Exp Ophthalmol. 2010;248(10):1447–56.

101. Sugar A, Bokosky JE, Meyer RF. A randomized trial of topical corticosteroids in epithelial healing after keratoplasty. Cornea. 1984;3:268–71.

102. Sundmacher R, Reinhard T, Heering P. Six years' experience with systemic cyclosporin A prophylaxis in high-risk perforating keratoplasty patients. A retrospective study. Ger J Ophthalmol. 1992;1:432–6.

103. Takahashi N, Hayano T, Suzuki M. Peptidyl-prolyl cis-trans isomerase is the cyclosporin A-binding protein cyclophilin. Nature. 1989;337:473–5.

104. Tambasco FP, Cohen EJ, Nguyen LH, Rapuano CJ, Laibson PR. Oral acyclovir after penetrating keratoplasty for herpes simplex keratitis. Arch Ophthalmol. 1999;117(4):445–9.

105. Tan DT, Janardhanan P, Zhou H, Chan YH, Htoon HM, Ang LP, Lim LS. Penetrating keratoplasty in Asian eyes: the Singapore Corneal Transplant Study. Ophthalmology. 2008;115(6):975–82.

106. Tandon R, Verma K, Chawla B, Sharma N, Tiliyal JS, Kalaivani M, Vajpayee RB. Intravenous dexamethasone vs methylprednisolone pulse therapy in the treatment of acute endothelial graft rejection. Eye (Lond). 2009;23(3):635–9.

107. Thiel MA, Ross CA, Coster DJ. Corneal allograft rejection: has the time come for intravenous pulsed methylprednisolone? A debate. Clin Experiment Ophthalmol. 2000;28:398–404.

108. Unal M, Yücel I. Evaluation of topical ciclosporin 0.05 % for prevention of rejection in high-risk corneal grafts. Br J Ophthalmol. 2008;92(10):1411–4.

109. van Rooij J, Rijneveld WJ, Remeijer L, Völker-Dieben HJ, Eggink CA, Geerards AJ, Mulder PG, Doornenbal P, Beekhuis WH. Effect of oral acyclovir after penetrating keratoplasty for herpetic keratitis: a placebo-controlled multicenter trial. Ophthalmology. 2003;110(10):1916–9.

110. Vail A, Gore SM, Bradley BA, Easty DL, Rogers CA, Armitage WJ. Influence of donor and histocompatibility factors on corneal graft outcome. Transplantation. 1994;58:1210–6.

111. Varssano D, Russ V, Linhart Y, Lazar M. Air transportation of corneal tissue: experience with local compared to transatlantic donor corneas. Cornea. 2005;24:674–7.

112. Volker-Dieben HJ, Claas FH, Schreuder GM, Schipper RF, Pels E, Persijn GG, Smits J, D'Amaro J. Beneficial effect of HLA-DR matching on the survival of corneal allografts. Transplantation. 2000; 70:640–8.

113. Völker-Dieben HJ, Kok-van Alphen CC, Kruit PJ. Advances and disappointments, indications and restrictions regarding HLA-matched corneal grafts in high-risk cases. Doc Ophthalmol. 1979;46:219–26.

114. Williams KA, Lowe M, Bartlett C, Kelly TL, Coster DJ. Risk factors for human corneal graft failure within the Australian corneal graft registry. Transplantation. 2008;86(12):1720–4.

115. Williams KA, Muehlberg SM, Lewis RF, Coster DJ. Influence of advanced recipient and donor age on the outcome of corneal transplantation. Australian Corneal Graft Registry. Br J Ophthalmol. 1997; 81:835–9.

116. Yalcindag FN, Incel O, Ozdemir O. Effectiveness of tacrolimus in high-risk limbal allo-graft transplantation. Ann Ophthalmol (Skokie). 2008;40(3–4):152–6.

117. You IC, Yoon KC. Therapeutic effect of intravitreal injection of triamcinolone in the treatment of endothelial graft rejection: a pilot study. Cornea. 2012;31(10):1135–40.

118. Young AL, Rao SK, Cheng LL, Wong AK, Leung AT, Lam DS. Combined intravenous pulse methylprednisolone and oral cyclosporine A in the treatment of corneal graft rejection: 5-year experience. Eye (Lond). 2002;16(3):304–8.

Immunomodulation Against Inflammatory Postkeratoplasty Neovascularisation

7

Björn Bachmann and Claus Cursiefen

Contents

B. Bachmann, MD, FEBO
Department of Ophthalmology,
University of Cologne,
Kerpener Str 62, Cologne 50928, Germany
e-mail: bjoern.bachmann@uk-koeln.de

C. Cursiefen, MD (✉)
Department of Ophthalmology,
University of Cologne, Kerpener Str 62,
Cologne 50928, Germany
e-mail: claus.cursiefen@uk-koeln.de

7.1 Definition

Corneal neovascularisation after corneal transplantation is described as the ingrowths of blood and lymphatic vessels from the physiological limbal vessel arcade or from pathological pre-existing corneal neovascularisation into the physiologically avascular cornea. Corneal neovascularisation can be superficial at the epithelial or subepithelial level or deep within the corneal stroma. The extent of corneal neovascularisation can be clinically graded into clock hours or quadrants involved and by the extension of blood vessels from the limbal arcade towards the corneal centre. The most accurate method of grading corneal blood vessels is performed by a computer-aided morphometrical analysis [1]. Although morphometrical methods require a certain technical setup and experienced technical assistant, this approach helps to identify even minor changes in corneal neovascularisation.

Corneal neovascularisation is frequently observed after low-risk as well as after high-risk corneal transplantation [2–6]. Preoperative corneal neovascularisation has long been identified as a risk factor for immune rejection after keratoplasty. The role of additional ingrowths of blood vessels and clinically invisible lymphatic vessels *after* keratoplasty has been evaluated extensively in animal models demonstrating the contribution of postoperative hem- and lymphangiogenesis in the initiation and perpetuation of an allogenic graft rejection.

U. Pleyer et al. (eds.), *Immune Modulation and Anti-Inflammatory Therapy in Ocular Disorders*,
DOI 10.1007/978-3-642-54350-0_7, © Springer-Verlag Berlin Heidelberg 2014

7.2 Aetiology

The aetiology of postkeratoplasty neovascularisation is diverse. Hem- and lymphangiogenesis after corneal transplantation is often suture related. The ingrowths of blood vessels directing towards the sutures anchoring the graft to the host cornea are common [7]. Even though most sutures after low-risk corneal transplantation remain non-reactive for an almost unlimited period, they can also cause a subtle chronic inflammatory stimulus thus promoting corneal hem- and lymphangiogenesis. Other conditions causing postkeratoplasty corneal neovascularisation are dry eye syndrome, corneal endothelial decompensation, limbal stem cell deficiency or infectious inflammation like in recurrent herpes keratitis.

7.3 Clinical Symptoms and Signs of the Underlying Condition/Disorder

Peripheral corneal vascularisation passing the physiological limbal arcade can be frequently seen without causing any symptoms [7]. The main complaint in patients with corneal vascularisation approaching the optical zone is blurred vision. Some patients also observe haloes due to corneal oedema. Especially newly formed blood vessels tend to leak facilitating the transfer of fluid into the corneal stroma. Depending on the degree of the underlying vascularisation, this kind of corneal oedema can involve the whole or only parts of the cornea which is the case after focal ingrowths of blood vessels. This can induce changes to the corneal curvature leading to corneal astigmatism which further impairs the patient's vision and can cause symptoms like monocular diplopia. In addition to corneal oedema, vessel leakage can also lead to the deposition of fatty materials in the superficial or deeper corneal stroma which is clinically recognised as secondary lipid keratopathy. Particularly new corneal blood vessels can also bleed leading to an intrastromal haemorrhage which can be recognised by the patient as an acute worsening of vision.

Both preoperative blood and lymphatic vessels are important contributors to an allogenic graft rejection following keratoplasty [8]. The process of graft rejection is described by the immune reflex arc where lymphatic vessels serve as the afferent arm which allows antigen-presenting cells to reach the corresponding lymph nodes where they promote the formation of effector T cells. These effector T cells are directed against the graft's antigens and use the blood vessels as the efferent arm of the immune reflex arc to reach the corneal transplant. Different anatomical structures of the cornea can be involved depending on whether the immunological reaction is directed against the corneal epithelium, stroma or endothelium. Endothelial rejection, which is the most common form, is characterized by inflammatory cells in the anterior chamber and by precipitates on the endothelial surface. In addition, the eye can show unspecific general symptoms of inflammation and corneal oedema such as redness or photophobia.

7.4 Differential Diagnosis

Different types of corneal vascularisation can be distinguished. Corneal vascularisation can result from the sole ingrowths of blood and lymphatic vessels. In addition, superficial or stromal scarring can be caused by accompanying ingrowths or formation of fibrotic tissue which is then called fibrovascular tissue or pannus when covering the cornea. In superficial or anterior vascularisation, concomitant ingrowths of conjunctival tissue can be observed in limbal stem cell deficiency. In this situation the physiological barrier between the cornea and the conjunctiva maintained by the limbus is abolished resulting in a conjunctival overgrowth over the cornea which is termed conjunctivalisation.

Conditions which can mimic progression of corneal vascularisation or a higher state of vessel activity are diseases causing an increase in the pressure of the venous system which results in an enlargement of the conjunctival and episcleral veins surrounding the cornea. Thrombosis of the cavernous sinus and fistulisation between the internal carotid artery or its branches and the cavernous sinus are examples of diseases causing a rise in the pressure of the ocular venous system.

7.5 Treatment

Corneal neovascularisation is a risk factor for graft rejection and graft failure after keratoplasty [8]. There are two different ways to address the problem of postkeratoplasty corneal neovascularisation. The first aims on the reduction of postoperative angiogenesis by postoperative antiangiogenic treatment. The second approach aims on the improvement of the preoperative situation in terms of preconditioning the host cornea by reducing the preoperative neovascularisation. Reducing the preload of corneal neovascularisation before corneal transplantation can positively influence the postoperative formation of additional blood and lymphatic vessels and thus contributes to a reduction in risk of graft rejection and graft failure [9].

Several therapeutic strategies are or were in clinical use for restoring corneal clarity or reducing the risk of graft rejection after keratoplasty caused by corneal neovascularisation including steroids, radiation, cryotherapy and conjunctival recession. Depending on the degree and the anatomical position of corneal neovascularisation, surgical techniques like laser coagulation, fine-needle diathermy, lamellar keratectomy or corneal lamellar or perforating keratoplasty can improve the patient's vision or reduce the risk of graft rejection. New pharmaceutical antiangiogenic treatment options offer the opportunity to reduce or prevent corneal neovascularisation without or in combination with a surgical approach.

7.5.1 Pharmaceutical Antiangiogenic Treatment

New pharmaceutical treatments aiming on decreasing a VEGF-mediated angiogenic stimulus are most effective in preventing or reducing the formation of freshly grown blood and lymphatic vessels. Old corneal blood vessels have

established vessel walls coated by pericytes and show much less response to a gap in VEGF supply. Thus, a pure pharmaceutical treatment can be performed in active and progressive vascularisation rather than in established blood vessels.

The potency of various antiangiogenic agents on corneal neovascularisation has been shown in numerous animal studies and has also been examined in humans [10–16]. However, so far only one study addressed this issue in a randomised, controlled and multicenter setting where GS-101, an antisense oligonucleotide with antiangiogenic properties, was applied topically bid and reduced corneal neovascularisation in patients with progressive vascularisation [13]. Up to now the effect of a pharmaceutical antiangiogenic treatment after keratoplasty has only been evaluated in animal models. Here, the postkeratoplasty administration of VEGF-Trap, a potent inhibitor of angiogenesis, has shown a reduction in postoperative angiogenesis as well as a prolonged graft survival of allogenic corneal grafts after low- and high-risk keratoplasty [2–4, 17]. No systemic or topical antiangiogenic drug is approved for the treatment of corneal neovascularisation. Bevacizumab is the drug most widely used because of its low price and its well known antiangiogenic effect in ocular neovascularisation other than corneal neovascularisation.

Side effects under local antiangiogenic treatment with bevacizumab eyedrops (5 mg/ml) are rare and mainly comprise wound healing defects of the corneal surface [10]. However, even under antiangiogenic treatment, closure of corneal erosions has been described [15].

7.5.2 Surgical Antiangiogenic Treatment

Superficial corneal neovascularisation can be treated by mechanically removing the vascularised tissue (pannectomy or lamellar keratectomy). Stromal vascularisation is amenable to coagulation of the vessels which can be performed with a focal destruction of tissue using a yellow dye laser (577 nm) or by fine-needle diathermy [18, 19]. The latter utilises a stainless steel needle attached to a 10-00 nylon suture. The needle is introduced into or nearby the vessel lumen, and the tip of a coagulation probe is then attached to the needle until a white blanching of the corneal stroma indicates coagulation of the blood vessels.

Even though lamellar or penetrating keratoplasty itself is a treatment for vascularised corneas, a postoperative vascularisation into the grafted cornea is likely if the angiogenic stimulus persists. This, in addition to the higher risk of graft rejection, will contribute to an accelerated failure of the graft. For example, in case of recurrent herpes keratitis, a postoperative prophylactic antiviral therapy has to be conducted (aciclovir 400 mg BID for 12 months) [20]. Dry eye syndrome has to be treated according to the guidelines of the dry eye workshop, and limbal stem cell deficiency should be treated by transplantation of epithelial stem cells before keratoplasty takes place [21–24]. Generally, these measures have to be performed months till years before the intended optical corneal transplantation. Increasing the chance of a lasting avascular graft, the patient's cornea must not have signs of chronic ongoing vascularisation or inflammation during this prekeratoplasty period.

Both the surgical approach and the pharmaceutical treatment can be combined to maximise the antiangiogenic effect.

References

1. Bock F, Onderka J, Hos D, Horn F, Martus P, Cursiefen C. Improved semiautomatic method for morphometry of angiogenesis and lymphangiogenesis in corneal flatmounts. Exp Eye Res. 2008;87(5):462–70.
2. Cursiefen C, Cao J, Chen L, Liu Y, Maruyama K, Jackson D, Kruse FE, Wiegand SJ, Dana MR, Streilein JW. Inhibition of hemangiogenesis and lymphangiogenesis after normal-risk corneal transplantation by neutralizing VEGF promotes graft survival. Invest Ophthalmol Vis Sci. 2004;45(8):2666–73.
3. Bachmann BO, Bock F, Wiegand SJ, Maruyama K, Dana MR, Kruse FE, Luetjen-Drecoll E, Cursiefen C. Promotion of graft survival by vascular endothelial growth factor a neutralization after high-risk corneal transplantation. Arch Ophthalmol. 2008;126(1):71–7.
4. Bachmann BO, Luetjen-Drecoll E, Bock F, Wiegand SJ, Hos D, Dana R, Kruse FE, Cursiefen C. Transient postoperative vascular endothelial growth factor (VEGF)-neutralisation improves graft survival in corneas with partly regressed inflammatory neovascularisation. Br J Ophthalmol. 2009;93(8):1075–80.
5. Regenfuss B, Bock F, Parthasarathy A, Cursiefen C. Corneal (lymph)-angiogenesis–from bedside to bench and back: a tribute to Judah Folkman. Lymphat Res Biol. 2008;6:191–201.
6. Regenfuss B, Bock F, Bachmann B, König Y, Hos D, Parthasarathy A. Cursiefen C [Topical inhibition of angiogenesis at the cornea. Safety and efficacy]. Ophthalmologe. 2009;106:399–406.
7. Cursiefen C, Wenkel H, Martus P, Langenbucher A, Nguyen NX, Seitz B, Kuchle M, Naumann GO. Impact of short-term versus long-term topical steroids on corneal neovascularization after non-high-risk keratoplasty. Graefes Arch Clin Exp Ophthalmol. 2001;239(7):514–21.
8. Bachmann B, Taylor RS, Cursiefen C. Corneal neovascularization as a risk factor for graft failure and rejection after keratoplasty: an evidence-based meta-analysis. Ophthalmology. 2010;117(7):1300–5, e1307.
9. Nirankari VS, Baer JC. Corneal argon laser photocoagulation for neovascularization in penetrating keratoplasty. Ophthalmology. 1986;93(10):1304–9.
10. Koenig Y, Bock F, Horn F, Kruse F, Straub K, Cursiefen C. Short- and long-term safety profile and efficacy of topical bevacizumab (Avastin) eye drops against corneal neovascularization. Graefes Arch Clin Exp Ophthalmol. 2009;247(10):1375–82.
11. Doctor PP, Bhat PV, Foster CS. Subconjunctival bevacizumab for corneal neovascularization. Cornea. 2008;27(9):992–5.
12. Bahar I, Kaiserman I, McAllum P, Rootman D, Slomovic A. Subconjunctival bevacizumab injection for corneal neovascularization. Cornea. 2008;27(2):142–7.
13. Cursiefen C, Bock F, Horn FK, Kruse FE, Seitz B, Borderie V, Fruh B, et al. GS-101 antisense oligonucleotide eye drops inhibit corneal neovascularization: interim results of a randomized phase II trial. Ophthalmology. 2009;116(9):1630–7.
14. Dastjerdi MH, Al-Arfaj KM, Nallasamy N, Hamrah P, Jurkunas UV, Pineda 2nd R, Pavan-Langston D, Dana R. Topical bevacizumab in the treatment of corneal neovascularization: results of a prospective, open-label, noncomparative study. Arch Ophthalmol. 2009;127(4):381–9.
15. Kim SW, Ha BJ, Kim EK, Tchah H, Kim TI. The effect of topical bevacizumab on corneal neovascularization. Ophthalmology. 2008;115(6):e33–8.
16. You IC, Kang IS, Lee SH, Yoon KC. Therapeutic effect of subconjunctival injection of bevacizumab in the treatment of corneal neovascularization. Acta Ophthalmol. 2009;87(6):653–8.
17. Dietrich T, Bock F, Yuen C, Hos D, Bachmann BO, Zahn G, Wiegand S, Chen L, Cursiefen C. Cutting edge: lymphatic vessels, not blood vessels, primarily mediate immune rejections after transplantation. J Immunol. 2010;184:535–9.

18. L'Esperance Jr FA. Clinical photocoagulation with the organic dye laser. A preliminary communication. Arch Ophthalmol. 1985;103(9):1312–6.

19. Pillai CT, Dua HS, Hossain P. Fine needle diathermy occlusion of corneal vessels. Invest Ophthalmol Vis Sci. 2000;41(8):2148–53.

20. van Rooij J, Rijneveld WJ, Remeijer L, Volker-Dieben HJ, Eggink CA, Geerards AJ, Mulder PG, Doornenbal P, Beekhuis WH. Effect of oral acyclovir after penetrating keratoplasty for herpetic keratitis: a placebo-controlled multicenter trial. Ophthalmology. 2003;110(10):1916–9; discussion 1919.

21. Rama P, Matuska S, Paganoni G, Spinelli A, De Luca M, Pellegrini G. Limbal stem-cell therapy and long-term corneal regeneration. N Engl J Med. 2010;363(2):147–55.

22. Kenyon KR, Tseng SC. Limbal autograft transplantation for ocular surface disorders. Ophthalmology. 1989;96(5):709–22; discussion 722–3.

23. Inatomi T, Nakamura T, Kojyo M, Koizumi N, Sotozono C, Kinoshita S. Ocular surface reconstruction with combination of cultivated autologous oral mucosal epithelial transplantation and penetrating keratoplasty. Am J Ophthalmol. 2006;142(5):757–64.

24. Nakamura T, Inatomi T, Cooper LJ, Rigby H, Fullwood NJ, Kinoshita S. Phenotypic investigation of human eyes with transplanted autologous cultivated oral mucosal epithelial sheets for severe ocular surface diseases. Ophthalmology. 2007;114(6):1080–8.

Carolina Arruabarrena Sánchez
and Marta S. Figueroa

Contents

C.A. Sánchez, MD (✉)
Retina Section, Hospital Príncipe de Asturias,
Alcalá de Henares, Carretera de Meco s/n,
Alcalá de Henares, Madrid 28050, Spain
e-mail: carruabarrenas@gmail.com

M.S. Figueroa, MD, PhD
Retina Section, Vissum Madrid, Santa Hortensia 58,
Madrid 28002, Spain
e-mail: figueroa@servicom2000.com

8.1 Introduction

Vitreoretinal surgery is comprised of a number of techniques, and any of them can cause inflammation for different reasons. This chapter will focus on the treatment of inflammation caused by scleral buckling, pars plana vitrectomy, and combined procedure phacovitrectomy.

To aid comprehension, we will describe the inflammatory complications secondary to each procedure and then address methods of prevention and treatment.

8.1.1 Pars Plana Vitrectomy

Sutureless microincisional surgery with 23- and 25-gauge instruments has significantly reduced postoperative inflammation. Nevertheless, it remains a significant complication in vitrectomy.

8.1.1.1 Ocular Surface Inflammation

Traditional 20-gauge vitrectomy causes severe inflammation in the sclerotomies sites and conjunctiva. Microincisional surgery with 23- and 25-g. instruments can now minimize ocular surface trauma with the use of sutureless transconjunctival cannulas. However, when sclerotomies are sutured with transconjunctival sutures, local inflammation is more severe than if the sclera and conjunctiva are sutured separately (Fig. 8.1). One way of reducing this inflammation is to perform a temporary transconjunctival suture that can be removed the day after surgery under the slit lamp.

U. Pleyer et al. (eds.), *Immune Modulation and Anti-Inflammatory Therapy in Ocular Disorders*,
DOI 10.1007/978-3-642-54350-0_8, © Springer-Verlag Berlin Heidelberg 2014

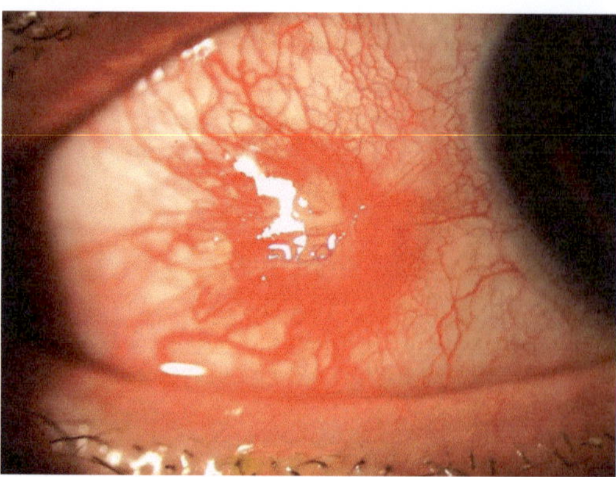

Fig. 8.1 Conjunctival inflammation secondary to a transconjunctival suture of the sclerotomy

8.1.1.2 Anterior Chamber Inflammation

In a recent study with the use of a flare meter, no differences in anterior chamber inflammation were found between 20-g. vitrectomy and sutureless microincisional vitrectomy [1].

Although anterior chamber inflammation following a vitrectomy is usually mild, inflammatory cells may occlude the trabecular network and lead to an inflammatory glaucoma in the early postoperative period.

This increase in intraocular pressure (IOP) may be worsened if either silicon oil or a gas tamponade is used. This IOP increase has been described with SF6 and C3F8 [2]. It has been suggested that the expansion of the gas causes an anterior displacement of the iridocrystalline diaphragm and a closed-angle glaucoma, either with or without a pupillary block. The IOP increase is more frequent when there are fibrinous exudates in the anterior chamber [3].

Silicone oil causes an IOP increase through a number of mechanisms, including inflammation. Others include pupillary block, synechial angle closure, iridis rubeosis, and the migration of emulsified silicone oil into the anterior chamber [4–6].

8.1.1.3 Choroidal Detachment

Choroidal detachment is unusual with current microincisional techniques because intraocular pressure is kept quite stable throughout the procedure [7]. However, a recent report describes a high incidence of subclinical choroidal detachment with an anterior segment OCT following 25-g. vitrectomies. This has been related to a higher percentage of postoperative hypotony due to a leak through the sclerotomies [8].

This complication is more common in younger patients, myopic patients, and following vitrectomy for retinal detachment with scleral indentation at 360° to shave the vitreous base.

Choroidal detachment, whether intraoperative or postoperative, alters the blood-ocular barrier and induces intraocular inflammation in both the anterior and posterior segments.

8.1.1.4 Alteration of Extraocular Muscles

Alteration in extraocular muscles is rare following vitrectomy, although it is more frequent when associated with scleral buckling. Many factors can cause diplopia, for which sensorial fusion loss is equally as important as mechanical causes related to muscular damage. This type of damage is more common when extended scleral indentation is performed in vitrectomy for retinal detachment. In our experience with 128 vitrectomies for retinal detachment without buckling, only one patient developed temporary diplopia following surgery.

8.1.1.5 Persistent Macular Edema Following Vitrectomy

Vitrectomy is useful in the treatment of tractional macular edema [9, 10]. However, macular edema may persist after vitrectomy in diseases like diabetic macular edema [9, 10], epiretinal membranes, Irvine-Gass Syndrome, and retinal vein occlusions.

A recent study with OCT of a number of retinal diseases that have been treated with pars plana vitrectomy shows a persistence of macular edema in 47 % of cases 1 month after surgery (Fig. 8.2). In the study, macular thickness was related to an inflammatory reaction 1 month after surgery [11].

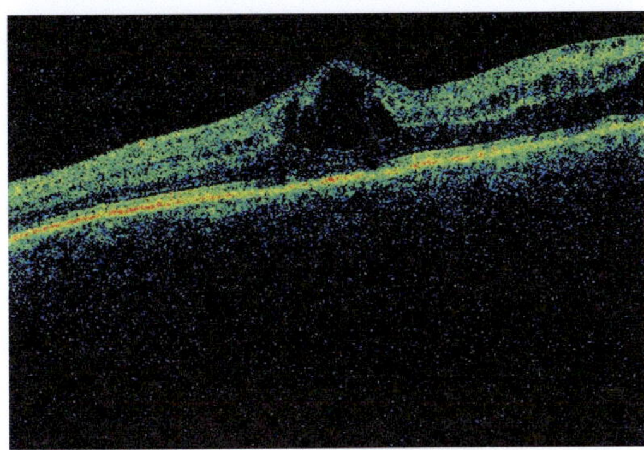

Fig. 8.2 Optical coherence tomography showing macular edema in a vitrectomized diabetic eye

Refractory macular edema following vitrectomy is usually treated with steroids. Good results have been described in the treatment of persistent diabetic macular edema with sub-Tenon and intravitreal triamcinolone [12–14]. A meta-analysis of the literature comparing the results of a placebo versus intravitreal or sub-Tenon triamcinolone has found that either method of administering triamcinolone reduces refractory macular edema and improves visual acuity more than a placebo. This visual acuity improvement is significantly better when triamcinolone is administered intravitreally, although the effect will only last 3 months in either case, with no differences compared to baseline at 6 months. Independently of the method of administration, the most frequent secondary effects are intraocular hypertension, cataract progression, and endophthalmitis [15].

Recently, an intravitreal dexamethasone delivery system has been developed to reduce the secondary effects of intraocular steroids [16–18]. The system is also useful in reducing refractory diabetic macular edema following surgery.

8.1.2 Scleral Buckling

Scleral buckling can be performed on its own or in combination with pars plana vitrectomy to treat retinal detachment. It causes inflammation in the early postoperative period owing to the more extensive surgical maneuvers involved. It can also cause long-term inflammation due to the extrusion and infection of the silicone buckle.

8.1.2.1 Early Postoperative Inflammation

Surface Inflammation

Following scleral buckling, inflammation can often be found in the conjunctiva, Tenon capsule, or muscle insertions affected by surgical maneuvers. Reducing the intensity of this inflammation requires a careful conjunctival peritomy, a precise dissection of the Tenon capsule, and a careful manipulation of extraocular muscles, while avoiding unnecessary trauma. A continuous suture of the conjunctiva and Tenon capsule will reduce postoperative scarring and simplify any reoperation. If postoperative inflammation persists, the conjunctiva suture can be removed 7–10 days after surgery.

Anterior Chamber Inflammation

Although inflammation in the anterior chamber after scleral buckling is usually mild, it may contribute to increasing IOP. Inflammatory cells and fibrin in the anterior chamber can occlude the trabecular network and cause an inflammatory glaucoma, although the glaucoma will respond well to topical hypotensive treatment with beta-blockers and steroids. Increased IOP may also result from steroid treatment.

Another factor that can contribute to higher IOP following scleral buckling is the narrowing of the anterior chamber, which usually persists for 1 year [19]. Anterior segment inflammation may also give rise to anterior and posterior iris synechiae.

Choroidal Detachment

Choroidal detachment after scleral buckling is not uncommon: incidence of up to 40 % has been described [20].

The risk factors for choroidal detachment can include the following: the length of the buckle; the position of the buckle; the age of the patient, with a higher risk in older patients; hypotony; and pathologic myopia [21].

Peripheral choroidal detachment has no effect on vision, although it does increase the risk of retinal re-detachment. In contrast, in massive choroidal detachment, kissing choroidal detachment, or if the macula is affected, the reduction in visual acuity is usually severe. If the detachment is peripheral, topical, systemic steroids and rest are recommended. However, more severe cases will require transscleral drainage.

A special case is annular choroidal detachment of the ciliary body, which causes an anterior displacement of the ciliary body and a secondary angle closure. Postoperative closed-angle glaucoma has an incidence of 1.4–4 % following scleral buckling [22–24]. This complication usually occurs between 2 and 7 days after surgery. Gonioscopy may be difficult to perform because of the corneal edema. Ultrasound is used for the diagnosis, particularly ultrasound biomicroscopy.

The first step in treatment is to control inflammation and IOP. This can be achieved as follows: topical hypotensive drugs to reduce aqueous humor production, oral steroids to control inflammation, and cycloplegic drugs to tighten the zonula and deepen the anterior chamber. Only in cases of coexistence of the detachment with a pupillary blockage, can a laser ND: YAG iridotomy be performed to facilitate circulation of the aqueous humor.

If the angle closure persists, more aggressive treatment may be needed to prevent iridocorneal synechiae. If these synechiae develop, an iridoplasty or laser gonioplasty must be performed to open the angle [25]; if this technique fails to achieve results, drainage of supraciliary fluid is necessary.

Cystoid Macular Edema

Cystoid macular edema is a response to inflammation caused by surgical maneuvers during scleral buckling, transscleral cryotherapy, or laser photocoagulation to achieve retinopexy [21]. It is known that certain mediators like prostaglandins and vascular endothelial growth factor (VEGF) are involved in its development. These mediators increase microvascular permeability by altering the inner blood-retinal barrier in the perifoveal capillaries [26]. This results in an accumulation of intraretinal fluid in the intra- and extracellular space.

The incidence of macular edema following scleral buckling, as revealed in angiography, affects between 30 and 65 % of cases [27, 28], with the higher percentage found among aphakic and older patients. New diagnostic techniques like optical coherence tomography can reveal subclinical macular edema with no visual impact after scleral buckling [29]. Unlike fluorescein angiography, OCT is a noninvasive technique that can also measure the thickness of the retina, which is highly useful in following up anti-inflammatory treatment [30].

Even though macular edema is occasionally mild and self-limited, most cases require anti-inflammatory treatment.

One of the most common treatments is nonsteroidal anti-inflammatory drugs (NSAIDs) that inhibit the synthesis of prostaglandins by blocking cyclooxygenase. These drugs have been used both systemically and topically to prevent or treat macular edema or to facilitate the drainage of residual subretinal fluid after scleral buckling. Topical indomethacin would seem to minimize the incidence of postoperative macular edema diagnosed in angiography [31], while studies with oral valdecoxib (a selective inhibitor of cyclooxygenase 2) show that it does not prevent macular edema, although it does improve the reabsorption of residual subretinal fluid [32].

Steroids inhibit the inflammatory pathway of prostaglandins prior to the use of NSAIDs, thus inhibiting the formation of arachidonic acid from membrane lipids [33]. They can be administered topically, periocularly, intravitreally, orally, or intravenously.

Inhibitors of carbonic anhydrase (oral acetazolamide) facilitate the transport of fluid through the retinal pigment epithelium to the choroid and minimize edema. They also cause acidification in the subretinal space, which increases retinal adhesiveness [34]. They are useful in treating macular edema in retinitis pigmentosa and Irvine-Gass syndrome.

8.1.2.2 Delayed Postoperative Inflammation

Epiretinal Membranes

The development of epiretinal membranes following scleral buckling is common (3–17 %), and it is one of the main causes of visual acuity loss [21, 35].

The most significant risk factors are postoperative inflammation, vitreal hemorrhage, and vitreous loss during drainage of subretinal fluid. Suitable anti-inflammatory treatment in the immediate postoperative period can reduce the incidence of this complication, which may otherwise require surgery.

Alteration of Extraocular Muscles

In the first 6 weeks of the postoperative period, more than 50 % of patients present diplopia, which can be minimized by treatment of extraocular muscle inflammation. In 5–25 % of cases, this diplopia becomes permanent [36]. The risk factors for permanent diplopia are the position and size of the scleral buckle – the larger the buckle, the greater the risk of diplopia [37] – and fibrosis around the buckle and extraocular muscles.

The best treatment for diplopia is prevention. Retinal surgeons must take great care during muscle dissection to prevent exposure to the sub-Tenon fat in order to prevent the development of postoperative adherences; they should avoid excessive traction or direct cryotherapy of the muscles, as this will lead to atrophy and, over time, muscular tearing. Debate continues about whether muscular disinsertion during surgery increases the risk of diplopia [37].

Initial treatment of diplopia is conservative, as anti-inflammatory treatment is usually sufficient to achieve resolution. If diplopia persists for 2 months or longer, treatment is necessary. If the deviation is concomitant and small – that is, less than 15 prismatic deviations – it can be treated with prisms. If the deviation angle is larger, either the buckle can be removed or muscle surgery can be performed [37].

Orbital Inflammation

Chronic low-grade inflammation caused by rejection of the buckle or of the sutures can lead to foreign body granulomas, inflammatory pseudotumors, or buckle extrusion. These complications have been more frequently described in hydrogel explants than in solid silicone bands [38, 39]. Treatment usually involves surgical removal of the buckle, which is easier when the band is made of silicone than of hydrogel, which tends to fragment [38].

Buckle Extrusion and Infection

Chronic erosion of the Tenon and conjunctiva caused by scleral buckling can be complicated by extrusion and infection of the buckle. It has been described in 0.2–1.2 % of silicone buckles, but the incidence is higher in segmental buckles [40].

This complication does not usually respond to topical antibiotics or anti-inflammatory drugs. Treatment consists of removing the buckle and suturing the Tenon and conjunctiva. Removal of the implant poses a risk of retinal detachment in 4–33 % of cases [41–44]. The re-detachment rate is higher in cases of buckle infection, vitreous traction, large retinal detachment at baseline, and shorter postoperative periods [45]. This risk can be minimized by photocoagulation of retinal tears 2 weeks prior to buckle removal.

8.1.3 Combined Procedure: Phacovitrectomy

8.1.3.1 Anterior Chamber Inflammation

A combined procedure of phacoemulsification of the lens and pars plana vitrectomy can achieve quicker visual recovery in a single procedure, but it increases the duration of surgery and causes greater inflammation in the anterior chamber. It increases the risk of ciliary body effusion (80 % of cases) and the risk of narrowing of the anterior chamber, complications revealed in ultrasound biomicroscopy [46]. A more severe reaction in the anterior chamber and a greater tendency to develop fibrin and posterior synechiae have also been reported [47, 48]. These can induce postoperative tension peaks and IOL displacement (Fig. 8.3). The fibrinous reaction in the anterior chamber has been described in up to 7 % of combined procedures and more frequently in diabetic, young, or uveitis patients [49]. The treatment of choice is steroids while avoiding the use of long-duration mydriatic drugs to prevent posterior synechiae of the iris to the lens.

8.1.3.2 Irvine-Gass Syndrome

In 1953, Irvine described a syndrome of macular alteration following cataract surgery and associated it with ocular irritation [50]. In 1966,

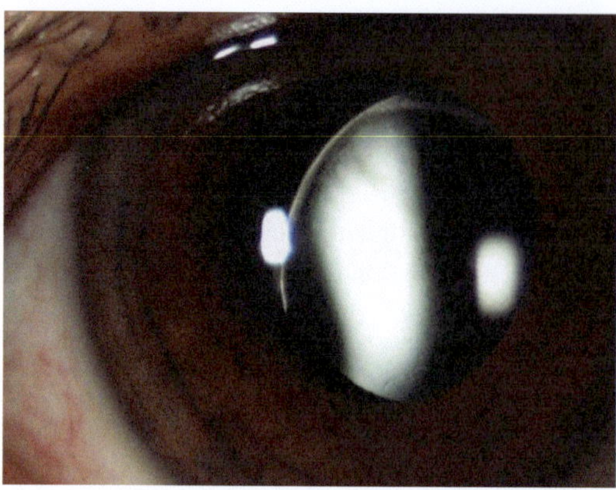

Fig. 8.3 IOL dislocation after phacovitrectomy surgery

Gass described cystic macular changes associated with an angiographic leak following cataract surgery [51]. These findings are now known as pseudophakic cystoid macular edema. Although the etiology is not well understood, it has been related to inflammation induced by surgery and vitreous traction in the macular area.

There are three ways of diagnosing macular edema: fluorescein angiography, ophthalmoscopy, and optical coherence tomography (OCT), where the last of these is the most sensitive.

Although the incidence of macular edema following combined retina and cataract surgery was reported in early studies to be 43 % [52], more recent studies have found an incidence of approximately 9 % [47, 49].

No specific studies of macular edema following phacovitrectomy have been reported.

## 8.2	Prevention of Postoperative Inflammation

We will now discuss the drugs used to prevent inflammation following vitreoretinal surgery.

### 8.2.1	Preoperative Use of Nonsteroidal Anti-inflammatory Drugs

NSAIDs have been used preoperatively in cataract surgery, and it is known that they reduce pain, inflammation, and myosis, thus facilitating surgery

and recovery. Indeed, they prevent the development of macular edema following surgery.

They have been administered in different ways prior to vitreoretinal surgery.

There are indications that intravenous administration of ketorolac during vitreoretinal surgery reduces pain and nausea in the postoperative period [53, 54]. A study comparing topical ketorolac used 4 times a day for 3 days prior to surgery and 4 weeks postoperatively with placebo has shown a reduction in pain and inflammation in the postoperative period and better visual results in the treatment group. No differences were found in the level of mydriasis achieved during the procedure [55].

### 8.2.2	Heparin in Irrigation Solution

Heparin is a derivative of heparan sulfate that has an anticoagulant effect. It has been used in vitreoretinal surgery for two purposes: to prevent proliferative retinopathy and to minimize fibrinous reaction.

Low-molecular-weight heparin (LMWH) has been used in vitrectomy irrigation infusion in association with 5 fluorouracil to prevent proliferative retinopathy because it also inhibits fibroblast adhesion and collagen polymerization, which is synergistic with the antimetabolite [56–58].

LMWH has been used in irrigation infusion to minimize fibrinous response to surgery. In animals, it has successfully been used in combined procedure phacovitrectomy [59]. However, the use of intravenous heparin combined with heparin in irrigation infusion was associated with bleeding [60]. Studies have progressively increased the dose of LMWH in irrigation infusion, resulting in a reduction of the anterior chamber reaction without increasing the risk of bleeding at a dosage of 6.0 IU/ml of enoxaparin in the infusion [61]. This approach may be useful in combined procedures in diabetic patients.

### 8.2.3	5-Fluorouracil in Irrigation Solution

5-Fluorouracil is an antimetabolite that has been used in vitrectomy irrigation infusion combined with low-molecular-weight heparin in an attempt

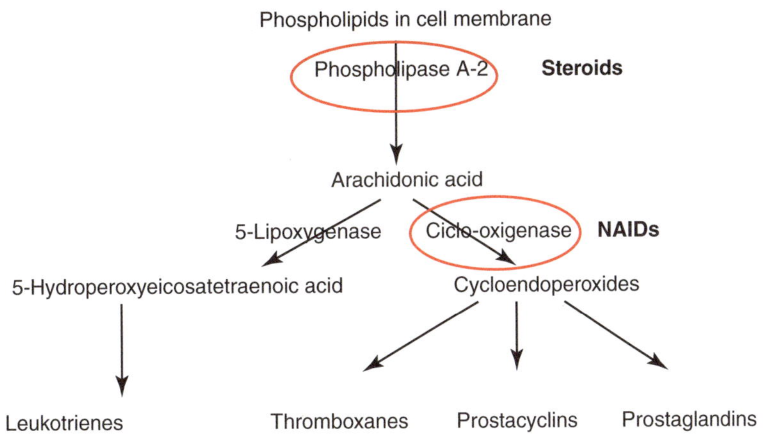

Fig. 8.4 Mechanism of action of anti-inflammatory drugs

to minimize proliferative retinopathy in retinal detachment surgery. Results from clinical trials would suggest that this treatment does not improve surgical outcomes [56–58].

8.2.4   Steroids in Irrigation Infusion

In 1996, Williams and Chang reported using steroids in irrigation solution during vitrectomy for PVR [62].

In 2001, we started a prospective, randomized, masked pilot study to evaluate the effectiveness of 2 mg of dexamethasone in 500 ml of BSS irrigation solution during combined procedure phacovitrectomy.

On the first postoperative day, eyes that received intravitreal dexamethasone showed less alteration of the blood-ocular barrier. By 1 week after surgery, the findings were the opposite: that is, treated eyes showed a higher flare level than untreated eyes, and this remained unchanged 1 month later. This may be a rebound effect after administration of intravitreal steroids. Nevertheless, this difference was not statistically significant at any time during the follow-up period. Intraocular pressure during follow-up was above 20 mmHg in 22 % of treated eyes, compared to 5.3 % of controls, a difference that was not significant. High intraocular pressure was successfully reduced with temporary topical hypotensive treatment.

Another method for administering steroids during surgery is vitrectomy assisted by triamcinolone. This has the advantage facilitating

visualization and complete removal of the vitreous gel, with a reduction of anterior chamber inflammation measured by laser flare meter 8 days after surgery [63].

8.3   Treatment of Postoperative Inflammation

8.3.1   Mechanism of Action of Anti-inflammatory Drugs

Anti-inflammatory drugs act on the arachidonic acid pathway, as shown in Fig. 8.1. NSAIDs inhibit cyclooxygenase (Fig. 8.4), in some cases specifically cyclooxygenase-2, which is the predominant form in retinal pigment epithelial cells [64]. Steroids inhibit phospholipase A-2, thus inhibiting the synthesis of prostaglandins and leukotrienes. Steroids also have other effects: locally, they block the activity of macrophages and minimize the production of lymphokines and the migration of lymphocytes. Triamcinolone acetate has a beneficial effect on macular edema by stabilizing the blood-retinal barrier [63], reducing vascular leakage and reducing the synthesis of vascular endothelial growth factor [65].

8.3.2   Topical and Systemic Nonsteroidal Anti-inflammatory Drugs (NSAIDs)

NSAIDs inhibit cyclooxygenase and, thus, the synthesis of prostaglandins. Prostaglandins are produced in the ciliary body and the iris in response to surgery, causing myosis, pain, and inflammation [66]. Several studies have shown that NSAIDs are successful in minimizing these effects and preventing cystoid macular edema and improving visual results in cataract surgery. Nevertheless, few studies have evaluated the usefulness of NSAIDs in vitreoretinal surgery.

NSAIDs can be used either topically or systemically. The following drugs can be used topically: ketorolac, diclofenac, nepafenac, and bromfenac.

They are useful in vitreoretinal surgery in a number of ways. First, they can be used to treat acute inflammation as in cataract surgery. Bromfenac, nepafenac, and ketorolac can penetrate the vitreous cavity and reduce prostaglandin E2, which mediates inflammation. The most effective topical NSAID is ketorolac [67]. One clinical study has shown that ketorolac administered both before and after vitrectomy can minimize inflammation [55].

It has been used in treating pseudophakic macular edema and as a prophylaxis for inflammation following cataract surgery [68–70].

It has been found that combining NSAIDs with steroids has a synergistic effect that is quite beneficial in the treatment of pseudophakic macular edema [71, 72].

The most frequent secondary effects are alteration of the ocular surface and foreign body sensation, with punctate keratitis or epithelial defects occasionally appearing [73, 74]. There have also been reports of severe corneal melting [75–80], although we have found that toxic keratolysis would appear to be more frequent when NSAIDs are combined with steroids [81].

Selective inhibitors of cyclooxygenase have been used intravenously in scleral buckling, but no significant differences have been found in macular thickness or visual acuity compared to a placebo [32]. Intravenous ketorolac during vitrectomy minimizes postoperative pain and nausea [53, 54].

8.3.3 Topical Steroids

Commercially available steroids for topical application include medium-strength drugs like fluorometholone and hydrocortisone and high-strength

drugs like dexamethasone, prednisolone, and rimexolone. Medium-strength steroids reach only low levels of concentration in the aqueous humor and are thus not very effective in treating intraocular inflammation, although they are useful in treating conjunctival and episcleral inflammation, with a lower incidence of secondary high intraocular pressure [82, 83]. High-strength steroids are used in isolation or in association with NSAIDs in treating surface and anterior chamber inflammation secondary to vitrectomy. They have also been used in prophylaxis and to treat postsurgical macular edema.

The secondary effects of topical steroids are more severe than with NSAIDs, as they not only cause corneal melting but can also predispose to infection, slow down wound closure, induce cataract formation, and increase IOP [84]. Rimexolone has the lowest hypertensive effect.

8.3.4 Periocular Steroids

After depot injection, corticosteroid action peaks at 1 week, with residual activity persisting for 3–6 months. Periocular injections reduce the risk of serious complications such as endophthalmitis and retinal detachment, but the duration of the effect is shorter than in the intravitreal pathway [33].

These steroids have been used in both the prophylaxis of pseudophakic macular edema and in treating the edema with good results, but they are less effective than intravitreal triamcinolone [15].

This pathway has also been useful in the treatment of post-vitrectomy refractory macular edema [12].

8.3.5 Intravitreal Steroids

The most frequently used intravitreal steroid is triamcinolone, which has been beneficial in cases of post-vitrectomy refractory macular edema and of pseudophakic macular edema. It can also be used intraoperatively to enable identification of the posterior hyaloids and the interior-limiting membrane.

The effect of intravitreal triamcinolone is of a limited duration, estimated at between 2 and 4 months in non-vitrectomized eyes and an even shorter duration in vitrectomized eyes [85].

The complications of intravitreal triamcinolone therapy include secondary ocular hypertension in about 40 % of the eyes injected, medically uncontrollable high intraocular pressure leading to glaucoma surgery in about 1–2 % of eyes [86], posterior subcapsular cataracts and nuclear cataracts leading to cataract surgery in about 15–20 % in elderly patients within 1 year after injection [87], postoperative infectious endophthalmitis with a rate of about 1:1,000 [88, 89], noninfectious endophthalmitis [90] that may be due to a reaction to the solvent agent, and pseudoendophthalmitis with triamcinolone acetonide crystals appearing in the anterior chamber [91], in addition to possible complications arising from the injection technique.

8.3.6 Steroid Sustained-Release Devices

As the effect of intravitreal triamcinolone is temporary and its duration in vitrectomized eyes is low, devices to release steroids in a sustained manner have been developed.

Permanent or biodegradable devices for steroid delivery to the vitreous are becoming more commonly used (i.e., Retisert, Bausch & Lomb Pharmaceuticals, Tampa, FL; Ozurdex and Posurdex, Allergan, Inc., Irvine, CA). These implants show promise in both the prophylaxis and treatment of pseudophakic cystoid macular edema [92]. Ozurdex is effective in treating refractory diabetic macular edema in vitrectomized eyes, uveitis cases, or Irvine-Gass syndrome [16–18].

8.3.7 Systemic Steroids

Oral steroids were previously used following scleral buckling, but comparative studies have shown no beneficial effects in terms of visual acuity, macular edema, choroidal detachment, or proliferative retinopathy compared to placebo [93].

Systemic steroids are used in only selected cases. Evidence exists that oral prednisolone (at a dosage of 1 mg per Kg per day) in cases of retinal detachment complicated by choroidal detachment increases the rate of retinal reattachment following vitrectomy [94]. They are also used in cases of severe intraocular inflammation such as endophthalmitis or uveitis.

References

1. Hikichi T, Matsumoto N, Ohtsuka H, et al. Comparison of one-year outcomes between 23- and 20-gauge vitrectomy for preretinal membrane. Am J Ophthalmol. 2009;147(4):639–43 (C).
2. Steven J, Gedde MD. Management of glaucoma after retinal detachment surgery. Curr Opin Ophthalmol. 2002;13:103–9 (B).
3. Abrams GW, Swanson DE, Sabates WI. The results of sulfur hexafluoride gas in vitreous surgery. Am J Ophthalmol. 1982;94:165–71 (D).
4. Ichhpujani P, Jindal A, Jay KL. Silicone oil induced glaucoma: a review. Graefes Arch Clin Exp Ophthalmol. 2009;247(12):1585–93 (B).
5. Budenz DL, Taba KE, Feuer WJ, et al. Surgical management of secondary glaucoma after pars plana vitrectomy and silicone oil injection for complex retinal detachment. Ophthalmology. 2001;108:1628–32 (D).
6. Jonas JB, Knorr HL, Rank RM, Budde WM. Intraocular pressure and silicone oil endotamponade. J Glaucoma. 2001;10:102–8 (D).
7. Fujikawa A, Kitaoka T, Miyamura N, Amemiya T. Choroidal detachment after vitreous surgery. Ophthalmic Surg Lasers. 2000;31(4):276–81 (D).
8. Guthoff R, Riederle H, Meinhardt B, Goebel W. Subclinical choroidal detachment at sclerotomy sites after 23-gauge vitrectomy: analysis by anterior segment optical coherence tomography. Ophthalmologica. 2010;224(5):301–7 (D).
9. Lewis H, Abrams GW, Blumenkranz MS, Campo RV. Vitrectomy for diabetic macular traction and edema associated with posterior hyaloid traction. Ophthalmology. 1992;99:753–9 (D).
10. Tachi N, Ogino N. Vitrectomy for diabetic macular edema in cases of diabetic retinopathy. Am J Ophthalmol. 1992;122:258–60 (D).
11. Kim SJ, Martin DF, Hubbard III GB, Srivastava SK. Incidence of postvitrectomy macular edema using optical coherence tomography. Ophthalmology. 2009;116:1531–7 (D).
12. Sato H, Naito T, Matsushita S, Takebayashi M, Shiota H. Efficacy of sub-Tenon's capsule injection of triamcinolone acetonide for refractory diabetic macular edema after vitrectomy. J Med Invest. 2008;55:279–82 (D).
13. Wada M, Ogata N, Minamino K, Koriyama M, Higuchi A, Matsumura M. Trans-Tenon's retrobulbar

injection of triamcinolone acetonide for diffuse macular edema. Jpn J Ophthalmol. 2005;49:509–15 (D).

14. Figueroa MS, Contreras I, Noval S. Surgical and anatomical outcomes of pars plana vitrectomy for diffuse nontractional diabetic macular edema. Retina. 2008;28:420–6 (D).

15. Yilmaz T, Weaver CD, Gallagher MJ, et al. Intravitreal triamcinolone acetonide injection for treatment of refractory diabetic macular edema: a systematic review. Ophthalmology. 2009;116:902–13 (B).

16. Haller JA, Kuppermann BD, Blumenkranz MS, Williams GA, et al., Dexamethasone DDS Phase II Study Group. Randomized controlled trial of an intravitreous dexamethasone drug delivery system in patients with diabetic macular edema. Arch Ophthalmol. 2010;128(3):289–96. (C).

17. Williams GA, Haller JA, Kuppermann BD, et al., on behalf of the Dexamethasone DDS Phase II Study Group. Dexamethasone posterior-segment drug delivery system in the treatment of macular edema resulting from uveitis or Irvine-Gass syndrome. Am J Ophthalmol. 2009;147:1048–54. (C).

18. Kuppermann BD, Blumenkranz MS, Haller JA, et al., for the Dexamethasone DDS Phase II Study Group Randomized Controlled Study of an Intravitreous. Dexamethasone drug delivery system in patients with persistent macular edema. Arch Ophthalmol. 2007;125:309–17. (C).

19. Goezinne F, La Heij EC, Berendschot TT, et al. Anterior chamber depth is significantly decreased after scleral buckling surgery. Ophthalmology. 2010;117(1):79–85 (D).

20. Burton TC, Stevens TS, Harrison TJ. The influence of subconjunctival depot corticosteroid on choroidal detachment following retinal detachment surgery. Trans Sect Ophthalmol Am Acad Ophthalmol Otolaryngol. 1975;79(6):OP845–9 (D).

21. Williams GA, Aaberg TM. Técnicas de identación escleral. En Retina. Ryan. 4ª ed. New York: Elsevier Inc., 2009 (C).

22. Kawana K, Okamoto F, Hiraoka T, Oshika T. Ciliary body edema after scleral buckling surgery for rhegmatogenous retinal detachment. Ophthalmology. 2006;113(1):36–41 (D).

23. Kreiger AE, Hodgkinson BJ, Frederick AR, et al. The results of retinal detachment surgery. Analysis of 268 operations with a broad scleral buckle. Arch Ophthalmol. 1971;86:385–94 (C).

24. Perez RN, Phelps CD, Burton TC. Angle-closure glaucoma following scleral buckling operations. Trans Sect Ophthalmol Am Acad Ophthalmol Otolaryngol. 1976;81:247–52 (D).

25. Burton TC, Folk JC. Laser iris retraction for angle-closure glaucoma after retinal detachment surgery. Ophthalmology. 1988;95:742–8 (D).

26. Zur D, Fischer N, Tufail A, Monés J, Loewenstein A. Postsurgical cystoid macular edema. Eur J Ophthalmol. 2010;21(S6):62–8 (C).

27. Lobes Jr LA, Grand MG. Incidence of cystoid macular edema following scleral buckling procedure. Arch Ophthalmol. 1980;98(7):1230–2 (D).

28. Meredith TA, Reeser FH, Topping TM, Aaberg TM. Cystoid macular edema after retinal detachment surgery. Ophthalmology. 1980;87(11):1090–5 (D).

29. Wilkinson CP. Mysteries regarding the surgically reattached retina. Trans Am Ophthalmol Soc. 2009;107:55–7 (D).

30. Huang D, Swanson EA, Lin CP, et al. Optical coherence tomography. Science. 1991;254:1178–81 (B).

31. Miyake K. Indomethacin in the treatment of postoperative cystoid macular edema. Surv Ophthalmol. 1984;28(Suppl):554–68 (C).

32. Benson SE, Ratcliffe S, VAN Raders P, Schlottmann PG, Khan I, Newsom R, Langford RM, Charteris DG. A randomised comparison of parecoxib/valdecoxib and placebo for the prevention of cystoid macular edema after scleral buckling surgery. Retina. 2009;29: 387–394 (C).

33. Rotsos TG, Moschos MM. Cystoid macular edema. Clin Ophthalmol. 2008;2(4):919–30 (B).

34. Kita M, Marmor MF. Effects on retinal adhesive force in vivo of metabolically active agents in the subretinal space. Invest Ophthalmol Vis Sci. 1992;33:1883–7 (C).

35. Sabates NR, Sabates FN, Sabates R, Lee KY, Ziemianski MC. Macular changes after retinal detachment surgery. Am J Ophthalmol. 1989;108(1):22–9 (D).

36. Spencer AF, Newton C, Vernon SA. Incidence of ocular motility problems following scleral buckling surgery. Eye (Lond). 1993;7(Pt 6):751–6 (C).

37. Farr AK, Guyton DL. Strabismus after retinal detachment surgery. Curr Opin Ophthalmol. 2000;11: 207–10 (B).

38. Le Rouic JF, Bettembourg O, d'Hermies F, Azan F, Renard G, Chauvaud D. Late swelling and removal of miragel buckles a comparison with silicone indentations. Retina. 2003;23:641–6 (D).

39. Bernardino CR, Mihora LD, Fay AM, Rubin PAD. Orbital complications of hydrogel scleral buckles. Ophthal Plast Reconstr Surg. 2006;22(3):206–8 (D).

40. Brown DM, Beardsley RM, Fish RH, Wong TP, Kim RY. Long-term stability of circumferential silicone sponge scleral buckling exoplants. Retina. 2006;26:645–9 (D).

41. Flindall RJ, Norton EW, Curtin VT, et al. Reduction of extrusion and infection following episcleral silicone implants and cryopexy in retinal detachment surgery. Am J Ophthalmol. 1971;71:835–7 (D).

42. Russo CE, Ruiz RS. Silicone sponge rejection: early and late complications in retinal detachment surgery. Arch Ophthalmol. 1971;85:647–50 (D).

43. Hilton GF, Wallyn RH. The removal of scleral buckles. Arch Ophthalmol. 1978;96:2061–3 (D).

44. Lindsey PS, Pierce LH, Welch RB. Removal of scleral buckling elements causes and complications. Arch Ophthalmol. 1983;101:570–3 (D).

45. Schwartz PL, Pruett RC. Factors influencing retinal redetachment after removal of buckling elements. Arch Ophthalmol. 1977;95:804–7 (D).

46. Park SP, Ahn JK, Lee GH. Morphologic changes in the anterior segment after phacovitrectomy for proliferative diabetic retinopathy. J Cataract Refract Surg. 2009;35(5):868–73 (D).

47. Lahey JM, Francis RR, Kearney JJ. Combining phacoemulsification with pars plana vitrectomy in patients with proliferative diabetic retinopathy: a series of 223 cases. Ophthalmology. 2003;110:1335–9 (C).

48. Shinoda K, O'hira A, Ishida S. Posterior synechia of the iris after combined pars plana vitrectomy, phacoemulsification, and intraocular lens implantation. Jpn J Ophthalmol. 2001;45:276–80 (D).

49. Li W, Sun G, Wu R, Wang X, Xu M, Sun C. Longterm results after phacovitrectomy and foldable intraocular lens implantation. Acta Ophthalmol. 2009;87(8):896–900 (D).

50. Irvine S. A newly defined vitreous syndrome following cataract surgery. Am J Ophthalmol. 1953;36:599–619 (D).

51. Gass JDM, Norton EW. Cystoid macular edema and papilledema following cataract extraction. Arch Ophthalmol. 1966;76:646–60 (D).

52. Miller JH, George JM, Hoskings JC. Combined macular hole and cataract surgery. Am J Ophthalmol. 1997;123:705–7 (D).

53. Fekrat S, Marsh MJ, Elsing SH. Intraoperative ketorolac and eye pain after vitreoretinal surgery: a prospective, randomized, placebo-controlled study. Retina. 2003;23(1):8–13 (C).

54. Vlajkovic G, Sindjelic R, Stefanovic I. Ketorolac as a pre-emptive analgesic in retinal detachment surgery: a prospective, randomized clinical trial. Int J Clin Pharmacol Ther. 2007;45(5):259–63 (B).

55. Kim SJ, Lo WR, Hubbard III GB, et al. Ketorolac in vitreoretinal surgery: a prospective, randomized, placebo-controlled, double-masked trial. Arch Ophthalmol. 2008;126(9):1203–8 (B).

56. Sundaram V, Barsam A, Virgili G. Intravitreal low molecular weight heparin and 5-Fluorouracil for the prevention of proliferative vitreoretinopathy following retinal reattachment surgery. Cochrane Database Syst Rev. 2010;(7):CD006421. (A).

57. Wickham L, Bunce C, Wong D, McGurn D, Charteris DG. Randomized controlled trial of combined 5-Fluorouracil and low-molecular-weight heparin in the management of unselected rhegmatogenous retinal detachments undergoing primary vitrectomy. Ophthalmology. 2007;114(4):698–704 (A).

58. Garcia RA, Sanchez JG, Arevalo JF. Combined 5-fluorouracil, low-molecular-weight heparin, and silicone oil in the management of complicated retinal detachment with proliferative vitreoretinopathy grade C. Ophthalmic Surg Lasers Imaging. 2007;38(4):276–82 (B).

59. Iverson DA, Katsura H, Hartzer MK, Blumenkranz MS. Inhibition of intraocular fibrin formation following infusion of low-molecular-weight heparin during vitrectomy. Arch Ophthalmol. 1991;109:405–9 (D).

60. Johnson RN, Blankenship G. A prospective, randomized, clinical trial of heparin therapy for postoperative intraocular fibrin. Ophthalmology. 1988;95:312–7 (D).

61. Lane RG, Jumper MJ, Nasir MA, MacCumber MW, McCuen II BW. A prospective, open-label, dose-escalating study of low molecular weight heparin during repeat vitrectomy for PVR and severe diabetic retinopathy. Graefe's Arch Clin Exp Ophthalmol. 2005;243:701–5 (C).

62. Williams RG, Chang S, Comaratta MR, Simoni G. Does the presence of heparin and dexamethasone in the vitrectomy infusate reduce reproliferation in proliferative vitreoretinopathy? Graefes Arch Clin Exp Ophthalmol. 1996;234(8):496–503 (D).

63. Sakamoto T, Miyazaki M, Hisatomi T, Nakamura T, Ueno A, Itaya K, Ishibashi T. Triamcinolone-assisted pars plana vitrectomy improves the surgical procedures and decreases the postoperative blood–ocular barrier breakdown. Graefe's Arch Clin Exp Ophthalmol. 2002;240:423–9 (D).

64. Chin MS, Nagineni CN, Hooper LC, Detrick B, Hooks JJ. Cyclooxygenase-2 gene expression and regulation in human retinal pigment epithelial cells. Invest Ophthalmol Vis Sci. 2001;42:2338–46 (C).

65. Cheng T, Cao W, Wen R, Steinberg RH, LaVail MM. Prostaglandin E2 induces vascular endothelial growth factor and basic fibroblast growth factor mRNA expression in cultured rat Muller cells. Invest Ophthalmol Vis Sci. 1998;39:581–91 (C).

66. Ambache N, Kavanagh L, Whiting J. Effect of mechanical stimulation on rabbits' eyes: release of active substance in anterior chamber perfusates. J Physiol. 1965;176:378–408 (C).

67. Heier JS, Awh CC, Busbee BG, et al. Vitreous nonsteroidal antiinflammatory drug concentrations and prostaglandin E2 levels in vitrectomy patients treated with ketorolac 0.4%, bromfenac 0.09%, and nepafenac 0.1%. Retina. 2009;29:1310–3 (C).

68. Burnett J, Tessler H, Isenberg S, et al. Double-masked trial of fenoprofen sodium: treatment of chronic aphakic cystoid macular edema. Ophthalmic Surg. 1983;14:150–2.

69. Jampol LM, Sanders DR, Kraff MC, et al. Prophylaxis and therapy of aphakic cystoid macular edema. Surv Ophthalmol. 1984;28(Suppl):535–9 (D).

70. Shelsta HN, Jampol LM. Pharmacologic therapy of pseudophakic cystoid macular edema 2010 Update. Retina. 2011;31:4–12.

71. Heier JS, Topping TM, Baumann S, et al. Ketorolac versus prednisolone versus combination therapy in the treatment of acute pseudophakic cystoid macular-edema. Ophthalmology. 2000;107:2034–8.

72. Flach AJ. Discussion: ketorolac vs prednisolone vs combination therapy in the treatment of acute pseudophakic CMD. Ophthalmology. 2000;107:2039 (C).

73. Sher NA, Krueger RR, Teal P, Jans RG, Edmison D. Role of topical corticosteroids and nonsteroidal antiinflammatory drugs in the etiology of stromal infiltrates after excimer photorefractive keratectomy. J Refract Corneal Surg. 1994;10:587–8 (D).

74. Shimazaki J, Saito H, Yang HY, Toda I, Fujishima H, Tsubota K. Persistent epithelial defect following penetrating keratoplasty: an adverse effect of diclofenac eyedrops. Cornea. 1995;14:623–7 (D).

75. Lin JC, Rapuano CJ, Laibson PR, Eagle Jr RC, Cohen EJ. Corneal melting associated with use of topical nonsteroidal anti-inflammatory drugs after ocular surgery. Arch Ophthalmol. 2000;118:1129–32 (D).

76. Asai T, Nakagami T, Mochizuki M, Hata N, Tsuchiya T, Hotta Y. Three cases of corneal melting after instillation of a new nonsteroidal anti-inflammatory drug. Cornea. 2006;25:224–7 (D).
77. Isawi H, Dhaliwal DK. Corneal melting and perforation in Stevens Johnson syndrome following topical bromfenac use. J Cataract Refract Surg. 2007;33:1644–6 (D).
78. Wolf EJ, Kleiman LZ, Schrier A. Nepafenac-associated corneal melt. J Cataract Refract Surg. 2007;33:1974–5 (D).
79. Bekendam PD, Narvaez J, Agarwal M. Case of corneal melting associated with the use of topical nepafenac. Cornea. 2007;26:1002–3 (D).
80. Flach AJ. Corneal melts associated with topically applied nonsteroidal anti-inflammatory drugs. Trans Am Ophthalmol Soc. 2001;99:205–10 (D).
81. Alvarez MT, Figueroa MS, Teus MA. Toxic keratolysis from combined use of nonsteroid anti-inflammatory drugs and topical steroids following vitreoretinal surgery. Eur J Ophthalmol. 2006;16(4):582–7.
82. McGhee CN. Pharmacokinetics of ophthalmic corticosteroids. Br J Ophthalmol. 1992;76(11):681–4 (B).
83. Akingbehin AO. Comparative study of the intraocular pressure effects of fluorometholone 0.1% versus dexamethasone 0.1%. Br J Ophthalmol. 1983;67(10):661–3.
84. Awan MA, Agarwal PK, Watson DG, McGhee CN, Dutton GN. Penetration of topical and subconjunctival corticosteroids into human aqueous humour and its therapeutic significance. Br J Ophthalmol. 2009; 93(6):708–13 (B).
85. Chin HS, Park TS, Moon YS, Oh JH. Difference in clearance of intravitreal triamcinolone acetonide between vitrectomized and nonvitrectomized eyes. Retina. 2005;25(5):556–60 (B).
86. Jonas JB, Degenring RF, Kreissig I, Akkoyun I, Kamppeter BA. Intraocular pressure elevation after intravitreal triamcinolone acetonide injection. Ophthalmology. 2005;112:593–8 (A).
87. Jonas JB, Degenring RF, Vossmerbaeumer U, Kamppeter BA. Frequency of cataract surgery after intravitreal injection of high-dosage triamcinolone acetonide. Eur J Ophthalmol. 2005;15: 462–4 (B).
88. Jonas JB, Kreissig I, Degenring RF. Endophthalmitis after intravitreal injection of triamcinolone acetonide. Arch Ophthalmol. 2003;121:1663–4 (B).
89. Westfall AC, Osborn A, Kuhl D, Benz MS, Mieler WF, Holz ER. Acute endophthalmitis incidence: intravitreal triamcinolone. Arch Ophthalmol. 2005;123: 1075–7 (C).
90. Jonas JB, Kreissig I, Spandau UH, Harder B. Infectious and non-infectious endophthalmitis after intravitreal triamcinolone acetonide. Am J Ophthalmol. 2006;141:579–80 (C).
91. Moshfeghi AA, Scott IU, Flynn Jr HW, Puliafito CA. Pseudohypopyon after intravitreal triamcinolone acetonide injection for cystoid macular edema. Am J Ophthalmol. 2004;138:489–92 (D).
92. Williams GA, Haller JA, Kuppermann BD, et al. Dexamethasone posterior-segment drug delivery system in the treatment of macular edema resulting from uveitis or Irvine-Gass syndrome. Am J Ophthalmol. 2009;147:1048–54 (B).
93. Dehghan MH, Ahmadieh H, Soheilian M, Azarmina M, Moradian S, Ramezani AR, Tavallal A, Naghibozakerin J. Effect of oral prednisolone on visual outcomes and complications after scleral buckling. Eur J Ophthalmol. 2010;20(2):419–23 (A).
94. Sharma T, Gopal L, Reddy RK, et al. Rhegmatogenous retinal detachment and choroidal detachment with or without oral corticosteroids: a pilot study. Retina. 2005;25:152–7 (D).

Treatment of Intermediate Uveitis

9

Elisabetta Miserocchi, Umberto De Benedetto,
and Giulio Modorati

Contents

9.1 Introduction

9.1.1 Definition

The term intermediate uveitis (IU) was introduced by the International Uveitis Study Group (IUSG) to define an idiopathic inflammatory syndrome, mainly involving the anterior vitreous, the peripheral retina, and the ciliary body to replace previously used terms such as posterior cyclitis, hyalitis, vitritis, and basal uveoretinitis [8]. The term intermediate uveitis was also suggested to replace that of pars planitis. However, both terms continue to be used adding to the confusion in the literature.

E. Miserocchi, MD (✉) • U. De Benedetto, MD
G. Modorati, MD
Ophthalmology – Ocular Immunology
and Uveitis Service, San Raffaele Scientific Institute,
Via Olgetina 60, Milan 20123, Italy
e-mail: miserocchi.elisabetta@hsr.it;
debenedetto.umberto@hsr.it; modorati.giulio@hsr.it

U. Pleyer et al. (eds.), *Immune Modulation and Anti-Inflammatory Therapy in Ocular Disorders*,
DOI 10.1007/978-3-642-54350-0_9, © Springer-Verlag Berlin Heidelberg 2014

The term intermediate uveitis was used synonymously with pars planitis by IUSG, and thus most of the intermediate uveitis was assumed to be idiopathic in etiology. The Standardization of Uveitis Nomenclature (SUN) Working Group defined IU as that subset of uveitis where vitreous is the major site of inflammation, irrespective of the presence of peripheral vascular sheathing or macular edema [44]. The diagnostic term *pars planitis* should be used only for that subset of intermediate uveitis where there is snowbank or snowball formation occurring in the absence of an associated infection or systemic disease (i.e., "idiopathic"). If there is an associated infection (e.g., Lyme disease) or systemic disease (e.g., sarcoidosis), then the term intermediate uveitis should be used.

9.1.2 Epidemiology

The etiology of intermediate uveitis is not well known and is mostly believed to be autoimmune, although it may be associated with systemic diseases such as sarcoidosis, multiple sclerosis, and several infectious conditions. The etiology may vary in different parts of the world as it could be influenced by the geographic location and ethnicity [12, 14, 34, 41, 70].

Intermediate uveitis is the least common form of uveitis affecting about 8–22 % of patients with uveitis, and most of the cases are idiopathic [12, 14, 34, 41, 70].

There is limited data on the incidence of intermediate uveitis. In the Northern California Epidemiology Study, the reported rate of intermediate uveitis was of 1.5 per 100,000 population years [34]. Pars planitis is much more common among Caucasians and is very rare in other races. Pars planitis usually presents in childhood or young adulthood and rarely presents after 40 years of age. In fact, some authors [35, 66] have insisted on an age of onset below 40 years for inclusion.

In the population-based study by Donaldson, the authors used the resources of the Rochester Epidemiology Project database over a period of 20 years (from 1985 to 2004) [21]. The annual incidence of pars planitis adjusted to the age and gender distribution in this study was 2.08 per 100,000 population. This is slightly higher than

that of Northern California of 1.5 per 100,000 [34], which may be the result of the higher proportion of Caucasians in Minnesota.

A relationship between smoking and pars planitis was observed in Donaldson's study, with 52 % of patients with pars planitis being smokers. This was the first study that linked pars planitis with an increased rate of smoking. More recently, Lin and colleagues have confirmed the strong correlation between smoking and cystoid macular edema in patients with intermediate uveitis compared to patients with other anatomic location of uveitis [62].

9.1.3 Clinical Features

There is a wide variation in clinical presentation of intermediate uveitis. At one end of the spectrum, there are patients totally asymptomatic that present for other reasons and are noted to have vitreous cells and old snowbanks; at the other end of the spectrum, there are patients with severe, progressive inflammatory disease resulting in severe vision loss because of macular edema or retinal complications [109].

Hence, patients with IU may be completely asymptomatic or present with minimal symptoms such as floaters, blurred vision, and photopsia without pain. In more severe cases, the visual acuity may be significantly reduced due to intense vitreitis or to vitreous hemorrhage or retinal complications [109]. In Donaldson's study, the most common presenting symptoms of pars planitis were blurred vision (73.9 %) and floaters (60.9 %) [21].

The anterior chamber is usually quiet or may have discrete signs of inflammation in the form of sparse keratic precipitates, low-grade flare, and cells. Posterior synechia are rarely seen. Vitreitis is the most characteristic feature of intermediate uveitis, ranging from 1+ to 4+ vitreous haze. The typical yellow-white inflammatory aggregates, snowballs, and the exudates of the pars plana, snowbanks, are mostly found in the inferior periphery of the retina and in the midvitreous. In 10–32 % of cases, signs of peripheral retinal vasculitis and periphlebitis are seen in intermediate uveitis [5, 21].

9.1.4 Complications

Most patients with intermediate uveitis develop few ocular complications and maintain good vision, thanks to the benign nature of this cause of uveitis. Deane and colleagues showed that 63 % of patients followed for a period of 2 years maintained a visual acuity of 20/20 or better [15]. However, severe complications can occur if chronic, indolent inflammation is allowed to persist. It rarely may also lead to blindness.

The incidence of secondary glaucoma and cataract has been reported to be approximately 8 and 50 %, respectively, in patients with intermediate uveitis [5].

Macular edema and maculopathy are the most common causes of visual loss in intermediate uveitis, occurring in 12–50 % of patients, and this incidence seems to increase with severity and duration of inflammation [66].

In the Rochester Epidemiology study on the outcome of pars planitis, the most common complications were epiretinal membrane (36 %), cataract (30.4 %), and cystoid macular edema (26.1 %) [21]. The mean interval between onset of pars planitis and development of epiretinal membrane varied between 7.9 years [21] and 6.5 years [18].

Retinal vasculitis may induce the formation of epiretinal membranes, cyclitic membranes, and neovascularization in 15–36 % of patients. Vitreous hemorrhage resulting from vitreoretinal traction and peripheral neovascularization is an uncommon complication occurring in 3–5 % of cases in countries with a well-developed health system. Retinal detachment may be exudative (in 5–17 % of patients) or tractional (in 3–22 % of patients) secondary to vitreoretinal traction. These membranes can progress to cause retinal breaks [109].

Optic nerve involvement is common in patients with intermediate uveitis associated to multiple sclerosis and is more commonly observed in children manifesting as hyperemia and disk edema [66].

9.1.5 Differential Diagnosis

The differential diagnosis of intermediate uveitis includes both infectious causes and autoimmune causes of vitreous inflammation. The most commonly associated systemic diseases are multiple sclerosis (MS), sarcoidosis, and intraocular lymphoma [109].

Among the infectious causes mimicking intermediate uveitis, the most common entities identified are syphilis, Lyme disease, tuberculosis, toxocariasis, Whipple's disease, human T-cell leukemia virus type 1 (HTLV-1), Epstein-Barr virus, and cat scratch disease. The probability of a given diagnosis depends on the prevalence of disease in a given region. Tuberculosis, for example, is an important cause of IU in India where the disease accounts for approximately 46.7 % of cases [86].

9.1.6 Intermediate Uveitis and Multiple Sclerosis

Several studies show a strong association between multiple sclerosis and pars planitis. The association between the two has been reported to have a significant female preponderance. It is found most commonly in young adult or middle-aged Caucasians. Recent large studies have found the prevalence of uveitis in patients with MS to be 1.1–2.4 % and the prevalence of MS in patients with uveitis to be 1–1.3 % [69]. This is ten times the predicted prevalence of uveitis for the general population. In a study by Donaldson, the incidence of MS in pars planitis was 2.077 per 100,000 person, and this value was much higher than the incidence of multiple sclerosis in the Olmsted County population during the same period, which had been measured to be 7.5 per 100,000 persons [21].

There appears to be no temporal association between the development of uveitis and MS. The diagnosis of MS may occur before, concurrently, or after the diagnosis of uveitis.

If one looks specifically at intermediate uveitis, the prevalence figures are much higher as one could expect. Between 3 and 27 % of patients with MS develop intermediate uveitis, and 7.8–14.8 % of patients with intermediate uveitis develop MS [66]. IU in patients with associated MS typically presents with bilateral snowbank and retinal periphlebitis.

9.1.7 Intermediate Uveitis in Children

IU occurs in up to 42 % of the pediatric uveitis population and is the second most common form of uveitis in childhood. The course of IU in children can be worsened by many sight-threatening complications [102]. However, while the incidence is high, most children and young adults with IU will maintain good visual acuity in the absence of ongoing therapy; their disease often resolves spontaneously. However, while the visual outcome in most children is favorable, one-fifth of patients (19 %) develop unilateral legal blindness [102]. In a study of 35 patients with IU, younger age at onset of IU was associated with a worse visual outcome during a 3-year follow-up [49]. In the present study, children with earlier onset of IU were found at increased risk of vitreous hemorrhage, secondary glaucoma, and cataract surgery; the presence of papillitis and snowbanking, at the onset of IU, was associated with a later development of cystoid macular edema [49].

In a large Italian series of 116 children with uveitis, IU was more frequently bilateral (84 %) and idiopathic in nature (97 %). The most common ocular complications were macular edema (74 %) and cataract (25.9 %). The prevalence of MS in children is low, ranging between 3 and 5 %, with an onset before 10 years of age considered exceptionally rare [88].

9.2 Treatment

The most commonly proposed approach to treat intermediate uveitis consists in a stepwise approach based on disease severity. Very mild cases with normal visual acuity and no vision-threatening complications such as macular edema may require no treatment. In a large study on the 20-year outcome of pars planitis, one-third of patients maintained normal visual acuity without requiring treatment [21] (EBM 2++ B). This is an important message considering the side effects of systemic treatment, including corticosteroid-induced cataract, glaucoma, and the potentially life-threatening complications of systemic corticosteroids.

9.2.1 Indication for Treatment

The decision to treat a patient with intermediate uveitis depends on the presence of several factors such as active inflammation, active retinal vasculitis, the presence of macular edema and the extent or degree of pars plana inflammatory exudation, the laterality of the disease, the age of patient, systemic-associated diseases, and comorbidities.

The current consensus suggests that treatment should be started when there is a reduction in visual acuity [84], although some authors [109] do not subscribe to this view and treat patients regardless of the vision.

Some authors have suggested a visual acuity of 20/40 as a threshold for treatment [84], although others [109] do not wait based on the premise that treating inflammation early and aggressively is more effective in preserving vision. In 20 % of patients with IU, who are treated when visual loss already has occurred, there is no restoration to a normal vision [109]. Before starting with anti-inflammatory treatment, infectious causes and malignancies need to be excluded and treated with specific therapies.

The treatment regimen proposed by Kaplan consists in a four step starting with a series of periocular corticosteroid injections, followed by oral prednisone for patients with recurrent and aggressive disease and followed by vitrectomy or immunosuppressive therapy [50].

Foster has suggested a modification (Table 9.1) and uses a five-step program as follows: (1) topical corticosteroids in the presence of anterior segment inflammation, together with regional corticosteroid injections (triamcinolone acetonide, 40 mg; no more than 6 injections); (2) oral nonsteroidal anti-inflammatory drugs (NSAIDs), if the inflammation recurs following the third injection, and topical NSAIDs in the presence of macular edema; (3) a short course of systemic corticosteroids should inflammation persist or recur despite the previous interventions; (4) peripheral retinal cryopexy or indirect laser photocoagulation of the inferior pars plana should the pars planitis recur following the sixth periocular corticosteroid injection; and (5) therapeutic pars plana

Table 9.1 Step-ladder approach by Foster for intermediate uveitis

Step-ladder approach	Treatment	Indication
Step 1	Topical corticosteroids	Active anterior uveitis
	Regional periocular corticosteroid injections	Active intermediate-posterior uveitis and macular edema
Step 2	Oral NSAIDs + topical NSAIDs	Recurrence of inflammation after the 3rd injection, macular edema
Step 3	Short-course systemic corticosteroids	Recurrence-persistence of inflammation despite steps 1–2
Step 4	Cryopexy or laser photocoagulation	Recurrence of inflammation despite 6th periocular injection
Step 5	Pars plana vitrectomy or systemic immunosuppression	Inflammation recalcitrant to previous steps

vitrectomy or systemic immunosuppressive treatment when the inflammation is recalcitrant to previous therapeutic strategies [109].

9.3 Local Treatment

9.3.1 Corticosteroids

Corticosteroids are still the gold standard of treatment for patients with intermediate uveitis. Although topical corticosteroids may be partially effective in aphakic eyes with moderate degree of inflammation of the pars plana and vitreous, generally peribulbar, systemic, or intravitreal corticosteroids are required.

9.3.2 Periocular Corticosteroids

Periocular injections are an effective alternative in the treatment of intermediate uveitis because they have the advantage of delivering a large amount of corticosteroid to the posterior segment of the eye via trans-scleral absorption minimizing the risk of systemic corticosteroid side effects.

There are essentially three types of commercially available preparations of injectable corticosteroids:

- The water-soluble short-acting dexamethasone
- The aqueous suspension of triamcinolone acetonide (TA)
- The long-acting depot of methylprednisolone

The short-acting dexamethasone needs repeated injections, while the duration of action of the depot preparation of methylprednisolone is much longer.

Thus, a triamcinolone suspension is a better therapeutic choice in many clinical situations.

Different routes of periocular corticosteroid administration have been described based on the type and severity of uveitis.

In particular, two methods for periocular corticosteroid injections have been described:

1. The Smith and Nozik method (posterior sub-Tenon injection), the most common employed method, consists in the injection of triamcinolone acetonide in the posterior sub-Tenon space in the superotemporal quadrant. This method has recently been modified with the development of a cannula method, by which the corticosteroid is placed closer to the macula with a soft polytetrafluoroethylene cannula which reduces the chance of globe perforation during the procedure [95].
2. The orbital floor injection method [107].

Venkatesh et al. have compared three different methods of periocular injections. Patients were randomized into three treatment groups of ten eyes each. Each group received PST injection of triamcinolone acetonide 0.5 ml (20 mg) by one of three methods: cannula method (group 1), Smith and Nozik method (group 2), or orbital floor injection method (group 3). In this prospective randomized comparative trial, no differences in visual acuity or retinal thickness were detected at 12 months of follow-up. However, orbital floor injections were associated with a slightly slower onset of action (EBM: 2+D) [107]. The authors did not report any serious complications such as globe perforation. Inadvertent globe perforation with the Smith and Nozik method has been previously described.

Posterior sub-Tenon corticosteroid injection has been proven effective for inflammation of the posterior segment in another retrospective study, of 58 eyes with intermediate uveitis; 80 % of the treated eyes showed an improvement of at least 2 Snellen lines, and 20 % of the eyes had an improvement of more than 5 Snellen lines at long-term follow-up (EBM: 2–D) [59].

Complications with posterior sub-Tenon corticosteroid injections such as high intraocular pressure were reported in 30–36 % of patients. In 9 % of cases, topical antiglaucoma treatment and glaucoma-filtering surgery were required (EBM: 2–D) [40, 59].

Leder and colleagues evaluated the efficacy of a single periocular TA injection, in a series of 156 eyes. In 53 % of cases, cystoid macular edema resolved after 1 month of follow-up. However, 15 % of patients were refractory to treatment and had persistent edema, while 53 % of cases had recurrent macular edema despite multiple injections [61] (EBM: 2–D).

A recent non-randomized comparative study (EBM: 2–D) [25] compared the effectiveness of posterior sub-Tenon versus orbital floor injections for intermediate uveitis. No significant differences in control of macular edema and vitritis were found between the two techniques.

9.3.3 Intraocular Vitreal Injections of Triamcinolone Acetonide (IVTA)

Triamcinolone acetonide is a commercially available corticosteroid that is inexpensive and has been for several decades via periocular injections to treat uveitic macular edema. More recently, TA has been administered by intravitreal injection, allowing for maximal bioavailability in the vitreous cavity. As TA is only slightly soluble in water [97], a 4-mg dose provides therapeutic levels in the vitreous for up to 3 months [71] compared with dexamethasone sodium phosphate which clears from the vitreous in about 3 days [58].

In a retrospective review on 16 patients (20 eyes), Androudi and colleagues reported a significant improvement in visual acuity by 1 month persisting to the end of follow-up of 34 weeks (EBM: 3D) [4].

Similar results were reported by Hogewind et al. who observed an improvement in visual acuity at 1- and 3-month follow-up, but this improvement was absent at 12-month postinjection (EBM: 3D) [43].

In a recent large review, these results were confirmed and it was reported that the maximum duration of the TA effect (4 mg in 0.1 ml) was 4–5 months and the maximum effect on visual acuity of a single injection was found between 1 and 6 months after injection [106]. Hence, in chronic ocular inflammatory disease, 57 % of the eyes required repeated injections. In another series, cystoid macular edema was still present in 50 % of cases at the end of follow-up (EBM: 3D) [4]. And in the remaining patients, despite resolution of edema, there was only a slight improvement in visual acuity.

Cataract progression was noted in 20 % of the eyes, one patient had retinal detachment, and another necessitated filtering surgery for uncontrolled high intraocular pressure [106].

Galor, in a retrospective review, evaluated the rate of adverse events after IVTA injections comparing patients with and without uveitis. The IOP increase ranged from 9.3 to 16 % for non-uveitic eyes and from 17 to 83 % for the uveitic eyes (EBM: 3D) [28].

Other rare reported adverse events related to IVTA are bacterial, sterile, and pseudo-endophthalmitis (1.1 %) [106].

In conclusion, in cases of decreased visual acuity in patients affected by uveitic cystoid macular edema (CME) refractory to topical and/or systemic treatment, IVTA may be considered. However, the duration of the effects is limited, and final visual outcome is unpredictable (EBM: 3D) [4]. One should also mention that while many studies suggest a positive effect of IVTA on visual acuity and macular edema, this treatment remains an off-label use of the drug and a randomized controlled trial is lacking to confirm these findings.

9.3.4 Intraocular Implant Device: Fluocinolone

A fluocinolone acetonide (FA) intravitreal implant (Retisert®) was the first FDA-approved implantable device for the treatment of severe, noninfectious, posterior uveitis [63]. This device is surgically placed in the vitreous cavity at the pars plana. The implant, which contains 0.59 mg of fluocinolone acetonide, slowly releases corticosteroid over the course of 30 months [10]. When inflammation recurs around the 30-month time point, a supplemental FA implant can be placed adjacent to the original implant in the pars plana [45]. This tandem placement avoids the need to remove the original implant which has an increased risk of vitreoretinal complications.

Several studies have reported on the benefits of the implant in the management of patients with noninfectious posterior uveitis [10, 46, 63]. The rate of recurrence was reported with the implant. Recurrence rates of inflammation changed from 62 % before implant to 4, 10, and 20 %, respectively, at 1, 2, and 3 years of follow-up [10, 46]. However, from the results of this study, it is impossible to extrapolate data only on intermediate uveitis. Similar results were reported by Pavesio et al. in a multicenter randomized controlled study (EBM: 1+B) [90], which demonstrated that the recurrences of uveitis after implantation were significantly reduced compared to the year before implantation and were statistically significantly lower in the implant study eye versus the study eye of patients treated with oral corticosteroids. In addition, the rate of CME reduction was statistically higher in the implanted eyes compared to the eyes treated with oral corticosteroid. However, at the end of follow-up, the two groups were comparable with regard to final visual acuity.

FA implants have marked effect on cataract formation; in a long-term clinical study within 3 years of implantation, 100 % of patients required cataract extraction (EBM: 1++A) [46].

High intraocular pressure is one of the major complications observed with FA implants: 51.1 and 78 % of patients required topical antiglaucoma treatment at 34-week and 3-year follow-up. Moreover, about 40 % of patients that received the implant required glaucoma-filtering surgery within 3 years following implantation due to uncontrolled increases in IOP (EBM: 1++A) [32].

9.3.5 Intraocular Implants Device: Dexamethasone

The anti-inflammatory potency of dexamethasone is five times higher than triamcinolone acetonide. Being hydrophilic, its solubility in vitreous is greater allowing for higher concentrations. Higher solubility also implies higher clearance rates, and hence its half-life is only 3–6 h [24]. These limitations have been solved by the use of a biodegradable delivery system containing 0.7 mg of dexamethasone which can be injected into the eye through a 22-gauge single-use applicator. It is injected through the pars plana similar to other intravitreal injections [57].

A recent randomized clinical trial has focused on the use and safety of the dexamethasone implant as monotherapy for the treatment of noninfectious intermediate and posterior uveitis. Lowder et al. evaluated the efficacy of 0.35-mg or 0.7-mg dexamethasone intravitreal implant versus sham (1:1:1 randomization) in patients with noninfectious intermediate or posterior uveitis (EBM: 1+B) [64]. A total of 229 patients (81 % of patients in the study had intermediate uveitis) were observed for 26 weeks.

The dexamethasone implant was effective in reducing vitreous haze and resulted in visual acuity improvement in treated eyes compared to the sham starting at week 3 with the difference persisting through the 26-week study period. The dexamethasone implant was well tolerated and had a favorable safety profile. Less than 10 % of the eyes had an IOP of 25 mmHg or greater. Throughout the duration of the study, 23 % of the eyes in the 0.7-mg dexamethasone implant group required IOP-lowering medications and no eyes required surgical or laser therapy for elevated IOP.

Cataract formation was reported as an adverse event in 15 % of the eyes in the 0.7-mg dexamethasone implant group, 12 % of the eyes in the 0.35-mg dexamethasone implant group, and 7 % in the sham group. These differences were not statistically significant. There were no systemic side effects noted in the DEX implant groups.

9.3.6 Comparison Between the Different Implants

There are currently no randomized controlled trials to compare the devices. Moreover, existing studies have different follow-up periods and inclusion criteria making it difficult to draw conclusions given the different half-lives, pharmacokinetic properties, and duration of the two corticosteroid implants.

In terms of visual acuity, 21 % of patients treated with the FA implant had improvement of 15 letters or more at 34 weeks, while 38 % of the eyes with the dexamethasone implant obtained 15-letter improvement at 26 weeks. Based on available data, the FA implant may lead to additional eye surgery for the management of cataract and/or glaucoma within a 30-month period. Fewer patients treated with the dexamethasone implant required additional ocular surgery for the management of adverse effects, but follow-up was limited to 6 months (EBM: 1++A) [32, 99].

The biodegradable nature of the dexamethasone implant may be an important advantage in comparison to other corticosteroid implants. Repeated injections do not leave a nonbiodegradable shell in the vitreous cavity which might require removal at a later time. As compared to a soluble formulation, its half-life remains stable whether a vitrectomy has been performed or not.

9.3.7 The Multicenter Uveitis Steroid Treatment (MUST) Trial

Recently, the results of a randomized controlled parallel superiority clinical trial comparing the relative effectiveness of systemic corticosteroids plus immunosuppression versus fluocinolone acetonide implant for noninfectious uveitis were published. This study compared two groups of patients as regards visual outcome, control of inflammation, incidence of local and systemic complications, and quality of life. Bilateral implants were allowed if required.

The authors reported no differences in final visual acuity and visual field sensitivity between the systemic corticosteroid and FA implanted groups (180 eyes with intermediate uveitis) in a total of 255 patients.

Among the complications reported, nearly all phakic eyes receiving an implant required cataract surgery and about 25 % of implanted eyes underwent glaucoma surgery in the 24 months of follow-up. The risk of retinal detachment or endophthalmitis was low or zero in both groups. Systemic therapy was responsible for a few systemic complications and a slightly increased number of clinic visits. Little differences were found in the incidence of elevated blood pressure and infections requiring treatment. No statistically significant differences were reported regarding body weight and diabetes. They concluded that the choice of treatment in a specific patient should be guided by the relative importance of cost/benefit profile of the treatment alternatives for a particular patient and his clinical condition (EBM: 1++A) [52].

> **Core Message**
> - Periocular injections of corticosteroids are an effective therapy in patients with IU in particular those with unilateral or asymmetric disease.
> - IVTA is effective in reducing CME and in improving visual acuity in patients with IU. However, the effectiveness is limited in time, and the treatment is an off-label.
> - Corticosteroid intraocular implants are superior to direct drug injections as they release medication over a longer period of time, even in vitrectomized eyes.
> - Fluocinolone acetonide intraocular device (Retisert®) is effective in improving

intraocular inflammation and visual acuity, but it is associated with a high incidence of cataract and IOP increase over the 3 years of drug release.

- The dexamethasone intraocular implant (Ozurdex®) is a biodegradable device that is effective at suppressing intraocular inflammation with a shorter duration of action than the fluocinolone implant but which does not require surgical removal at the end of its life cycle.
- The MUST trial showed similar efficacy between fluocinolone acetonide implant and strict systemic treatment.

9.4 Systemic Treatment

9.4.1 Systemic Corticosteroids

Oral prednisone is started at the dose of 1 mg/kg daily. Tapering should be started 2 weeks after the start of treatment and guided by the clinical response (improvement of visual acuity, reduction of active inflammation). Treatment with corticosteroids at a dose above 5 mg/kg is rarely extended beyond 3 months. In case of persistent inflammation, corticosteroid-sparing agents should be considered. When macular edema is present, periocular corticosteroid injections or acetazolamide 250 mg bid can be used as adjunctive treatment [109].

Core Message
- Based on current evidence, corticosteroids remain the gold standard of treatment for intermediate uveitis.
- Exclusion of infections and masquerade syndromes before starting corticosteroids is mandatory.
- Systemic corticosteroids (prednisone 1 mg/kg/day) are preferred in bilateral or severe cases for a period of 3 months.

9.4.2 Cyclosporine

Cyclosporine is a potent immunosuppressive agent that selectively inhibits the activation of T cells. The most common side effects associated with the use of cyclosporine are nephrotoxicity and hypertension. Renal toxicity occurs more commonly at dosages greater than 5 mg/kg of body weight per day and with increasing age. Daily dosages of cyclosporine between 2.5 and 5.0 mg/kg alone or in combination with corticosteroids appear to reduce this risk of nephrotoxicity [109]. Several studies have shown the efficacy of cyclosporine in the treatment of various forms of vision-threatening intermediate uveitis [83]. The largest retrospective study to date was conducted by the Systemic Immunosuppressive Therapy for Eye Diseases Cohort Study Research Group [53], where the authors of four tertiary ocular inflammation clinics in the United States observed 373 patients that used cyclosporine as a single immunosuppressive agent between 1979 and 2007 [48] (EBM 2++; B). In this study, 99 patients were affected by intermediate uveitis. In this study, the demographic characteristics of the IU patients were as follows: 60 % female, 11 % aged less than 18 years of age, and 57 % between 18 and 39 years of age, mainly with bilateral intermediate uveitis (88 % of patients). Complete control of inflammation with no activity of uveitis was achieved by 39.3 % of patients at 6 months of follow-up and in 51.8 % at 12 months. Control of inflammation with prednisone less than 5 mg was achieved by 19 % of patients at 6 months. After 1 year of follow-up, these corticosteroid-sparing values raised to 38 % with prednisone ≤10 mg/day and 32 % with prednisone ≤5 mg/day. Only 3.7 % of patients at 6 months and 9.2 % at 1 year achieved control of inflammation without the need of systemic corticosteroids.

Cyclosporine doses of 151–250 mg/day were associated with an increased likelihood of control of inflammation (adjusted relative risk (RR) = 1.89, CI 1.15–3.09) with respect to 150 mg/day or less, but the likelihood of corticosteroid-sparing success was similar across all dosage groups. Doses higher than 250 mg/day were not associated with further therapeutic advantage.

Renal toxicity and hypertension were the most frequently observed side effects leading to cessation of therapy, contributing to 4.3 and 3.2 % of drug discontinuations, respectively, by 1 year of therapy.

Patients older than 55 years of age were several fold more likely to develop treatment-limiting side effects than patients aged 18–39, suggesting that cyclosporine may not be a good choice for many older patients and that such patients should be carefully monitored [48] (EBM 2++; B).

Studies regarding long-term risks of cyclosporine therapy from comprehensive literature review suggest that cancer risk is not substantially elevated with cyclosporine treatment for autoimmune diseases [54, 55] (2++ B).

In another study by Walton and coauthors evaluating the safety and efficacy of cyclosporine in children with severe bilateral uveitis, seven patients were affected by intermediate uveitis. All children were younger than 18 years of age, and the mean total duration of cyclosporine treatment was 45 months. Side effects observed in these children were transient increases in serum creatinine of more than 30 % of baseline value (5 patients), hypertension [1], gingival hyperplasia [2], hirsutism [2], and nausea [1, 110] (EBM 3, D).

The results of Walton's study suggest that cyclosporine is a safe and effective agent in the treatment of severe bilateral intermediate uveitis in children who do not respond to systemic corticosteroids or cytotoxic agents or both. However, children treated with cyclosporine should be treated in cooperation with a pediatric rheumatologist because of differences in the pharmacokinetics of many drugs and immunosuppressives in children including a potential for many different drug interactions which could lead to toxicities [110] (EBM 3, D). Frequent monitoring of blood cyclosporine levels, serum creatinine, creatinine clearance, hemoglobin, and blood pressure may minimize the risk that adverse effects may occur. Increases in serum creatinine or decreases in creatinine clearance of more than 30 % of baseline levels should prompt reductions in cyclosporine dosages. Using these guidelines, children with severe forms of intermediate uveitis can be treated safely while the risk of adverse effects is minimized [110] (EBM 3, D).

In a prospective, randomized, open-label study, Murphy and coworkers compared the efficacy and tolerability of tacrolimus and cyclosporine in posterior and intermediate uveitis. In this study, eight patients with intermediate uveitis were treated with tacrolimus and six patients with cyclosporine and followed up for a median time of 7 months (range 4–18, tacrolimus group) and 4 months (range 3–13, cyclosporine group). The median maintenance drug dose was 4 mg [3–5] for tacrolimus and 250 mg (200–344) for cyclosporine [80] (EBM 2-, D). Overall, the efficacy of tacrolimus and cyclosporine was comparable, with response rates of 67 and 68 % respectively. Tacrolimus and cyclosporine were similar with regard to efficacy for posterior segment intraocular inflammation, but the results suggested a more favorable safety profile for tacrolimus therapy. These findings are similar to those reported in the transplantation literature, in which tacrolimus has been shown to cause significantly fewer toxic effects, particularly with regard to systemic hypertension and hyperlipidemia [80] (EBM 2-, D).

> **Core Message**
> - Dosing regimens of cyclosporine for intermediate uveitis should be between 2.5 and 5 mg/kg/day.
> - Based on current evidence from a large retrospective study (SITE), cyclosporine is effective in controlling intermediate uveitis. Inflammation is absent in 39.3 % of patients at 6 months and in 51.8 % at 12 months (EBM 2++; B).
> - In only 9.2 % of patients treated with cyclosporine was the inflammation controlled without systemic corticosteroids at the end of 12 months.
> - Cyclosporine is also a safe and effective agent in children with severe bilateral intermediate uveitis. However, careful monitoring and collaboration with a pediatric rheumatologist is warranted to reduce the risk of potential systemic side effects (EBM 3, D).

9.4.3 Tacrolimus

Tacrolimus, also called FK506, is a macrolide widely used in organ transplantation. Although structurally different from cyclosporine, the mechanism of action of tacrolimus is similar in that it binds to an intracellular-binding protein (FK) which then associates with calcineurin, thus inhibiting the activation of T cells and production of cytokines. Tacrolimus is significantly more potent than cyclosporine and is given at initial oral doses of 0.05–0.15 mg/kg/day in patients with uveitis. Despite the evidence of tacrolimus' efficacy as a rescue therapy for patients with cyclosporine-refractive uveitis [100] (EBM 3 D), use in ocular inflammation has been limited because early studies demonstrated significant side effects, but target serum levels were double compared to those advocated today. In a recent retrospective study of 62 patients with noninfectious uveitis, Hogan et al. have evaluated the long-term efficacy and tolerance of tacrolimus [42] (EBM 2- D). In this cohort, 16 patients (25.8 %) had intermediate uveitis. There was an 85 % probability of a successful prednisone taper to 10 mg daily after 1 year of treatment; this corticosteroid-sparing success was achieved with a median tacrolimus trough level of 5.2 ng/ml and a median total daily tacrolimus dose of 3 mg. Tacrolimus in this series was discontinued due to intolerance at a rate of 0.13/PY, predominantly due to non-cardiovascular adverse events [42] (EBM 2- D).

Core Messages
- Dosing regimen of tacrolimus for intermediate uveitis should be between 0.05 and 0.15 mg/kg/day.
- Tacrolimus has a similar mechanism of action as cyclosporine but is significantly more potent than cyclosporine.
- A prospective-comparative study between tacrolimus and cyclosporine showed that overall the efficacy of the two drugs in treating intermediate uveitis is similar, but tacrolimus had a superior adverse event profile (EBM 2- D).

9.4.4 Methotrexate

Methotrexate, an antimetabolite drug, has been the most commonly employed immunosuppressive agent for ocular inflammation for several decades. The principal mechanism of action is the reduction of cell proliferation, increasing the rate of T-cell apoptosis, increasing endogenous adenosine concentrations, and altering cytokine production and humoral responses. First introduced as an antineoplastic agent, it was approved by the FDA for the treatment of rheumatoid arthritis in 1988.

In a recent retrospective cohort study [30] (EBM, 2+ C), 38 patients with intermediate uveitis managed at four tertiary ocular inflammation clinics were observed. Patients initiating methotrexate as a sole (non-corticosteroid) immunosuppressive agent during observation constitute the study population reported. All patients were seen between 1979 and 2007.

The majority of patients with intermediate uveitis included in this study were Caucasians (76.3 %), female (73.7 %), with a median age of 32 years and with bilateral inflammation (65.8 %). The highest dose of methotrexate given was 12.5 mg weekly or less in 60 % of patients; only 5.3 % of patients was taking doses greater than 22.5 mg/week. Among patients with active or slightly active inflammation at the start of methotrexate therapy, complete control of inflammation was achieved at 6 months in 47.4 % of patients and at 12 months for 74.9 %. Prednisone could be tapered to $\leq$10 mg/day in 41.3 % of patients at 6 months, and this success rate continued to improve with time and was achieved by 68.8 % of patients at 12 months. Only 7.4 % of patients with intermediate uveitis at 6 months and 15 % at 12 months were able to stop systemic corticosteroids completely. Prior use of other immunosuppressive agents was not associated with significantly different rates of treatment success. No difference in success rates was observed with alternative dosages of methotrexate or with the use of oral versus parenteral therapy. Regarding the tolerability of methotrexate, in this study, 16 % of patients discontinued the treatment because of side effects and 13 % because of ineffectiveness.

Overall, data from this large retrospective study suggest that methotrexate is likely to be well tolerated in patients with intermediate uveitis and adverse reactions are usually reversible and seem to be rare when careful monitoring of liver function test is appropriate [30] (EBM, 2+ C).

In another large retrospective cohort study of 257 patients [27] (EBM 2++, C) comparing the relative effectiveness of antimetabolite drugs, 36 patients included were affected by intermediate uveitis. Among patients with intermediate uveitis, 17 (19 %) were treated with methotrexate, 3 (8 %) with azathioprine, and 16 (12 %) with mycophenolate mofetil. Treatment success was evaluated by various doses of methotrexate: 70 % of treatment success occurred with a dosage between 15 and 20 mg/week and 90 % of success with a dosage between 12.5 and 20 mg/week, suggesting that dosages less than 15 mg/week are less effective. By using incidence curves to evaluate the time to corticosteroid-sparing success, a significant difference was seen between the mycophenolate and methotrexate groups ($p=0.002$) but not between the mycophenolate and azathioprine groups. After 6 months of treatment, corticosteroid-sparing success was achieved in more patients receiving mycophenolate (79 %) than in patients receiving azathioprine (58 %) or methotrexate (42 %). More patients discontinued therapy because of insufficient effect in the methotrexate group. The proportion of patients able to discontinue prednisone after 6 months of antimetabolite therapy was higher in the mycophenolate group (12 %) than in the azathioprine (6 %) or methotrexate (6 %) groups, although this difference was not statistically significant. The rate of side effects (gastrointestinal upset, hematologic abnormalities, liver dysfunction) and the rate of discontinuing therapy because of side effect in azathioprine-treated patients were higher than in the other groups. Data from this study suggests that mycophenolate mofetil was better at achieving a treatment success and did so more rapidly than azathioprine or methotrexate [27] (EBM 2++, C).

In a small retrospective case review of ten children with chronic uveitis (four patients with intermediate uveitis), low-dose methotrexate was shown to be effective and safe in controlling intraocular inflammation for a mean of 22.5 months [65] (EBM 3, D).

In a retrospective non-comparative study of 160 patients [96] (EBM 2+ C), 18 patients with intermediate uveitis were included (11.3 %); the rate of control of inflammation among this group of patients was 88.9 % ($p=0.23$). A corticosteroid-sparing effect was achieved in 64 % of patients treated with an average maintenance dose of methotrexate of 12.3 mg weekly (range, 7.5–40 mg weekly). In 18 % of patients, the drug was discontinued because of adverse events, mainly increased liver function tests, nausea, malaise, and leucopenia [96] (EBM 2+ C).

Core Message

- The dosing regimen of methotrexate for intermediate uveitis should be between 7.5 mg and 20 mg/week. Treatment success of 90 % is achieved with dosage between 12.5 and 20 mg/week, suggesting that dosages less than 15 mg/week are less effective (EBM 2++ C).

- Based on current evidence from the largest retrospective study (SITE), methotrexate is likely to be well tolerated in patients with intermediate uveitis, and important long-term adverse effects are usually reversible and seem to be rare when monitoring is appropriate (EBM 2+ C).

- In the SITE study, control of intraocular inflammation in intermediate uveitis was 47.4 % at 6 months and 74.9 % at 12 months; no differences in success rate were observed with alternative dosages of methotrexate or with the use of oral versus parenteral therapy (EBM 2+ C).

- A comparative study between methotrexate, azathioprine, and mycophenolate mofetil showed that mycophenolate mofetil achieved treatment success more frequently and more rapidly than the other two antimetabolites (EBM 2++ C).

9.4.5 Azathioprine

Azathioprine is a purine nucleoside analog which acts as an antimetabolite by interfering with DNA and RNA synthesis. Similar to methotrexate, it has been widely used in different ocular inflammatory diseases including chronic anterior uveitis, retinal vasculitis, Behcet's disease, and sympathetic ophthalmia as a monotherapy or in combination with other immunosuppressive agents. Randomized clinical trials are lacking and limited to the use of azathioprine for Behcet's disease [37, 113] and a small trial evaluating the efficacy of this drug in anterior uveitis [68, 78, 81].

In the SITE cohort study [89] (EBM, 2+ C) on the use of azathioprine in ocular inflammatory diseases, 18 patients with intermediate uveitis were included. The median age of patients was 44 years; the majority were female (67.3 %), Caucasian (88.9 %), and with bilateral inflammation (72.2 %). Complete control of inflammation was achieved in 69 % of patients at 6 months and 89 % at 12 months, while minimal activity was observed in 87 and 100 % of patients, respectively, at 6 and 12 months. Corticosteroid-sparing effect with less than 10 mg/day of prednisone was reached by 47 % of patients after 6 months and 68 % after 1 year of treatment. Compared to those with other sites of ocular inflammation, patients with intermediate uveitis were more likely to achieve both control of inflammation and corticosteroid-tapering success. Intermediate uveitis patients were seven times more likely to successfully taper corticosteroid as compared to anterior uveitis for both the ≤10 mg and the ≤5 mg levels. Use of higher dosages of azathioprine (125 mg or more per day) did increase the success rate. During a median follow-up of 230 days, 24 % of patients discontinued the drug because of adverse events and 17 % due to inefficacy. The most common side effects were gastrointestinal upset (9 %), bone marrow suppression (5 %), elevated liver enzymes (4 %), and infections (2 %). The results of the present study indicate that azathioprine may be especially favorable in patients with intermediate uveitis, since this degree of response was not observed in the SITE study in patients treated with methotrexate [30].

In another moderate-sized study of 257 patients (36 with intermediate uveitis on the use of azathioprine), 8 % of patients had intermediate uveitis; the proportion of patients with treatment success after 6 months of azathioprine therapy (95 % CI, 42–82 %) was 58 % [27] (EBM 2++, C).

> **Core Message**
> - Dosing regimen of azathioprine in intermediate uveitis: 1–3 mg/kg/day. Use of higher dosages of azathioprine (125 mg or more per day) does not seem to increase the likelihood of a treatment success.
> - Based on current evidence from the SITE study, control of inflammation at 6 months is 69 % and at 12 months is 89 % (EBM, 2+ C).
> - Patients with intermediate uveitis were more likely to achieve both control of inflammation and corticosteroid-tapering success compared to patients with other sites of ocular inflammation.
> - The results of the SITE study indicate that azathioprine may be especially favorable for patients with intermediate uveitis, since this pattern of response was not observed in the other SITE studies (EBM, 2+ C).

9.4.6 Mycophenolate Mofetil

Mycophenolate mofetil is an antimetabolite that selectively inhibits the purine biosynthesis enzyme inosine monophosphate dehydrogenase, causing depletion of guanosine nucleotides that are essential for purine synthesis uses in the proliferation of B and T lymphocytes. Several small- to medium-sized retrospective studies have evaluated the efficacy of mycophenolate mofetil in ocular inflammatory diseases suggesting that it is an effective corticosteroid-sparing agent and that its effectiveness is greater than methotrexate or azathioprine [27, 60] (EBM 2++, C).

In the SITE cohort study on mycophenolate mofetil in ocular inflammatory diseases, 28 patients with intermediate uveitis were included [13] (EBM 2+ C). The median age of patients was 44.3 years; 57 % were female, 71 % were Caucasians, and 67.9 % had bilateral intermediate uveitis. Control of inflammation with no residual activity was achieved in 65 % of patients at 6 months and in 76.7 % at 12 months. Corticosteroid-sparing effect with ≤10 mg of prednisone was achieved by 39 % at 6 months and 49.2 % at 12 months. Multiple regression analysis of time-to-treatment success showed that adults aged 18–39 years tended to respond less well than other age groups. Prior use of immunosuppressive agents tended to be associated with a lower likelihood of treatment success. Patients who had prior treatment with alkylating agents responded especially poorly to mycophenolate mofetil, with a 70 % lower likelihood of treatment success when compared with patients who had never been previously treated. However, patients who previously had receive different antimetabolites such as methotrexate had a likelihood of success similar to that of patients who had not taken immunosuppressive drugs previously [13] (EBM 2+ C). An extended report [103] (EBM 3 D) from one of the centers participating in the SITE cohort study confirmed that patients previously treated with methotrexate often respond to subsequent mycophenolate mofetil therapy, suggesting that mycophenolate mofetil is a reasonable next step for patients failing methotrexate.

About 12 % of patients in the SITE study discontinued treatment within the first year because of side effects such as gastrointestinal upset, but the toxicities were typically reversible with discontinuation of the drug [13] (EBM 2+ C).

In a retrospective non-comparative study of 54 patients treated with mycophenolate mofetil [6] (EBM 3 D), 4 patients were affected by pars planitis. Overall, control of inflammation was achieved in 75 % of patients with a daily dose of 2 g. Control of inflammation was independent of anatomic location. A corticosteroid-sparing effect was achieved in 41.6 % of cases, and adverse reactions were experienced by 44 % of patients [6] (EBM 3 D).

In a study of 17 children [22] (EBM 3 D) with a mean age of 8 years (range 2–13), 10 patients (58.8 %) with intermediate uveitis were treated with mycophenolate mofetil and followed up for a mean of 2.8 years. The dose of MMF given was that recommended in pediatric renal transplant recipients, 600 mg/m² twice daily. The average maintenance dose was 1 g (range 750 mg to 2 g daily). The drug was effective in 7/10 patients, and 5 patients (50 %) were able to discontinue systemic corticosteroids. Side effects during MMF treatment in these children were headache [3], gastrointestinal discomfort [1], rash [1], and leukopenia [1, 22] (EBM 3 D).

In a study of 18 patients with intermediate and posterior uveitis, Greiner and coauthors confirmed the efficacy of mycophenolate mofetil in controlling ocular inflammation in 13 out of 18 patients. Mycophenolate mofetil was given at a daily dose of 2 g in combination with cyclosporine and/or prednisone; corticosteroid-sparing effect was achieved in 14 patients, and 4 patients were able to discontinue corticosteroids. The most frequently observed side effects in this series were myalgia, fatigue, headache, and gastrointestinal discomfort [33] (EBM 3 D).

In a comparative study on effectiveness of antimetabolites in the treatment of intermediate uveitis, Galor et al. confirmed that mycophenolate mofetil was faster than methotrexate in reaching a treatment success and superior to azathioprine in its side effect profile. Nevertheless, other differences exist among antimetabolites including the cost of medication (mycophenolate's cost is higher), the dosing (methotrexate is weekly and more convenient), the availability of an injectable form (only for methotrexate), and the length of experience with children (longer for methotrexate). These factors should be taken into account when deciding on the appropriate immunosuppressive treatment for individual patients [27] (EBM 2++, C).

> **Core Message**
> - Dosing regimen of mycophenolate mofetil in intermediate uveitis is 1 g twice daily.
> - Based on current evidence from the SITE study, control of inflammation was achieved in 65 % of patients at 6 months and 76.7 % at 12 months (EBM 2+ C).
> - Patients between 18 and 39 years tended to respond less well than other age groups.
> - Prior use of immunosuppressive agents, in particular with alkylating agents, is

Table 9.2 Results of the SITE cohort study for cyclosporine, methotrexate, azathioprine, and mycophenolate mofetil referred to patients with only intermediate uveitis

	CSA	MTX	AZA	MMF
N. patients with IU	99	38	18	28
Median age year (range)		32.1 (7.6–63.3)	44.4 (19.6–68.3)	44.3 (19.8–75.4)
Gender, % female	60 (60.6 %)	28 (73.7 %)	13 (72.2 %)	16 (57.1 %)
Race				
% Caucasian	84 (84.8 %)	29 (76.3 %)	16 (88.9 %)	20 (71.4 %)
% Black	8 (8.1 %)	6 (15.8 %)	1 (5.6 %)	5 (17.9 %)
% Others	7 (7.1 %)	3 (7.9 %)	1 (5.6 %)	3 (10.7 %)
Duration of inflammation year (range)	3.2 (0–25.2)	3.3 (0.0–26.7)		5.9 (0.1–22.4)
Bilateral inflammation	88 (88.9 %)	25 (65.8 %)	13 (72.2 %)	19 (67.9 %)
Prednisone ≤10 mg/day		27 (71.1 %)		15 (53.6 %)
Treatment success at 6 months (%)				
No activity	39.3 %	47.4 %	69.3 %	65 %
Without systemic steroids	3.7 %	7.4 %	0 %	0 %
Treatment success at 12 months (%)				
No activity	51.8 %	74.9 %	89.8 %	100 %
Without systemic steroids	9.2 %	15 %	0 %	13.8 %
Discontinuation for				
Side effects	13 %	16 %	24 %	12 %
Ineffectiveness (data for overall anatomic types of uveitis)	6.7 %	13 %	15 %	9.7 %

associated with a lower likelihood of treatment success.

- In children with intermediate uveitis, MMF is effective in 70 % of cases and in 50 % has a corticosteroid-sparing effect (EBM 3 D).
- A comparative study showed that mycophenolate is superior to methotrexate with respect to rapidity of achieving treatment success and superior to azathioprine with respect to its side effect profile (EBM 2++ C).

The results of the SITE cohort study for cyclosporine, methotrexate, azathioprine, and mycophenolate mofetil referred to patients with only intermediate uveitis are summarized in Table 9.2.

9.4.7 Alkylating Agents

The alkylating agents, cyclophosphamide and chlorambucil, work by alkylating DNA resulting in DNA cross-linking and inhibition of DNA synthesis. Because of serious, life-threatening side effects, their use is limited to severe, sight-threatening uveitis that has not responded to less toxic therapy. In the era of new biologic drugs, the use of alkylating agents is reserved to recalcitrant forms of uveitis that have failed conventional treatment and treatment with biologic agents.

9.4.8 Cyclophosphamide

Most of the information on uveitis comes from small case reports on the efficacy of cyclophosphamide in scleritis, Wegener's granulomatosis, Behcet's disease, and serpiginous choroiditis.

The SITE study [93] (EBM, 2+ C) reported on 215 patients who achieved control of inflammation in 49 % of cases at 6 months and 76 % within 12 months but also showed a trend for slightly increased cancer-related mortality. This study demonstrated that cyclophosphamide is not associated with a statistically significant increase in overall mortality (adjusted HR = 1.14, $p = 0.45$), but found that cancer mortality tended to be higher with respect to unexposed cohort (adjusted cancer mortality $HR = 1.61$, $p = 0.17$) and in the US general population (cancer-specific $SMR = 1.42$, $p = 0.056$) [93] (EBM, 2+ C). However, in the SITE study, results on the efficacy of cyclophosphamide on uveitis are not presented based on different anatomic location of ocular inflammation. It is therefore impossible to extrapolate from this SITE study results concerning intermediate uveitis.

The use of intravenous cyclophosphamide therapy once a month has been evaluated in 11 patients refractory or intolerant to oral corticosteroids. Improvement in uveitis was found only in 5 patients, with sustained benefit without additional immunosuppressive agents in only 2 patients [94] (EBM 3 D).

The most common side effect is dose-dependent reversible myelosuppression, although clinicians monitor the degree of leukopenia and neutropenia as a marker for immunosuppressive effect. Other serious side effects include hemorrhagic cystitis and bladder cancer in patients who are unable to maintain adequate hydration. Cyclophosphamide also suppresses ovarian and gonadal function, and patients need to consider ways to maintain future fertility such as sperm or egg banking or the induction of temporary menopause. When given intravenously as a pulse therapy, there may be fewer side effects by avoiding prolonged exposure.

Commonly used doses for ocular inflammatory diseases are 1–3 mg/kg/day, with doses adjusted based on clinical response and degree of leukopenia. Alternatively, it can be given as IV pulse therapy at $1 \ g/m^2$ body surface area every 3–4 weeks.

9.4.9 Chlorambucil

Most of the evidence for chlorambucil comes from treatment series on patients with Behcet's disease.

In a retrospective study of 28 patients treated with chlorambucil, 2 patients with a diagnosis of pars planitis were treated at an initial dose of 6 mg. One was treated for 6 months and the other for 18 months. In both patients with pars planitis, the drug was effective and no other systemic immunosuppressants were required to control ocular inflammation after discontinuation of chlorambucil. One patient in this series had no side effects during treatment, and the other developed temporary amenorrhea [76] (EBM 2- D).

In another report on 53 patients (2 % with pars planitis), short-term (average duration 16 weeks) high-dose (average dose 20 mg/day) chlorambucil was effective in inducing remission in 77 % of patients. Dosing of chlorambucil was started at 2 mg/daily; if the white blood cell count was greater than $3,000/mm^3$, the dose was increased by 2 mg/day each week. Chlorambucil was discontinued if the blood cell count fell below $2,400/mm^3$ or if the platelet count fell below $100,000/mm^3$. Side effects in this retrospective study on chlorambucil were secondary amenorrhea, herpes zoster infection, testicular atrophy, and erectile dysfunction. Two dosing regimens have been used in ocular inflammatory disease. The first regimen for long-term therapy is chlorambucil at 0.1–0.2 mg/kg/day (6–12 mg/day) as a single oral dose, with gradual tapering of corticosteroids as inflammation is controlled. Chlorambucil is continued for 1 year after quiescence is achieved in an effort to induce prolonged remission. The second regimen is a short-term therapy with chlorambucil initiated at a dose of 2 mg/day for 1 week, with increasing the dose by 2 mg/week until inflammation is controlled; the duration of the short-term course is 3–6 months [31] (EBM 3 D).

> **Core Messages**
> - Dosing regimen of cyclophosphamide for intermediate uveitis: 1–3 mg/kg/day.
> - Dosing regimen of chlorambucil for intermediate uveitis:
> - Long term: 0.1–0.2 mg/kg/day (6–12 mg/day)
> - Short term: 2 mg/day and then 2 mg/week for 3–6 months
> - Based on current evidence from the literature, the use of alkylating agents in intermediate uveitis is very limited (EBM 3D).

- Alkylating agents are very potent drugs capable of inducing long-term remission of intraocular inflammation.
- Because of the potential for significant drug-related side effects, those agents should not be used as first-line agents, especially in young patients, and should be reserved for vision-threatening intermediate uveitis recalcitrant to other conventional and newer immunosuppressants.
- Patients treated with alkylating agents should be very carefully selected and monitored by expert hands.

9.4.10 TNF-α Blockers

Tumor necrosis factor (TNF)-α blockers are biologic immunomodulators that have been FDA approved for many systemic inflammatory conditions but are considered off-label for the treatment of ocular inflammatory disease. Although several small case series show promising results with respect to control of intraocular inflammation, there is a lack of randomized clinical trials on the efficacy of these drugs in uveitis. Among the TNF-α blockers, adalimumab and infliximab are the two more commonly used biologics in ocular inflammatory diseases.

A prospective clinical trial evaluated the efficacy of adalimumab in 19 patients with refractory uveitis; 3 patients with idiopathic intermediate uveitis were treated with 40-mg subcutaneous injections of adalimumab every other week during a 12-month follow-up study. All patients showed improvement in vitreous inflammation and visual acuity and had reduction of macular thickness after 12 months of therapy [20] (EBM 2++ C).

In a retrospective longitudinal case series of 43 patients describing the cortico-sparing effect of infliximab and adalimumab in patients with chronic uveitis, 10 patients with intermediate uveitis were included (eight treated with infliximab, two with adalimumab) [67]. Approximately 80 % of patients on infliximab or adalimumab were able to achieve sustained control of inflammation by 6 months. Control of inflammation and corticosteroid-sparing success at 12 months were achieved in 60.9 % of the infliximab group and 57.1 % of the adalimumab group. The overall discontinuation rate for infliximab was 0.26/PY, and the discontinuation rate due to adverse events was 0.11 /PY; two patients had serious pulmonary infections. The overall discontinuation rate for adalimumab was 0.26/PY, and there was no discontinuation due to adverse reactions in this group. This study suggests that infliximab and adalimumab are potentially more effective at controlling inflammation than conventional agents and that control may be achieved more quickly with these biologics agents. However, several months of treatment are required before sustained control of inflammation with corticosteroid sparing can be seen. Most of the patients included in this study received in addition to TNF-α blockers and corticosteroids an antimetabolite [67] (EBM 2- D).

Core Messages
- Dosing regimen of adalimumab for intermediate uveitis: 40-mg subcutaneous injections every 2 weeks.
- Dosing regimen of infliximab for intermediate uveitis: 3 to 10 mg/kg intravenously at 0, 2, and 6 weeks and then every 8 weeks.
- Based on current evidence, infliximab and adalimumab are potentially more effective at controlling intermediate uveitis than conventional agents; control of inflammation may be achieved more rapidly with biologics compared to conventional treatment (EBM 2- D).
- Regarding their corticosteroid-sparing effect, several months of treatment are required with biologics with sustained control of inflammation before successful taper of steroids is possible.

9.4.11 Interferon

Interferon (IFN) alpha is a cytokine belonging to the subgroup of type I interferons that have strong antiviral, antiproliferative, and various immunomodulatory effects. It is approved for the treatment of viral hepatitis, myeloproliferative disorders, and lymphomas. However, during the past years, IFN has also been employed with success in the treatment of patients with Behcet's disease [16, 17, 56] (EBM 3 D) with ocular involvement and for other types of refractory uveitis [9] (EBM 2-D). In a recent retrospective large study on the efficacy and tolerability of IFN alpha treatment in 24 consecutive patients with chronic cystoid macular edema, 18 patients (75 %) with intermediate uveitis were included [17] (EBM 3 D). The majority of patients had bilateral cystoid macular edema, and the median duration of the edema before IFN treatment was 36 months, and the median follow-up time was 21 months. INF treatment was very effective, demonstrating remission or partial remission of macular edema in 87.5 % of patients or 62.5 % of the eyes, and the vast majority of patients responded very quickly showing complete resolution of macular edema within 2 weeks. However, these data do not show any correlation between the grade of efficacy of IFN therapy and the duration of cystoid macular edema or the underlying uveitis condition (anterior, intermediate, or posterior). Although side effects occurred frequently in this series (mostly flu-like symptoms, fatigue, and increased liver enzymes), IFN treatment was generally well tolerated; most of the side effects were mild to moderate and dose dependent. The authors pointed out that the occurrence of flu-like symptoms after initiation of IFN therapy might be a positive sign with regard to the response of a patient. Thus, if a patient displays no flu-like symptoms or if therapy ceases to have an effect after the initial response, anti-TNF autoantibodies have to be excluded [17] (EBM 3 D).

In another report, in 13 patients with intermediate uveitis associated with multiple sclerosis, interferon beta (IFN-β) was reported to have beneficial effects on ocular inflammation. In this retrospective study, the median age of patients was 48 years, and the majority of them had bilateral uveitis recalcitrant to several immunosuppressive agents. After a median of 2.3 years following the onset of uveitis, patients were put on IFN-β treatment. During the median total observation time of 18.7 months, 71 % of the eyes improved their visual acuity, and in 21 % of patients, the visual acuity remained stable. Vitreous cell count also improved in 71 % of the eyes. At the last visit, 69 % of patients were not on systemic corticosteroids, and a reduction in the dose of prednisone to 10 mg/day or less had been documented in all patients. Side effects such as myopathy, depression, and dizziness were seen in 23 % of patients [7] (EBM 3 D).

> **Core Messages**
> - Dosing regimen of interferon α-2a for intermediate uveitis: initial dose three million (body weight ≤70 kg) or six million IU (body weight ≥70 kg) per day subcutaneously.
> - Dosing regimen of interferon β for intermediate uveitis:
>   - 22 or 44 µg, 3 times per week subcutaneously
>   - 30 µg once a week intramuscularly
> - Based on current evidence, interferon α-2a is very effective and rapid in resolution of macular edema associated with intermediate uveitis (EBM 3 D).
> - Side effects with interferon α-2a are frequent but usually mild to moderate and dose dependent.
> - Interferon β is effective in the treatment of intermediate uveitis associated with multiple sclerosis (EBM 3 D).

9.4.12 Daclizumab

Daclizumab is a humanized monoclonal antibody that binds to the CD25 portion of the IL-2 receptor on activated T cells that has been first used in patients undergoing renal transplantation showing an improvement of graft survival. A randomized, open-label study, phase I/II clinical trial showed that infusion of daclizumab every 4 weeks was effective in the treatment of intermediate and posterior noninfectious uveitis. In this study, three patients with intermediate uveitis were enrolled and the long-term administration of daclizumab drug was effective in controlling uveitis [82] (EBM 1- B).

In a more recent long-term study, Wroblewski et al. evaluated the efficacy and safety of daclizumab in 39 patients with noninfectious intermediate and posterior uveitis. Daclizumab was administered intravenously (1 mg/kg every 2 weeks for 1 month followed by monthly 1 mg/kg), subcutaneously (1 mg/kg monthly), or by high-dose intravenous injection (8 mg/kg IV followed by 4 mg/kg IV after 2 weeks). Six patients with idiopathic intermediate uveitis were included in this study. Daclizumab was effective in reducing concomitant immunosuppressive medication, in stabilizing visual acuity, and in preventing uveitis flares in most study patients. Cutaneous reactions were the most commonly observed adverse events with daclizumab therapy. Four out of 39 patients developed solid tumor *malignancies* during the 11-year period of observation. The side effect profile of daclizumab seems acceptable in the context of side effects associated with more conventional immunosuppressives, but the malignancy rate of this drug merits further review [112] (EBM 2- D).

> **Core Messages**
>
> - Dosing regimen of daclizumab for intermediate uveitis:
>   - Intravenously: 1 mg/kg every 2 weeks for 1 month followed by monthly 1 mg/kg
>   - Subcutaneously: 1 mg/kg/kg monthly
>   - High dose: 8 mg/kg IV followed by 4 mg/kg IV after 2 weeks
> - Based on current evidence, long-term daclizumab is effective in controlling intermediate uveitis, allowing a reduction of concomitant immunosuppressive medications, stabilization of visual acuity, and prevention of recurrences (EBM 1- B).
> - However, the side effect profile of daclizumab, particularly an increased risk of malignancies, merits further investigation and limits the use of this drug for intermediate uveitis, which is usually responsive to alternate medications (EBM 2- D).

9.5 Surgical Treatment

9.5.1 Cryotherapy

If the administration of local corticosteroids and systemic nonsteroidal anti-inflammatory drugs fails to control intraocular inflammation, cryotherapy (and laser photocoagulation) is a useful therapeutic alternative in patients with intermediate uveitis.

The exact mechanism is unknown. Josephberg and colleagues (EBM 3D) performed peripheral fluorescein angiography in 20 eyes affected by pars planitis before and after peripheral retinal cryotherapy. They showed that fluorescein leakage was reduced following treatment and postulated that it is secondary to a decrease in angiogenic factors by the ischemic peripheral retina in the areas of capillary dropout. They also suggested that the direct ablation of leaking vessels might also be a contributing factor in some cases [47].

Devenyi and associates (EBM 3D) recommended cryotherapy for neovascularization of the vitreous base in patients with pars planitis. They reported, in a series of patients affected by intermediate uveitis, inflammatory quiescence in 21 eyes (78 %), and intermittent inflammation in 5 eyes (18 %) after cryotherapy [19].

Similarly, favorable results were observed by Okinami (EBM 3D) with 61 % regression of inflammation after a single cryotherapy treatment in 28 eyes [85].

In a small randomized study (EBM 2-D) in which cryotherapy was compared with corticosteroids, cryotherapy was superior in improving visual acuity at 6 months [108].

Although favorable results have been reported with cryotherapy, this approach can promote the development of epiretinal membranes, cataract, and retinal detachments and can exacerbate macular edema [85].

9.5.2 Laser Photocoagulation

Panretinal photocoagulation has been shown to be effective for the treatment of peripheral neovascularization associated with IU. Park and associates (EBM 2-D) demonstrated the regression of neovascularization with stabilization of inflammation, reduction in cystoid macular edema, and improvement in visual acuity in six patients (ten eyes) presented with vitritis, cystoid macular edema, and neovascularization of the vitreous base, unresponsive to corticosteroid therapy. Three patients (five eyes) received scatter diode or argon photocoagulation treatment alone. The other three patients (five eyes) underwent pars plana vitrectomy coupled with argon or diode photocoagulation, placed in three rows, posterior to the area of inferior neovascularization of the vitreous base [87, 92].

Advantages of laser photocoagulation include ease of treatment delivery, fewer complications, and reduced ocular morbidity as compared to cryotherapy. In particular, Pulido et al. reported no cases of posttreatment tractional retinal detachments.

Incidence of epiretinal membrane formation after laser photocoagulation increases from 23 to 46 % (EBM 3D) [92], and it may be limited by the presence of vitreous opacity.

In conclusion, considering the apparent lack of significant complications, this treatment appears to be a viable therapeutic alternative in patients with pars planitis or may be used in place of or prior to the use of cryotherapy in patients unresponsive to corticosteroids.

9.5.3 Vitrectomy

Pars plana vitrectomy is usually required to manage complications such as vitreous opacities, hemorrhages, vitreoretinal tractions, and epireti-

nal membranes. Over the last decade, several reports have claimed that vitrectomy can have a beneficial effect on the natural history of the disease, in particular the grade of inflammation and macular. The reason for the anti-inflammatory effect is unknown, but some authors proposed that during vitrectomy, the vitreous cytokines and the removal of pro-inflammatory factors associated with the removal of inflammatory cells from the vitreous might be responsible for this amelioration [36, 39, 75, 111].

The positive effects of vitrectomy in 42 eyes of 32 patients have been reported by Wiechens and colleagues (EBM 3D). A regression of macular edema and an improvement in visual acuity of 59 % and 50 %, respectively, were observed after PPV [111].

Controversial results have been published on the outcome of the eyes affected by cystoid macula edema after PPV with some authors observing a success rate of 80 % and others reporting only minor effects. In a retrospective review, Heiligenhaus and associates (EBM 3D) observed 16 patients with IU who underwent PPV. In this review, the frequency and severity of inflammatory episodes decreased, and in three cases, macular edema resolved completely. Moreover, six patients were able to discontinue oral corticosteroids after vitrectomy [38].

Dugel and colleagues (EBM 3D) reported the visual acuity improvement and attenuation of macular edema unresponsive to corticosteroids in 7 of the 11 eyes that underwent vitrectomy [23].

Conversely, Schönfeld and coworkers (EBM 3D) reported that in 75 % of 42 eyes with IU undergoing PPV, visual acuity improved only to 20/200 suggesting that preexisting macular pathology limited the final visual outcome. The possible cause could be the presence of longstanding CME which can lead to retinal degeneration with permanent visual loss. Therefore, aggressive control of inflammatory activity by local and systemic anti-inflammatory and immunosuppressive therapy is mandatory to prevent serious long-term complications. However, it is still unclear whether aggressive treatment in the early stages can ameliorate the course of intermediate uveitis and thus the final visual outcome [98].

Epiretinal membrane formation is a frequent complication and cause of visual loss in patients with pars planitis [66]. Mieler and colleagues (EBM 3D) and Muralidhar and coauthors (EBM 3D) reported in two different case reports the positive effect of the epiretinal membrane peeling in improving visual acuity outcome [74, 79]. Moreover, Dev and associates demonstrated in a consecutive non-comparative study (EBM 3D) that the removal of the epiretinal membranes in seven patients affected by pars planitis was able to improve visual acuity over a 9-year follow-up time [18].

Vitrectomy is known to be a safe and effective procedure for non-cleaning vitreous hemorrhage caused by many conditions [101]. Two case reports and a case series of six eyes (EBM 3D) showed an improvement in visual acuity after vitrectomy without postoperative complications [75, 91, 101]. Molina-Prat and associates (EBM 3D) in another series of 7 eyes with vitreous hemorrhage observed vision improvement in all. Worsening of cataract and a postoperative increased ocular pressure in this series were present respectively in 40.9 % and in 18.2 % of treated eyes [77].

> **Core Message**
> - Cryotherapy and laser photocoagulation are useful therapeutic alternatives in patients with IU when local and systemic treatments have failed.
> - Vitrectomy may be considered in patients with IU and severe vitreous opacities or vitreous hemorrhages unresponsive to systemic treatment.
> - The efficacy of PPV remains an open question since no RCT is present in the literature.

9.5.4 Cataract Surgery

Cataract is a well-known complication in patients with pars planitis, secondary to chronic inflammation, long-term corticosteroids use, and vitrectomy surgery. Generally, cataract extraction is a safe procedure if intraocular inflammation is con-trolled with systemic treatment for a minimum of 3 months before surgery (EBM 3D) [1].

The safety of intraocular lens implantation in patients with IU was demonstrated in a prospective randomized study where no statistical significant differences were found at 1 year for visual acuity between the group with and without intraocular IOL implantation (EBM 2+C) [104].

Ganesh and associates evaluated a series of 100 eyes affected by pars planitis that underwent implantation with either polymethyl methacrylate (PMMA), heparin-surface-modified PMMA, or hydrophobic acrylic lens. The authors reported no statistically significant differences in postoperative visual outcome or surgery-related complications [29] (EBM 2+C). Kaufman and associates reported a postoperative visual acuity of 20/40 or better in 17 eyes (88 %) following cataract extraction in patients affected by intermediate uveitis. The factors that limited visual recovery in their series of patients were primarily macular edema, epiretinal membrane, and optic atrophy (EBM 2-D) [51].

To minimize vision-threatening complications in patients with IU, it is important to provide a close postsurgical follow-up and aggressively treat postoperative inflammation (EBM 3D) [1, 26]. Postoperative inflammation can lead to complications such as lens dislocation. In a series of 15 eyes with pars planitis that underwent extra-capsular cataract extraction with intraocular lens implantation, two eyes required lens explantation and five eyes required multiple laser or surgical procedures to clear posterior capsular membranes. Despite these complications, 50 % of the eyes achieved a postoperative visual acuity of 20/40 or better (EBM 3D) [73]. In a more recent retrospective study of 44 consecutive cases, Michaeli and associates reported that iris fixation is an effective method for treating subluxated IOLs (EBM 3D) [72].

Cataract extraction can be followed by PPV in a single- or two-step procedure (EBM 3D) [3, 26, 73]. The two approaches are equivalent for efficacy and safety, but the sequential surgery could be advantageous to minimize the postoperative anterior chamber inflammatory response [105]. Finally, a recent paper demonstrated that in 21 eyes with severe uveitis, a fluocinolone acetonide implant insertion can be combined safely with phacoemulsification plus IOL implantation during the same surgical session without any intraoperative complications. This technique seems to be useful in improving visual acuity and decreasing uveitic recurrences and the need for immunosuppression (EBM 3D) [11].

> **Core Message**
> - Cataract extraction may be performed in patients with IU when intraocular inflammation is controlled.
> - The safety of IOL implantation has been largely demonstrated.
> - Cataract extraction may be associated with PPV in one or two subsequent steps.

References

1. Akova YA, Küçükerdönmez C, Gedik S. Clinical results of phacoemulsification in patients with uveitis. Ophthalmic Surg Lasers Imaging. 2006;37(3):204–11.
2. Andrasch RH, Pirofsky B, Burns RP. Immunosuppressive therapy for severe chronic uveitis. Arch Ophthalmol. 1978;96:247–51.
3. Androudi S, Ahmed M, Fiore T, Brazitikos P, Foster CS. Combined pars plana vitrectomy and phacoemulsification to restore visual acuity in patients with chronic uveitis. J Cataract Refract Surg. 2005;31(3):472–8.
4. Androudi S, Letko E, Meniconi M, Papadaki T, Ahmed M, Foster CS. Safety and efficacy of intravitreal triamcinolone acetonide for uveitic macular edema. Ocul Immunol Inflamm. 2005;13(2–3):205–12.
5. Babu BM, Rathinam SR. Intermediate uveitis. Indian J Ophthalmol. 2010;58(1):21–7.
6. Baltatzis S, Tufail F, Yu EN, Vredeveld CM, Foster CS. Mycophenolate mofetil as an immunomodulatory agent in the treatment of chronic ocular inflammatory disorders. Ophthalmology. 2003;110(5):1061–5.
7. Becker MD, Heiligenhaus A, Hudde T, Storch-Hagenlocher B, et al. Interferon as a treatment for uveitis associated with multiple sclerosis. Br J Ophthalmol. 2005;89:1254–7.
8. Bloch-Michel E, Nussenblatt RB. International Uveitis study Group recommendations for the evaluation of intraocular inflammatory disease. Am J Ophthalmol. 1987;103:234–5.
9. Bodaghi B, Gendron G, Wechsler B, et al. Efficacy of interferon alpha in the treatment of refractory and sight threatening uveitis: a retrospective monocentric study of 45 patients. Br J Ophthalmol. 2007;91:335–9.
10. Callanan DG, Jaffe GJ, Martin DF, Pearson PA, Comstock TL. Treatment of posterior uveitis with a fluocinolone acetonide implant: three-year clinical trial results. Arch Ophthalmol. 2008;126(9):1191–201.
11. Chieh JJ, Carlson AN, Jaffe GJ. Combined fluocinolone acetonide intraocular delivery system insertion, phacoemulsification, and intraocular lens implantation for severe uveitis. Am J Ophthalmol. 2008;146(4):589–94.
12. Dandona L, Dandona R, John RK, et al. Population based assessment of uveitis in an urban population in southern India. Br J Ophthalmol. 2000;84:706–9.
13. Daniel E, Thorne JE, Newcomb CW, Pujari SS, et al. Mycophenolate mofetil for ocular inflammation. Am J Ophthalmol. 2010;149:423–32.
14. Darrell RW, Wegener HP, Kurlnand LT. Epidemiology of uveitis: incidence and prevalence in a small urban community. Arch Ophthalmol. 1962;68:502–14.
15. Deane JS, Rosenthal AR. Course and complications of intermediate uveitis. Acta Ophthalmol Scand. 1997;75:82–4.
16. Deuter CME, Kotter I, Wallace GR, et al. Behçet's disease: ocular effects and treatment. Prog Retin Eye Res. 2008;27:111–36.
17. Deuter CME, Kotter I, Gunaydin I, Stubiger N, et al. Efficacy and tolerability of interferon alpha treatment in patients with chronic cystoids macular oedema due to noninfectious uveitis. Br J Ophthalmol. 2009;93:906–13.
18. Dev S, Mieler WF, Pulido JS, Mittra RA. Visual outcomes after pars plana vitrectomy for epiretinal membranes associated with pars planitis. Ophthalmology. 1999;106(6):1086–90.
19. Devenyi RG, Mieler WF, Lambrou FH, Will BR, Aaberg TM. Cryopexy of the vitreous base in the management of peripheral uveitis. Am J Ophthalmol. 1988;106(2):135–8.
20. Diaz-Llopis M, Garcia-Delpech S, Salom D, Udaondo P, et al. Adalimumab therapy for refractory uveitis: a pilot study. J Ocul Pharmacol Ther. 2008;24:351–61.
21. Donaldson MJ, Pulido JS, Herman DC, Diehl N, Hodge D. Pars planitis: a 20-year study of incidence, clinical features, and outcomes. Am J Ophthalmol. 2007;144:812–7.
22. Doycheva D, Deuter C, Stuebiger N, et al. Mycophenolate mofetil in the treatment of uveitis in children. Br J Ophthalmol. 2007;91:180–4.
23. Dugel PU, Rao NA, Ozler S, Liggett PE, Smith RE. Pars plana vitrectomy for intraocular inflammation-related cystoid macular edema unresponsive to corticosteroids. A preliminary study. Ophthalmology. 1992;99(10):1535–41.
24. Edelman JL. Differentiating intraocular glucocorticoids. Ophthalmologica. 2010;224 Suppl 1:25–30.
25. Ferrante P, Ramsey A, Bunce C, Lightman S. Clinical trial to compare efficacy and side-effects of injection of posterior sub-Tenon triamcinolone versus orbital floor methylprednisolone in the management of posterior uveitis. Clin Exp Ophthalmol. 2004;32(6):563–8.

26. Fogla R, Biswas J, Ganesh SK, Ravishankar K. Evaluation of cataract surgery in intermediate uveitis. Ophthalmic Surg Lasers. 1999;30(3):191–8.

27. Galor A, Jabs DA, Leder HA, Kedhar SR, et al. Comparison of antimetabolite drugs as corticosteroid-sparing therapy for noninfectious ocular inflammation. Ophthalmology. 2008;115:1826–32.

28. Galor A, Margolis R, Brasil OM, Perez VL, Kaiser PK, Sears JE, Lowder CY, Smith SD. Adverse events after intravitreal triamcinolone in patients with and without uveitis. Ophthalmology. 2007;114(10):1912–8.

29. Ganesh SK, Babu K, Biswas J. Phacoemulsification with intraocular lens implantation in cases of pars planitis. J Cataract Refract Surg. 2004;30(10):2072–6.

30. Gangaputra S, Newcomb CW, Liesegang TL, Kaçmaz O, et al. Methotrexate for ocular inflammatory diseases. Ophthalmology. 2009;116:2188–98.

31. Goldstein DA, Fontanilla FA, Kaul S, Sahin O, Tessler HH. Long-term follow-up of patients treated with short-term high-dose chlorambucil for sight-threatening ocular inflammation. Ophthalmology. 2002;109:370–7.

32. Goldstein DA, Godfrey DG, Hall A, et al. Intraocular pressure in patients with uveitis treated with fluocinolone acetonide implants. Arch Ophthalmol. 2007; 125(11):1478–85.

33. Greiner K, Varikkara M, Santiago C, Forrester JV. Efficiency of mycophenolate mofetil in the treatment of intermediate and posterior uveitis. Ophthalmologe. 2002;99:691–4.

34. Gritz DC, Wong IG. Incidence and prevalence of uveitis in Northern California: the Northern California Epidemiology of Uveitis Study. Ophthalmology. 2004;111:491–500.

35. Guest S, Funkhouser E, Lightman S. Pars planitis: a comparison of childhood onset and adult onset disease. Clin Exp Ophthalmol. 2001;29:81–4.

36. Gutfleisch M, Spital G, Mingels A, Pauleikhoff D, Lommatzsch A, Heiligenhaus A. Pars plana vitrectomy with intravitreal triamcinolone: effect on uveitic cystoid macular oedema and treatment limitations. Br J Ophthalmol. 2007;91(3):345–8.

37. Hamuryudan V, Ozyazgan Y, Hizli N, et al. Azathioprine in Behcet's syndrome: effects on long-term prognosis. Arthritis Rheum. 1997;40:769–74.

38. Heiligenhaus A, Bornfeld N, Foerster MH, Wessing A. Long-term results of pars plana vitrectomy in the management of complicated uveitis. Br J Ophthalmol. 1994;78(7):549–54.

39. Heimann K, Schmanke L, Brunner R, Amerian B. Pars plana vitrectomy in the treatment of chronic uveitis. Dev Ophthalmol. 1992;23:196–203.

40. Helm CJ, Holland GN. The effects of posterior subtenon injection of triamcinolone acetonide in patients with intermediate uveitis. Am J Ophthalmol. 1995; 120:55–64.

41. Henderly DE, Genstler AJ, Smith RE, et al. Changing patterns of uveitis. Am J Ophthalmol. 1987;103:131–6.

42. Hogan AC, McAvoy CE, Dick AD, Lee RWJ. Long-term efficacy and tolerance of tacrolimus for the treatment of uveitis. Ophthalmology. 2007;114:1000–6.

43. Hogewind BF, Zijlstra C, Klevering BJ, Hoyng CB. Intravitreal triamcinolone for the treatment of refractory macular edema in idiopathic intermediate or posterior uveitis. Eur J Ophthalmol. 2008;18(3):429–34.

44. Jabs DA, Nussenblatt RB, Rosenbaum JT. Standardization of uveitis nomenclature for reporting clinical data: results of the First International Workshop, Standardization of Uveitis Nomenclature (SUN) Working Group. Am J Ophthalmol. 2005;140:509–16.

45. Jaffe GJ. Reimplantation of a fluocinolone acetonide sustained drug delivery implant for chronic uveitis. Am J Ophthalmol. 2008;145(4):667–75.

46. Jaffe GJ, Martin D, Callanan D, Pearson PA, Levy B, Comstock T. Fluocinolone acetonide implant (Retisert) for noninfectious posterior uveitis: thirty-four-week results of a multicenter randomized clinical study. Ophthalmology. 2006;113(6):1020–7.

47. Josephberg RG, Kanter ED, Jaffee RM. A fluorescein angiographic study of patients with pars planitis and peripheral exudation (snowbanking) before and after cryopexy. Ophthalmology. 1994;101(7):1262–6.

48. Kaçmaz O, Kempen JH, Newcomb CW, Daniel E, et al. Cyclosporine for ocular inflammatory diseases. Ophthalmology. 2010;117:576–84.

49. Kalinina Ayuso V, ten Cate HAT, van den Does P, Rothova A, de Boer JH. Young age as a risk factor for complicated course and visual outcome in intermediate uveitis in children. Br J Ophthalmol. 2011;95:646–51.

50. Kaplan HJ. intermediate uveitis (pars planitis, chronic cyclitis)-a four step approach to treatment. In: Saari KM, editor. Uveitis update. Amsterdam: Excerpta Medica; 1984. p. 169–72.

51. Kaufman AH, Foster CS. Cataract extraction in patients with pars planitis. Ophthalmology. 1993;100(8):1210–7.

52. Kempen JH, Altaweel MM, Holbrook JT, Jabs DA, Louis TA, Sugar EA, Thorne JE. 2011. Ophthalmology. 2011;118(10):1916–26.

53. Kempen JH, Daniel E, Gangaputra S, et al. Methods for identifying long-term adverse effects of treatment in patients with eye diseases: the Systemic Immunosuppressive Therapy for Eye Diseases (SITE) Cohort Study. Ophthalmic Epidemiol. 2008;15:47–55.

54. Kempen JH, Gangaputra S, Daniel E, et al. Long-term risk of malignancy among patients treated with immunosuppressive agents for ocular inflammation: a critical assessment of the evidence. Am J Ophthalmol. 2008;146:802–12.

55. Kempen JH, Daniel E, Dunn JP, Foster CS, Gangaputra S, Hanish A, Helzlsouer KJ, Jabs DA, Kaçmaz RO, Levy-Clarke GA, Liesegang TL, Newcomb CW, Nussenblatt RB, Pujari SS, Rosenbaum JT, Suhler EB, Thorne JE. Overall and cancer related mortality among patients with ocular inflammation treated with immunosuppressive drugs: retrospective cohort study. BMJ. 2009;339:b2480.

56. Kotter I, Gunaydin I, Zierhut M, et al. The use of interferon a in Behçet disease: review of the literature. Semin Arthritis Rheum. 2004;33:320–35.

57. Kuppermann BD, Blumenkranz MS, Haller JA, et al. Randomized controlled study of an intravitreous

dexamethasone drug delivery system in patients with persistent macular edema. Arch Ophthalmol. 2007; 125(3):309–17.

58. Kwak HW, D'Amico DJ. Evaluation of the retinal toxicity and pharmacokinetics of dexamethasone after intravitreal injection. Arch Ophthalmol. 1992;110(2):259–66.

59. Lafranco Dafflon M, Tran VT, Guex-Crosier Y, Herbort CP. Posterior sub-Tenon's steroid injections for the treatment of posterior ocular inflammation: indications, efficacy and side effects. Graefes Arch Clin Exp Ophthalmol. 1999;237(4):289–95.

60. Lau CH, Comer M, Lightman S. Long-term efficacy of mycophenolate mofetil in the control of severe intraocular inflammation. Clin Exp Ophthalmol. 2003;31:487–91.

61. Leder HA, Jabs DA, Galor A, Dunn JP, Thorne JE. Periocular triamcinolone acetonide injections for cystoid macular edema complicating noninfectious uveitis. Am J Ophthalmol. 2011;152(3):441–8.

62. Lin P, Loh AR, Margolis TP, Acharaya NR. Cigarette smoking as a risk factor for uveitis. Ophthalmology. 2010;117:585–90.

63. Lobo AM, Sobrin L, Papaliodis GN. Drug delivery options for the treatment of ocular inflammation. Semin Ophthalmol. 2010;25:283–8.

64. Lowder C, Belfort Jr R, Lightman S, et al. Dexamethasone intravitreal implant for noninfectious intermediate or posterior uveitis. Arch Ophthalmol. 2011;129(5):545–53.

65. Malik AR, Pavesio C. The use of low dose methotrexate in children with chronic anterior and intermediate uveitis. Br J Ophthalmol. 2005;89:806–8.

66. Malinowski SM, Pulido JS, Folk JC. Long-term visual outcome and complications associated with pars planitis. Ophthalmology. 1993;100:818–24.

67. Martel JN, Esterberg E, Nagpal A, Acharya NR. Infliximab and adalimumab for uveitis. Ocul Immunol Inflamm. 2012;20:18–26.

68. Mathews JD, Crawford BA, Bignell JL, Mackay IR. Azathioprine in active chronic iridocyclitis. A double-blind controlled trial. Br J Ophthalmol. 1969;53:327–30.

69. Mayr WT, Pittock SJ, McClelland RL, et al. Incidence and prevalence of multiple sclerosis in Olmsted County, Minnesota, 1985–2000. Neurology. 2003;61:1373–7.

70. Mc Cannel CA, Holland GN, Helm CJ, et al. Causes of uveitis in the general practice of ophthalmology, UCLA community-based Uveitis Study Group. Am J Ophthalmol. 1996;121:35–46.

71. McCuen 2nd BW, Bessler M, Tano Y, Chandler D, Machemer R. The lack of toxicity of intravitreally administered triamcinolone acetonide. Am J Ophthalmol. 1981;91(6):785–8.

72. Michaeli A, Soiberman U, Loewenstein A. Outcome of iris fixation of subluxated intraocular lenses. Graefes Arch Clin Exp Ophthalmol. 2012;250(9):1327–32.

73. Michelson JB, Friedlaender MH, Nozik RA. Lens implant surgery in pars planitis. Ophthalmology. 1990;97(8):1023–6.

74. Mieler WF, Aaberg TM. Vitreous surgery in the management of peripheral uveitis. Dev Ophthalmol. 1992;23:239–50.

75. Mieler WF, Will BR, Lewis H, Aaberg TM. Vitrectomy in the management of peripheral uveitis. Ophthalmology. 1988;95(7):859–64.

76. Miserocchi E, Baltatsis S, Ekong A, Roque M, Foster CS. Efficacy and safety of chlorambucil in intractable noninfectious uveitis. Ophthalmology. 2002;109:137–42.

77. Molina-Prat N, Adán AM, Mesquida M, Pelegrini L, Rey A, Alvarez G. Vitrectomy surgery for the treatment of the vitreo-retinal complications of the pars planitis. Arch Soc Esp Oftalmol. 2010;85(10):333–6.

78. Moore CE. Sympathetic ophthalmitis treated with azathioprine. Br J Ophthalmol. 1968;52:688–90.

79. Muralidhar NS, Playfair TJ, Gregory-Roberts JC. Surgery for pre-macular fibrosis. Aust N Z J Ophthalmol. 1990;18:91–3.

80. Murphy CC, Greiner K, Plskova J, et al. Cyclosporine vs tacrolimus therapy for posterior and intermediate uveitis. Arch Ophthalmol. 2005;123:634–41.

81. Newell FW, Krill AE. Treatment of uveitis with azathioprine (Imuran). Trans Ophthalmol Soc U K. 1967;87:499–511.

82. Nussenblatt RB, Fortin E, Schiffman R, Rizzo L, et al. Treatment of noninfectious intermediate and posterior uveitis with the humanized anti-Tac mAb: a phase I/II clinical trial. Proc Natl Acad Sci. 1999;96:7462–6.

83. Nussenblatt RB, Palestine AG, Chan CC, et al. Randomized, double-masked study of cyclosporine compared to prednisolone in the treatment of endogenous uveitis. Am J Ophthalmol. 1991; 112:13846.

84. Nussenblatt RB, Withcup SM, Palestine AG. Intermediate uveitis. In: Uveitis. Fundamentals and clinical practice. 2nd ed. St. Louis: Mosby; 1996. p. 279–88.

85. Okinami S, Sunakawa M, Arai I, Iwaki M, Nihira M, Ogino N. Treatment of pars planitis with cryotherapy. Ophthalmologica. 1991;202(4):180–6.

86. Parchand S, Tandan M, Gupta V, Gupta A. Intermediate uveitis in Indian population. J Ophthalmic Inflamm Infect. 2011;1:65–70.

87. Park SE, Mieler WF, Pulido JS. 2 peripheral scatter photocoagulation for neovascularization associated with pars planitis. Arch Ophthalmol. 1995;113(10):1277–80.

88. Paroli MP, Spinucci G, Monte R, Pesci FR, Abicca I, Pivetti Pezzi P. Intermediate uveitis in a pediatric Italian population. Ocul Immunol Inflamm. 2011;19:321–6.

89. Pasadhika S, Kempen JH, Newcomb CW, Liesegang TL, Pujari SS, Rosenbaum JT, Thorne JE, Foster CS, Jabs DA, Levy-Clarke GA, Nussenblatt RB, Suhler EB. Azathioprine for ocular inflammatory diseases. Am J Ophthalmol. 2009;148:500–9.

90. Pavesio C, Zierhut M, Bairi K, Comstock TL, Usner DW, Fluocinolone Acetonide Study Group. Evaluation of an intravitreal fluocinolone acetonide implant versus

standard systemic therapy in noninfectious posterior uveitis. Ophthalmology. 2010;117(3):567–75. 575.

91. Potter MJ, Myckatyn SO, Maberley AL, Lee AS. Vitrectomy for pars planitis complicated by vitreous hemorrhage: visual outcome and long-term follow-up. Am J Ophthalmol. 2001;131(4):514–5.

92. Pulido JS, Mieler WF, Walton D, Kuhn E, Postel E, Hartz A, Jampol LM, Weinberg DV, Logani S. Results of peripheral laser photocoagulation in pars planitis. Trans Am Ophthalmol Soc. 1998;96:127–37.

93. Pujari SS, Kempen JH, Newcomb CW, Gangaputra S, et al. Cyclophosphamide for ocular inflammatory diseases. Ophthalmology. 2010;117:356–65.

94. Rosenbaum JT. Treatment of severe refractory uveitis with intravenous cyclophosphamide. J Rheumatol. 1994;21:123–5.

95. Ryan SJ. Retina. 4th ed. New Delhi: Elsevier/Mosby; 2006. p. 1699–710.

96. Samson CM, Waheed N, Baltatsis S, Foster CS. Methotrexate therapy for chronic noninfectious uveitis: analysis of a case series of 160 patients. Ophthalmology. 2001;108:1134–9.

97. Scholes GN, O'Brien WJ, Abrams GW, Kubicek MF. Clearance of triamcinolone from vitreous. Arch Ophthalmol. 1985;103(10):1567–9.

98. Schönfeld CL, Weissschädel S, Heidenkummer HP, Kampik A. Vitreoretinal surgery in intermediate uveitis. Ger J Ophthalmol. 1995;4(1):37–42.

99. Sivaprasad S, McCluskey P, Lightman S. Intravitreal steroids in the management of macular oedema. Acta Ophthalmol Scand. 2006;84(6):722–33.

100. Sloper CM, Powell RJ, Dua HS. Tacrolimus (FK505) in the treatment posterior uveitis refractory to cyclosporine. Ophthalmology. 1999;106:723–8.

101. Smiddy WE, Isernhagen RD, Michels RG, Glaser BM, de Bustros SN. Vitrectomy for non-diabetic vitreous hemorrhage. Retinal and choroidal vascular disorders. Retina. 1988;8(2):88–95.

102. Smith JA, Mackensen F, Sen NH, et al. Epidemiology and course of disease in childhood uveitis. Ophthalmology. 2009;116:1544–51.

103. Sobrin L, Christen W, Foster CS. Mycophenolate mofetil after methotrexate failure or intolerance in the treatment of scleritis and uveitis. Ophthalmology. 2008;115:1416–21.

104. Tessler HH, Farber MD. Intraocular lens implantation versus no intraocular lens implantation in patients with chronic iridocyclitis and pars planitis. A randomized prospective study. Ophthalmology. 1993;100(8):1206–9.

105. Treumer F, Bunse A, Rudolf M, Roider J. Pars plana vitrectomy, phacoemulsification and intraocular lens implantation. Comparison of clinical complications in a combined versus two-step surgical approach. Graefes Arch Clin Exp Ophthalmol. 2006;244(7):808–15.

106. van Kooij B, Rothova A, de Vries P. The pros and cons of intravitreal triamcinolone injections for uveitis and inflammatory cystoid macular edema. Ocul Immunol Inflamm. 2006;14(2):73–85.

107. Venkatesh P, Kumar CS, Abbas Z, Garg S. Comparison of the efficacy and safety of different methods of posterior subtenon injection. Ocul Immunol Inflamm. 2008;16(5):217–23.

108. Verma L, Kumar A, Garg S, Khosla PK, Tewari HK. Cryopexy in pars planitis. Can J Ophthalmol. 1991;26(6):313–5.

109. Vitale AT, Zierhut M, Foster CS. Intermediate uveitis. In: Foster CS, Vitale AT, editors. Diagnosis and treatment of uveitis. Philadelphia: W.B. Saunders Company; 2002. p. 844–57.

110. Walton RC, Nussenblatt RB, Withcup SM. Cyclosporine therapy for severe sight-threatening uveitis in children and adolescents. Ophthalmology. 1998;105:2028–34.

111. Wiechens B, Nölle B, Reichelt JA. Pars-plana vitrectomy in cystoid macular edema associated with intermediate uveitis. Graefes Arch Clin Exp Ophthalmol. 2001;239(7):474–81.

112. Wroblewski K, Sen NH, Yeh S, Faia L, et al. Long-term daclizumab therapy for the treatment of noninfectious ocular inflammatory disease. Can J Ophthalmol. 2011;46:322–8.

113. Yazici H, Pazarli H, Barnes CG, et al. A controlled trial of azathioprine in Behcet's syndrome. N Engl J Med. 1990;322:281–5.

Posterior Uveitis

10

Piergiorgio Neri, Ilir Arapi, Uwe Pleyer,
Moncef Khairallah, Soumyava Basu, Michele Nicolai,
Vittorio Pirani, Alfonso Giovannini,
and Cesare Mariotti

Contents

P. Neri, BMedSc, MD, PhD (⊠)
A. Giovannini, MD • C. Mariotti, MD
Ospedali Riuniti "Umberto I-GM Lancisi-G Salesi",
The Eye Clinic-Polytechnic University of Marche,
Via Conca, n.71, Ancona 60020, Italy
e-mail: p.neri@univpm.it; alfgiovannini@hotmail.com;
c.mariotti@univpm.it

I. Arapi, MSc, MD • V. Pirani, MSc, MD
Department of Neuroscience,
Ospedali Riuniti di Ancona, Università Politecnica
delle Marche, Via Conca, n.71, Ancona 60126, Italy
e-mail: arapi_ilir@hotmail.com;
piranivittorio@virgilio.it

U. Pleyer, MD, FEBO • M. Nicolai, MSc, MD
Department of Ophthalmology, Charité,
Augustenburger Platz 1, Berlin 13353, Germany
e-mail: uwe.pleyer@charite.de,
michele.nicolai@hotmail.it

M. Khairallah, MD
Department of Opthalmology,
Fattouma Bourguiba University Hospital,
1st June Street, Monastir, 5019, Tunisia
e-mail: moncef.khairallah@rns.tn

S. Basu, MS
Retina-vitreous and Uvea Service, L V Prasad Eye
Institute, Patia, Bhubaneswar, Odisha 751024, India
e-mail: eyetalk@gmail.com

10.1   Infectious Posterior Uveitis

10.1.1 Viral Posterior Uveitis

10.1.1.1 Acute Retinal Necrosis Syndrome

Definition

Acute retinal necrosis (ARN) is a condition that was initially described in 1971 by Urayama [115]. It is a fulminant viral infection caused by members of the herpesvirus family. ARN is characterized by peripheral full-thickness retinitis with discrete borders, occlusive vasculopathy with arteriolar involvement, rapid progression with circumferential spread in untreated eyes, and marked vitritis. Late retinal detachment remains a serious complication despite prophylactic laser photocoagulation and vitreoretinal surgery.

ARN is generally diagnosed on the basis of its clinical features, as summarized by the diagnostic

U. Pleyer et al. (eds.), *Immune Modulation and Anti-Inflammatory Therapy in Ocular Disorders*,
DOI 10.1007/978-3-642-54350-0_10, © Springer-Verlag Berlin Heidelberg 2014

criteria established by the executive committee of the American Uveitis Society (Table 10.1).

Epidemiology/Etiology

Necrotizing retinitis from alpha herpesviruses HSV and VZV is a rare disease. The age of onset has a bimodal distribution with peaks occurring at ages of 20 and 50. The disease is prevalently diffused in the elderly population and in immune-deficient patients, through the fifth to seventh decade. HSV infection seems to involve early adulthood, while VZV dermatitis seems to involve the older population. The etiology of ARN was clarified in 1982 when it was shown

Table 10.1 AUS criteria for the diagnosis of acute retinal necrosis [1]

Characteristics required for diagnosis
Single or multiple areas of retinal necrosis with distinct borders
Necrotic foci usually located in the peripheral retina
Rapid disease progression if antiherpetic treatment is not instituted
Extension of foci of retinal necrosis in a circumferential fashion
Presence of occlusive vasculopathy with arteriolar involvement
Prominent anterior chamber and vitreous inflammation
Characteristics that support, but are not required for, diagnosis
Optic neuropathy or atrophy
Scleritis
Pain

that almost every member of the herpesvirus family could be implicated as a causative agent.

Clinical Symptoms and Signs

ARN is characterized by acute peripheral necrotizing retinitis with well-demarcated borders and a tendency to rapidly spread towards the posterior pole. ARN is commonly associated with mild to severe vitritis and retinal arteriolitis in the context of an occlusive vasculopathy [121] (EBM:2+, C). Subsequent optic neuropathy is a frequent consequence of vasculitis. ARN is usually a unilateral disease, but in almost one-third of patients, the second eye becomes involved within 6 weeks.

ARN may begin with an anterior granulomatous uveitis. Usually within 21 days, the retinal necrosis reaches its maximum extension, and the macula is often spared. The regression of ARN leads to retinal atrophy in a Swiss cheese-like pattern. The massive cellular infiltration of the vitreous body (Fig. 10.1) creates the conditions for membrane proliferation with subsequent PVD and rhegmatogenous retinal detachment and a subsequent proliferative vitreoretinopathy. If there is a severe inflammatory response, an exudative retinal detachment can occur.

Differential Diagnosis of Acute Retinal Necrosis (Fig. 10.2)

CMV retinitis mostly affects immunocompromised patients. Toxoplasmic retinochoroiditis is the most frequent disease simulating necro-

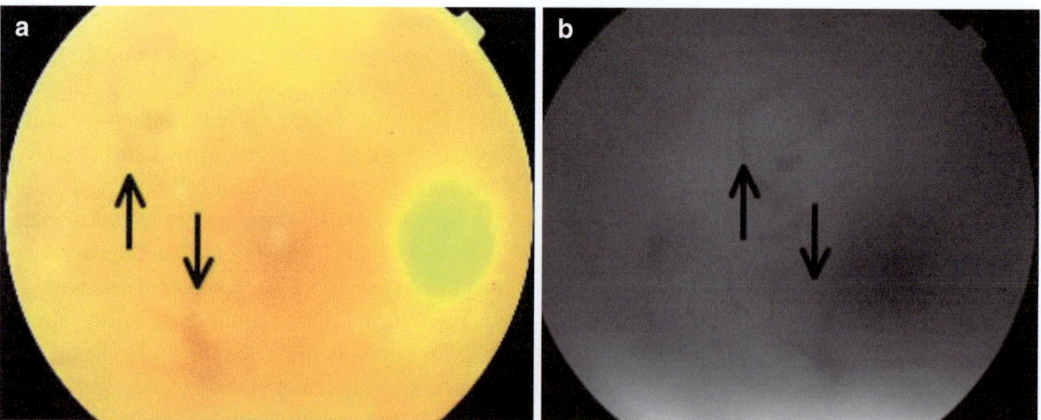

Fig. 10.1 Acute retinal necrosis: color fundus photograph showing a dense vitritis with retinal vasculitis (*black arrows*). Fluorescein angiography (**b**) proves the occlusive nature of the retinal vasculitis (*black arrows*)

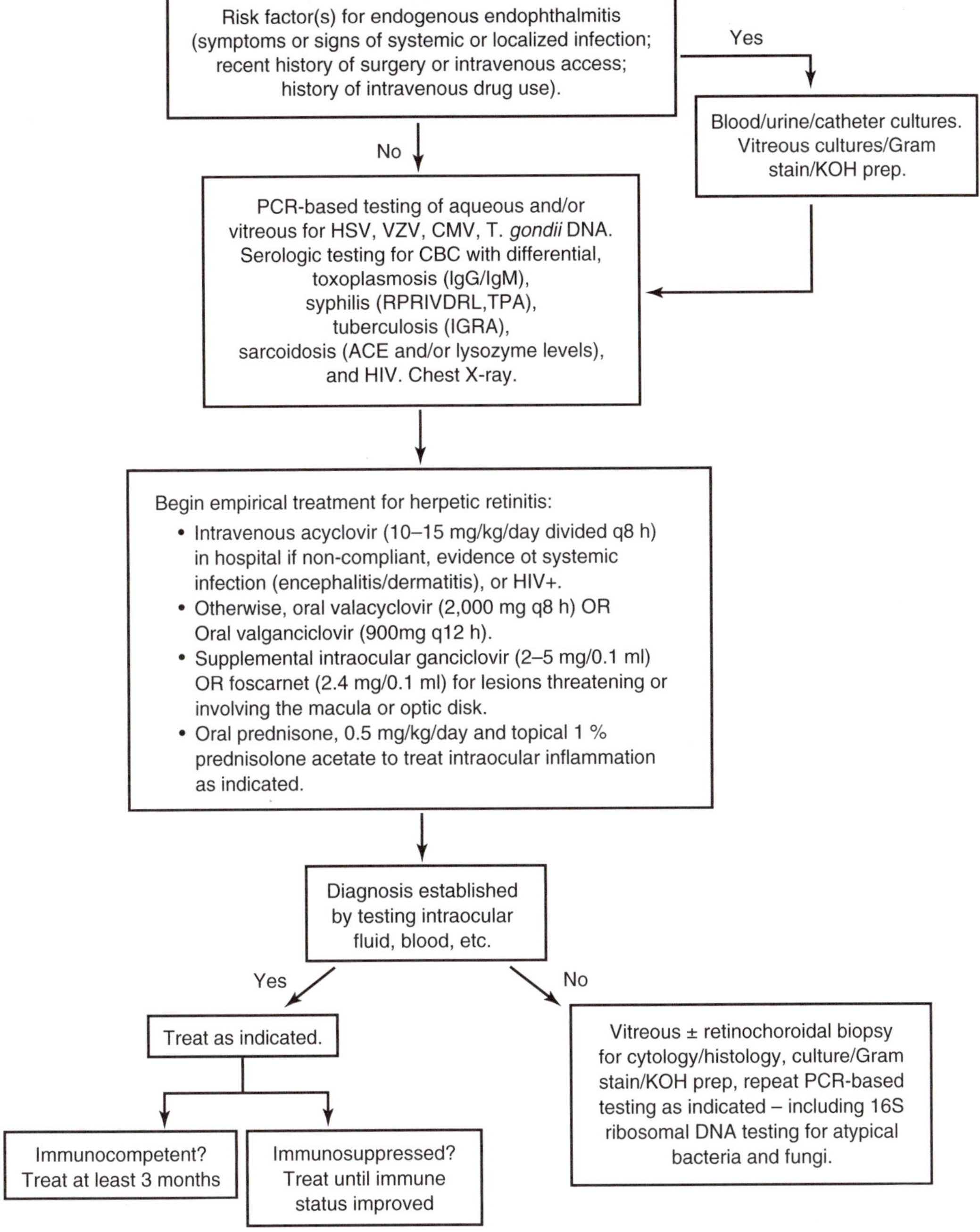

Fig. 10.2 Decision tree summarizing recommended approach to the patient with retinitis of unclear etiology [3]

tizing viral retinopathies; hemorrhage is not a characteristic of its lesions. Behcet's disease is a systemic disease associated with an inconstant course of remissions and exacerbations. Intraocular lymphoma is characterized by a slow course as compared to ARN.

Treatment

The therapeutic strategy of alpha herpesvirus retinitis includes antivirals, anti-inflammatories, and antiglaucomatous medications. Intravenous administration of acyclovir remains the main approach, in the light of its efficacy against both

Table 10.2 Agents commonly used in the treatment of acute retinal necrosis [188]

Drug	Route of administration	Adverse effects	Estimated cost[a]	Predicted relative efficacy
Acyclovir	15 mg/kg/day divided every 8 h IV for 7 days, followed by 800 mg five times daily po for 3–4 months	Common: GI symptoms, rash, headache Uncommon: renal/CNS toxicity	$7,834	HSV-2~HSV-1 >VZV>> CMV
Valacyclovir	1,000–2,000 mg po q8 h	Same as acyclovir	$4,551	HSV-2~HSV-1 >VZV>> CMV
Famciclovir	500 mg po q8 h	Common: headache, GI symptoms, rash	$4,570	HSV-1>HSV-2 >VZV
Ganciclovir	500 mg IV q12 h	Common: anemia, granulocytopenia, thrombocytopenia	$21,724	HSV-1~CMV >>HSV-2, VZV
	2–5 mg/0.1 ml IVT injection, three times per week	Uncommon: retinal detachment, hemorrhage, endophthalmitis	$3,891	
	Vitrasert surgical implant effective for Ð8 months	Uncommon: retinal detachment, hypotony, hemorrhage, endophthalmitis	$19,200	
Valganciclovir	900 mg twice daily po for 3 weeks induction, then 450 mg twice daily po for maintenance	Common: headache, GI symptoms Serious: bone marrow suppression, anemia, renal dysfunction	$16,331	HSV-1~CMV >> HSV-2, VZV
Foscarnet	For CMV: 60 mg/kg every 8 h IV for 2–3 weeks; for HSV: 40 mg/kg every 8 h IV for 2–3 weeks	Common: headache, GI symptoms Uncommon: renal/CNS toxicity	$32,850	HSV-1~HSV-2~ VZV>CMV
	2.4 mg/0.1 ml IVTT injection, weekly	Uncommon: retinal detachment, hemorrhage, endophthalmitis	$1,460	

[a]120 days of treatment; medications alone. 2011 average wholesale price as of 13 February 2012. Estimated additional costs for outpatient infusion (~$700/day) or inpatient hospital stay ($3,000–$5,000/day) are not included and may vary depending on the hospital institution and insurance status of the patient. Operating room, surgeon, and anesthesiologist fees not included

HSV and VZV. It is given for 14–21 days; after that, it is switched to 4 g of acyclovir or 3 g of valacyclovir daily per os for a period of 1–3 months. Usually, lesions stabilize within 48 h, but in resistant cases, intravenous foscarnet or ganciclovir is employed ([128] (EBM: 1-, A)). Acyclovir significantly decreases contralateral disease as compared with those untreated ([121] (EBM:2++, C), [128] (EBM: 1-, A), [188] (EBM:2++, C)). Recently, oral valacyclovir has been successfully used for the treatment of ARN, even though its role has still to be discussed ([250] (EBM: 3, C)). Anti-inflammatory drugs are still being discussed in ARN syndrome: they are employed to minimize damages to the optic nerve and retinal vessels. On the other hand, they have to be used only in conjunction with antivirals. Steroids must be started at 1 mg/kg and progressively tapered ([275] (EBM: 1-, A)). The role of anticoagulants and aspirin remains controversial, in particular, their effect on the occlusive vasculopathy. Retinal detachment in ARN syndrome remains a major problem with an incidence of 75 % in the untreated patients. Prophylactic vitrectomy and laser photocoagulation ([196] (EBM: 4, D)) are associated with a variable visual function and are still controversial.

Very recently, Wong et al. ([274] (EBM: 2++, B)) have proposed to treat ARN with intravitreal foscarnet. The authors evaluated 33 eyes with HSV-ARN and 48 with VZV-ARN. Visual acuity on presentation was similar ($p=0.48$), but a larger proportion had better vision (> or =20/60) in the HSV-ARN group (52 %) than the VZV-ARN group (35 %). A greater proportion of eyes with poor vision (< or =20/200) was found at the 12-month follow-up in the VZV-ARN group (60 %) compared with the HSV-ARN group

(35 %). A greater degree of visual loss in the VZV-ARN group compared with the HSV-ARN group was detected. Retinal detachment was 2.5-fold more commonly observed in VZV-ARN (62 %) compared with HSV-ARN (24 %). The eyes treated with ($n=56$) intravitreal foscarnet had 40 % lower rate in retinal detachment than those without ($n=25$) intravitreal treatment for VZV-ARN ($p=0.23$). Intravitreal foscarnet seemed to be a useful adjunct for the treatment of ARN in order to lower the rate of retinal detachment.

All commercially available antiviral drugs to date are virostatic, and this explains the frequent relapses, particularly, in absence of antiviral prophylaxis (Table 10.2).

10.1.1.2 Progressive Outer Retinal Necrosis

Definition

The designation of progressive outer retinal necrosis (PORN) generally describes patients with AIDS (CD4+ Tlymphocytes $\leq$50 cells/µl) or who are profoundly immunosuppressed.

PORN is a herpetic retinitis with less inflammation and a more aggressive clinical course than ARN. It is thought to be the second most frequent opportunistic retinal infection in patients with AIDS in North America.

Etiology

PORN is thought to be a variant necrotizing herpetic retinopathy in immunocompromised patients. There is sufficient evidence to identify VZV and HSV as causative factors of PORN. Very often, patients with PORN are infected with HIV (human immunodeficiency virus) and generally have advanced AIDS.

Clinical Symptoms and Signs

PORN is characterized by a sudden necrotizing retinitis of the deep retinal layers, starting at the posterior pole and arranged in a multifocal pattern. These inflammatory spots have a marked tendency towards peripheral spreading and confluence. Unlike ARN syndrome, retinal vasculitis, inflammatory reaction of the vitreous, and optic neuropathy are less common, particularly when associated with low Th-CD4+ cell counts.

The frequent occurrence of retinal detachment and the marked resistance to antivirals make the visual prognosis extremely poor.

Differential Diagnosis

The differential diagnosis for PORN is similar to that of ARN. It is very important to differentiate these two disorders on the basis of precise criteria, such as the pattern of distribution of retinal lesions, as well as the depth of the necrosis in the retinal layers (outer vs. full thickness), involvement of posterior pole vs. midperiphery, and presence of vitritis and vasculitis.

Treatment

Since viral replication is less prone to be controlled in patients affected by PORN syndrome, several combinations of intravenous and intravitreal antivirals have been tried in order to stop the progression of the necrosis ([137] (EBM D 3) and [284] (EBM D 3)), with little or even lack of evident efficacy. However, aggressive therapy based on intravenous foscarnet or ganciclovir and intravitreal ganciclovir remains the mainstay of therapy ([82], (EBM:3, D)). Several papers have reported that combination of antiviral therapy and highly active antiretroviral therapy (HAART) may improve long-term visual outcomes for VZV-PORN (Ferente [137] (EBM D 4) and [284] (EBM D 4)). Corticosteroids generally must be avoided in order to prevent complications resulting from viral replication.

Core Message

- The lytic reaction caused by herpetic ocular infection is accompanied by subsequent ocular inflammation.
- The diagnosis is based on clinical typical findings; recently, molecular techniques such as PCR have been applied to ocular fluids.
- Systemic antivirals are crucial in the control of viral replication. They should be used before corticosteroids.
- Antiviral prophylaxis is very important in preventing relapses.

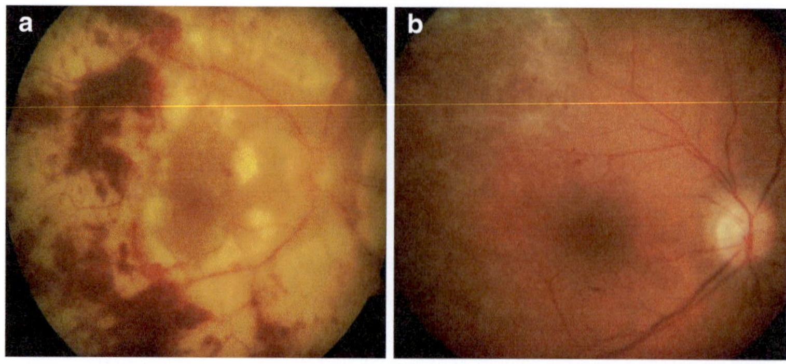

Fig. 10.3 Cytomegalovirus retinitis: "pizza pie" fundus (**a**) before the treatment. Note the improvement of the clinical picture after the treatment with ganciclovir and steroids (**b**)

10.1.1.3 Cytomegalovirus Retinitis

Definition

Cytomegalovirus (CMV) is a beta herpesvirus and contains double-stranded DNA. Commonly, CMV retinitis tends to occur in patients whose immune system has been significantly depressed, such as HIV [23]. In 1997, Whitcup et al. [269] reported that CMV retinitis did not progress in patients receiving HAART, albeit they were not receiving any anti-CMV therapy.

Etiology

CMV reaches the retina via bloodstream and infects the vascular endothelium which then spreads to the retinal cells. Infected cells show the pathognomonic cytomegalic inclusions with intracellular, large, and eosinophilic bodies.

Clinical Symptoms and Signs

Patients present blurred vision with acute visual impairment.

Histopathology shows a full-thickness retinal necrosis, associated with coagulative vasculitis and choroiditis. The typical chorioretinal lesions observed in CMV retinitis include:

- Hemorrhagic pattern which shows confluent area of full-thickness retinal necrosis with a yellow-white granular appearance, called "pizza pie" (Fig. 10.3)
- "Brush-fire" pattern showing a rapid spreading of the CNV in the retinal tissue
- "Granular pattern" which presents areas of retinal atrophy surrounded by whitish granular punctate lesions

Vitreous involvement can be variable in all the different retinal patterns.

One of the most severe complications of CMV retinitis is rhegmatogenous retina detachment. Persistent cystoid macular edema can occur.

Differential Diagnosis

Although the diagnosis of CMV retinitis is prevalently based on clinical criteria, the similarities between CMV retinitis and alpha herpesvirus retinitis cannot be easily distinguished. In order to make a correct diagnosis, both aqueous and vitreal polymerase chain reaction (PCR) analysis of intraocular antibody synthesis can confirm the diagnosis [245].

Treatment

The therapeutic approach to CMV retinitis is based on the patient's immune status, which requires an interdisciplinary approach.

Up to date, ganciclovir represents the drug used as the first line. The standard dose of ganciclovir is 5 mg/kg intravenously every 12 h for 2 weeks followed by maintenance at 10 mg/kg/day ([269], EBM: 1+A). Neutrophil count should be maintained higher than 500/μl.

Foscarnet is also used, particularly for those patients who have a low neutrophil count. The standard dose is 90 mg/kg twice daily, followed by maintenance therapy with 90–120 mg/kg [269]. Serum electrolytes should be regularly monitored.

Besides the traditional systemic approach, an intraocular ganciclovir implant seemed to be superior to intravenous ganciclovir in a large randomized controlled trials of HIV-associated CMV retinitis in the era before HAART ([174], EBM: B, 2++]). Unfortunately, the limitation of the intraocular ganciclovir implant to prevent CMV disease in the fellow eye represented its failure. As an alternative, oral valganciclovir has been proven as effective as initial intravenous ganciclovir for 4 weeks followed by oral valganciclovir. During the latter trial, most patients were also taking combination anti-HIV treatment. As the ocular penetration of systemically administered anti-CMV drugs is limited, current clinical guidelines include consideration of intraocular injection of anti-CMV drugs for patients who have sight-threatening CMV retinitis ([165], EBM: B, 2++).

> **Core Message**
> - CMV is a highly adapted opportunistic agent, which can induce a severe sight-threatening retinitis.
> - Although the diagnosis of CMV retinitis is based on clinical criteria, PRC of ocular fluids is useful to detect the specific viral agent involved in the pathogenesis of the disease.
> - For the treatment of CMV retinitis, the sustained-release ganciclovir implant is more effective than intravenous ganciclovir, but patients treated with a ganciclovir implant alone remain at greater risk for the development of CMV disease in the fellow eye ([245], EBM: B, 2++).
> - Orally administered valganciclovir appears to be as effective as intravenous ganciclovir for induction treatment and is convenient and effective for the long-term management of cytomegalovirus retinitis in immunocompromised patients ([269], EBM: B, 2++).

10.1.2 Human Immunodeficiency Virus (HIV) Retinal Microvasculopathy

10.1.2.1 Definition

Human immunodeficiency virus (HIV)-1 is a single-strand RNA virus and represents the most widespread type of HIV within the retrovirus family.

Until now, HIV infection remains a worldwide diffused disease, with different prevalences depending on both socioeconomic and geographic factors [189].

10.1.2.2 Etiology

HIV can be sexually transmitted, even though intravenous and perinatal infections can occur. Incubation lasts approximately 3 weeks after which an acute retroviral syndrome can occur. Symptomatology includes fever, rash, myalgias, headaches, and gastrointestinal involvement. However, acute symptoms are not frequently observed.

Acquired immunodeficiency syndrome (AIDS) is the most severe manifestation of immunodepression, secondary to the progressive reduction of T-helper CD4+. AIDS typically leads to a significantly higher risk of developing opportunistic infections, such as CMV retinitis, which can occur as soon as Th-CD4+ count is <50 cells/μl ([145] (EBM: B2++)). Other ocular opportunistic infections include syphilis, toxoplasmosis, tuberculosis, candidosis, herpes simplex virus, and herpes zoster virus ([189] (EBM: C2+), [23] (EBM: B2++)).

10.1.2.3 Clinical Symptoms and Signs

The most common ocular finding is retinal microvasculopathy, which is characterized by small retinal hemorrhages and cotton-wool spots ([23] (EBM: B2++)). Up to date, pathophysiology has not been clearly demonstrated.

10.1.2.4 Differential Diagnosis

HIV retinopathy should be differentiated from the cotton-wool spots observed in the diabetic retinopathy, as well as in the hypertensive retinopathy.

10.1.2.5 Treatment

Up to date, there are no meta-analyses or systematic reviews of randomized clinical trials available about HIV-related retinal microvasculopathy. The clinical course of HIV infection has been dramatically reduced as soon as highly active antiretroviral therapy (HAART) has been introduced. Unfortunately, the availability of HAART is limited in developing countries. The treatment of HIV-related retinopathy is substantially not indicated ([23] (EBM: B2++)).

> **Core Message**
> - Retinal microvasculopathy is the most common ocular manifestation that does not require treatment.
> - A significant higher risk of developing opportunistic infections when Th-CD4+ count is <50 cells/μl.
> - The clinical course of the disease has been dramatically improved since HAART was introduced.

10.1.3 Other Viral Uveitis

10.1.3.1 West Nile Virus
Definition

West Nile virus (WNV) is a zoonotic disease most often transmitted to humans by an infected Culex mosquito vector where wild birds serve as a vector. It is an enveloped single-stranded RNA flavivirus, member of the Japanese encephalitis virus serocomplex [87]. The disease has its peak in late summer.

Clinical Symptoms and Signs

About 80 % of human infections are apparently asymptomatic and the remaining 20 % become symptomatic manifesting almost always a self-limited febrile illness. The symptoms include high-grade fever, myalgia, arthralgia, malaise, nausea, headache, skin rash, weakness, and pharyngitis [13]. The acute illness typically lasts less than a week.

Since first described in 2002, several forms of ocular involvement have been recognized. Multifocal chorioretinitis [132], typically bilateral, with specific clinical and angiographic features is the most common finding, occurring in almost 80 % of patients with acute WNV infection. An associated mild to moderate vitreal inflammation is observed. Chorioretinal lesions involve the midzone and periphery in almost all eyes. The posterior pole is involved in nearly two-third of the eyes. Active lesions appear circular and creamy in ophthalmoscopy associated by early hypofluorescence and late staining in fluorescein angiography. Their size is variable. The linear cluster arrangement that the lesions take is a prominent feature. These streaks are typically oriented radially in the nasal and peripheral fundus or arranged in a curvilinear pattern in the temporal posterior fundus [131] (Fig. 10.4). ICGA tends to denote more choroidal lesions than those appreciated by fluorescein angiography. Diabetes

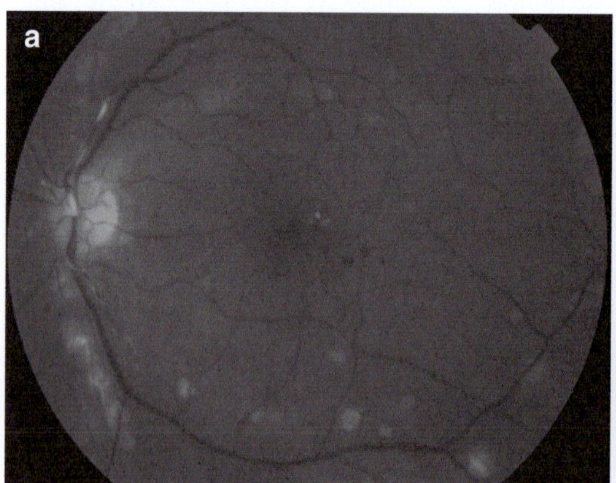
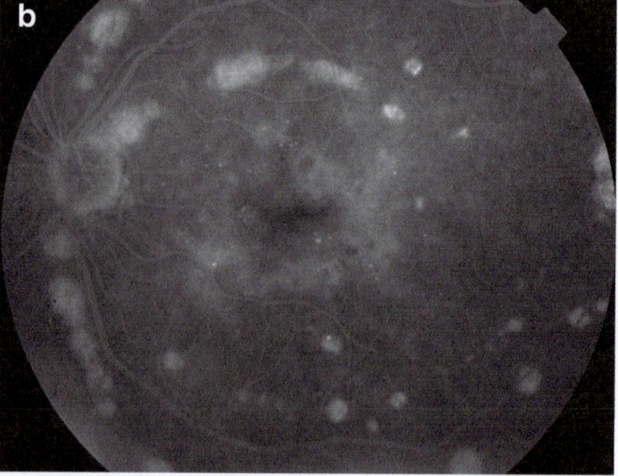

Fig. 10.4 Red-free fundus photograph (**a**) and fluorescein angiogram (**b**) of the left eye of a 64-year-old diabetic woman with West Nile virus infection show inactive multifocal chorioretinitis with a typical linear clustering of chorioretinal lesions. Note the presence of retinal arterial sheathing (**a**) and diabetic macular edema

mellitus appears being a risk factor for WNV-associated chorioretinitis [134].

Other ophthalmic manifestations include retinal hemorrhages, vascular sheathing and leakage, and occlusive vasculitis. Optic nerve involvement includes optic neuritis and optic disk swelling and staining [280].

Differential Diagnosis

The differential diagnosis of WNV systemic disease includes herpesvirus encephalitis, CNS involvement by legionella, rickettsioses, Epstein-Barr virus, hypertensive encephalopathy, and enteroviral aseptic meningitis. While the ocular involvement *can enter* in the differential diagnosis of syphilis, TBC, histoplasmosis, sarcoidosis, and idiopathic multifocal chorioretinitis.

Treatment

At present, there is no proven treatment for WNV infection ([87], EBM: C, 2-). Specific ophthalmic treatment such as topical steroids for anterior uveitis, peripheral retinal photocoagulation due to occlusive vasculitis, pars plana vitrectomy for vitreal hemorrhages or retinal detachment, and photodynamic therapy and anti-VEGF for choroidal neovascularization may be required in these specific situations ([226], EMB: 3, D).

> **Core Message**
> - The most common intraocular finding of West Nile virus is the bilateral multifocal chorioretinitis which is frequently self-limited and asymptomatic in the majority of patients where the CNS is affected.
> - Multifocal chorioretinitis manifests a unique pattern which is helpful for diagnosis.

10.1.3.2 Dengue Fever

Dengue fever (DF) is caused by any of the four immunologically related serotypes of the dengue virus, which belong to the genus *Flavivirus* of the family Flaviviridae. It is transmitted through the bite of an infected female *Aedes aegypti/Aedes albopictus* mosquito.

DF is considered to be one of the most important arthropod borne disease in the tropical and subtropical regions, being endemic in more than 100 countries, including America, Southeast Asia, Western Pacific, Africa, and the Eastern Mediterranean [276].

Clinical Presentation

Systemic Disease

The incubation period for DF varies from 3 to 14 days. The initial infection may be asymptomatic, may result in a nonspecific febrile illness, or may produce features of classic DF including sudden onset of high fever, severe headache, myalgias, arthralgias, nausea, vomiting, and a maculopapular rash. The majority of DF cases are self-limiting. A small proportion of affected patients may develop life-threatening dengue hemorrhagic fever syndrome, which is characterized by increased capillary permeability and hemostatic disturbances, or dengue shock syndrome, which is characterized by severe systemic hypotension. DF is often associated with a bleeding tendency secondary to thrombocytopenia [53, 107].

Ocular Disease

The ocular involvement was found to occur in 10 % of patients hospitalized for serologically confirmed DF. It usually occurs within one month after onset of symptoms of DF and is often bilateral. A subconjunctival hemorrhage, petechial in type and associated with a platelet count of less than 50,000/µl, was the most common ocular manifestation in an East Indian population with DF [133]. Numerous posterior segment changes have been associated with DF including retinal hemorrhages, retinal vasculitis, yellow subretinal dots, retinal pigment epithelial mottling, and foveolitis, seen clinically as a round yellowish lesion at the fovea with corresponding focal outer neurosensory retina-retinal pigment epithelium thickening on OCT. Other findings include macular edema, serous retinal detachment, retinal vascular occlusion, choroidal changes, optic disk swelling, optic neuritis, and neuroretinitis [53, 58, 62, 67, 125, 127, 150, 237].

Dengue-associated ocular disease usually has a self-limited course, with a significant improvement of visual acuity in 2–4 weeks. However, persistent visual impairment may occur in a subset of patients with maculopathy or neuropathy [58, 62, 150].

Laboratory Diagnosis

Within the first 2 days of fever, diagnosis is possible only by detecting the virion, RNA, or dengue proteins, such as nonstructural protein 1 (NS1).

Detection of newly formed antibodies (IgM) usually is not possible until after viremia ends or after fever subsides [270]. MAC-ELISA has become a widely used assay but seems to have a high rate of false-positive results [260]. Other tests, including immunochromatographic assay [33], complement fixation, neutralization test, hemagglutination inhibition, and IgG enzyme-linked immunosorbent assay (ELISA), are also helpful to confirm the diagnosis of DF [260].

Apart from the dengue-specific parameters, platelet count should be performed.

Treatment

To date, there is no specific treatment available for dengue virus infection. Any medicine that decreases the platelet level should be avoided ([107] EBM:C4, [58] EBM:D3). In cases of dengue hemorrhagic fever, hospitalization, prompt treatment with intravenous fluids, and close monitoring of vital signs, as well as hematologic parameters, are indicated ([107] EBM; C4).

There is no established treatment for ocular manifestations of DF. Topical, periocular, oral, and intravenous steroids, as well as intravenous immunoglobulins, have been advocated for the management of dengue ocular complications, based on the postulated immune-mediated pathogenesis of the disease. Indications for treatment may include dengue-associated uveitis and optic neuritis, visual acuity worse than 20/40, and deterioration of vision ([133] EBM:D 4, 58). Preventive measures by avoiding contact with infected mosquitoes are required to decrease the infection incidence. Vaccines targeting all the four serotypes of dengue virus hopefully will be available in the near future ([57] EBM C 2+, [240] EBM C 2+).

> **Core Message**
> - Dengue occurs in 10 % of patients hospitalized for serologically confirmed DF.
> - Ocular involvement can present different clinical patterns.
> - Treatment is still controversial.

10.1.3.3 Chikungunya

Chikungunya virus is a single-stranded RNA virus of the genus *Alphavirus* in the family Togaviridae which is transmitted to humans by the bite of infected *Aedes* mosquitoes (*A. aegypti* and *A. albopictus*). Since its first isolation in Tanzania in 1953, the virus has been associated with many epidemics in tropical regions of Africa, India, Southeast Asia, and South America. The infection which is endemoepidemic typically consists of an acute illness with fever, severe arthralgia, and skin rash [205].

Clinical Presentation

Systemic Disease

The incubation period ranges from 1 to 12 days, with an average of 2–4 days. Onset of the disease is abrupt and is characterized by high fever, severe arthralgia, and myalgia, along with headache and skin rash. Asymptomatic infections are rare (3–25 % of serologically proven infections) [47]. The debilitating polyarthralgia is very characteristic of chikungunya. Skin lesions may be seen in almost one-half of the patients. A pruriginous maculopapular rash, lasting for 2–3 days, is the most common feature [43, 202]. Rarely, severe infection associated with multiorgan failure, central neurological involvement, neonatal infection, and death occur [43, 202].

Ocular Disease

Ocular manifestations associated with chikungunya may be concomitant of the systemic disease or may follow its resolution [133]. Ocular involvement can be unilateral or bilateral. Acute anterior uveitis and retinitis are the most common ocular findings in chikungunya. The anterior uveitis is nongranulomatous or granulomatous and can be associated with increased intraocular pressure. Posterior synechiae are not common [133, 172]. The clinical course is typically benign.

Chikungunya retinitis presents in the form of areas of retinal whitening in the posterior pole with surrounding retinal and macular edema and associated mild vitritis [133]. FA usually shows early hypofluorescence and late hyperfluorescence of retinal lesions, along with focal areas of retinal vascular leakage and capillary non-perfusion [133]. OCT reveals increased reflectivity in the nerve fiber layer zone with aftershadowing corresponding to the areas of retinitis. It also helps in the detection and evaluation of associated retinal edema and exudative retinal detachment. Retinitis resolves gradually over a period of several weeks.

Other ophthalmic manifestations of chikungunya have been reported including conjunctivitis, episcleritis, keratitis, panuveitis, multifocal choroiditis, optic neuritis, neuroretinitis, central retinal artery occlusion, exudative retinal detachment, panophthalmitis, lagophthalmos, and sixth nerve palsy [133, 171].

Chikungunya-associated ocular disease is usually self-limiting, with most patients recovering good vision. However, permanent visual loss may occur mainly due to optic neuropathy.

Laboratory Diagnosis

In the acute phase of illness, diagnosis is based on the detection of viral nucleic acid in serum samples by RT-PCR, isolation of the virus, or detection of an antibody response. After resolution of the acute disease, the diagnosis is confirmed by the presence of an immune response. RT-PCR can detect viral nucleic acid from one day before onset of symptoms, up to day 7 after the beginning of the disease. Antigen capture ELISA may detect viral antigens as early as day 2 after onset. Indirect immunofluorescence and ELISA are rapid and sensitive techniques for the screening of IgM or IgG immune reaction. IgM antibody and IgG antibody response have been described to begin both by day 2 after onset [246].

Treatment

Nonsteroidal anti-inflammatory drugs are currently recommended for chikungunya-induced arthralgia. Ribavirin and interferon α may inhibit viral replication ([45] EBM C 2+), but further studies are needed to assess their efficacy in humans. Another potential treatment for chikungunya is chloroquine, but results of different studies have been inconclusive ([44] EBM C 2-, [69] EBM C 2 +).

Topical steroids and cycloplegic agents are used for anterior uveitis. Associated ocular hypertension is managed with topical beta-blockers and oral or topical carbonic anhydrase inhibitors. Systemic steroids may be used to control the inflammation in posterior uveitis, panuveitis, and optic neuritis ([133] EBM D 3). The use of acyclovir in association with corticosteroids has been described in some cases of chikungunya retinitis [133], but its efficacy remains doubtful. Efforts are to be made to prevent transmission of the virus and to develop efficient and safe vaccines against chikungunya ([47] EBM D 3).

> **Core Message**
> - Ocular involvement in chikungunya can occur after the systemic disease.
> - Ocular chikungunya can present various clinical patterns.
> - No valid treatment is available at this time.

10.1.4 Posterior Uveitis: Bacterial Infections

10.1.4.1 Intraocular Tuberculosis

Definition

Intraocular inflammation associated with *Mycobacterium tuberculosis* [29].

Etiology

This condition is caused by dissemination of *M. tuberculosis* to ocular tissues, from the lung. The exact sequence of events is not known. However, there is histopathologic and molecular (polymerase chain reaction, PCR) evidence of the presence of this organism in the diseased eyes [258].

Clinical Symptoms and Signs

Intraocular tuberculosis can affect virtually every tissue in the eye. The clinical manifestations can be broadly classified as follows (Adapted from Ref. [29]):

1. Anterior uveitis

Granulomatous, nongranulomatous, iris nodules, and ciliary body tuberculoma

2. Intermediate uveitis granulomatous
3. Posterior and panuveitis

Choroidal tubercle

Choroidal tuberculoma

Subretinal abscess

Multifocal serpiginoid choroiditis (previously called serpiginous-like choroiditis)

4. Retinitis and retinal vasculitis
5. Neuroretinitis and optic neuropathy
6. Endophthalmitis and panophthalmitis

In a high endemic population, the following clinical signs were statistically found to be predictive of intraocular tuberculosis, in patients with latent or manifest systemic tuberculosis ([104], EBM: C, 2+):

- Broad-based posterior synechiae
- Retinal vasculitis with or without choroiditis patches overlying the blood vessels (Fig. 10.5)
- Multifocal serpiginoid choroiditis

Infectious multifocal serpiginoid choroiditis: It is a form of superficial choroiditis characterized by multifocal lesions (Fig. 10.6) that are noncontiguous to the optic disk and show serpiginoid or ameboid spread ([26, 101], EBM:C, 2+). Lesions are often bilateral and have associated vitreous inflammation. The fovea is usually spared resulting in good final visual acuity. Fundus autofluorescence (FAF) and spectral domain optical coherence tomography (SD-OCT) are useful in following disease activity during the course of the disease. FAF usually shows hyperautofluorescence with ill-defined halo in acute stage with gradual stippling and progressive hypoautofluorescence as the lesions heal [102]. SD-OCT shows increased reflectivity from outer retinal layers in the acute stage followed by knobbly

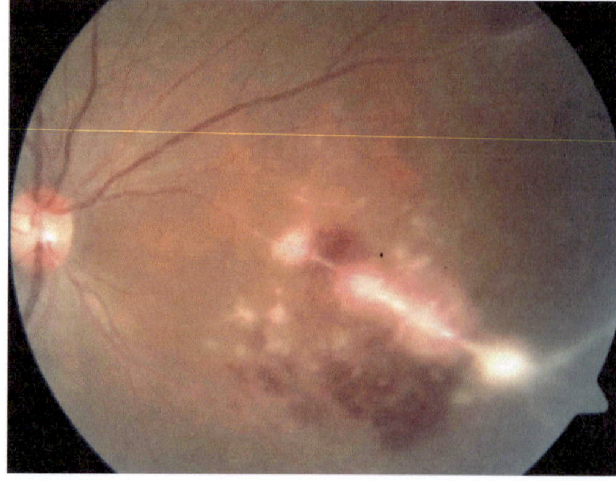

Fig. 10.5 Tubercular retinal vasculitis showing perivascular exudation and hemorrhages, associated with active chorioretinitis patch overlying the blood vessel

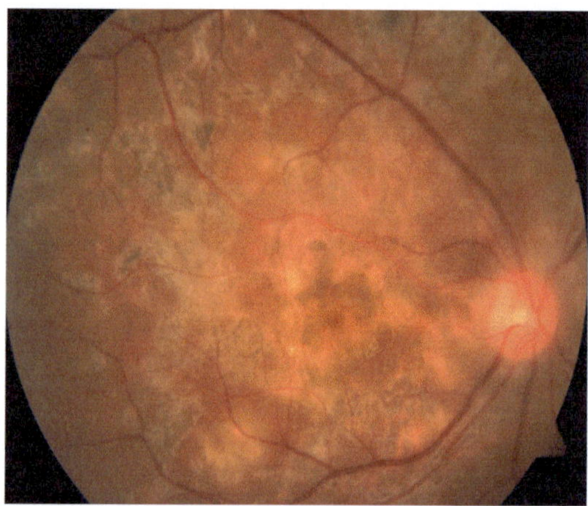

Fig. 10.6 Multifocal serpiginoid choroiditis showing multifocal areas of healed and active choroiditis

elevations in the outer retina and finally outer retinal atrophy and increased choroidal reflectivity [24]. Such lesions may also be observed in herpetic viral infections and syphilis in tuberculosis non-endemic regions [101].

Infectious multifocal serpiginoid choroiditis needs to be distinguished from classical serpiginous choroiditis that is seen in non-endemic populations and is characterized by large, peripapillary lesions that are rarely multifocal or associated with vitritis [101, 175].

Diagnosis

Currently, intraocular tuberculosis is mostly diagnosed based on characteristic clinical signs (mentioned above), associated ancillary tests (immunologic and radiological), and exclusion of other disease entities – infectious and noninfectious – that may have similar clinical presentation, in a given geographic region [29].

Immunologic tests include the tuberculin skin test (TST) and interferon-gamma release assays like the QuantiFERON-TB Gold test (QFT) and the T-SPOT test. Current evidence shows that while TST is more sensitive [278], QFT and T-SPOT are more specific for the diagnosis of presumed ocular tuberculosis ([11, 12], EBM: C, 2+). TST and T-SPOT test should be the investigation of choice in high and low endemic populations, respectively ([12], EBM:C, 2+).

However, the absence of systemic evidence of tuberculosis (immunologic and radiological) needs to be interpreted with caution while diagnosing intraocular tuberculosis. In a large series of 42 cases of histopathologically proven cases of ocular tuberculosis, 40 % of tested patients had negative TST and 57 % had normal chest radiograph [258]. Thus, there is a need for definitive diagnosis of this condition. PCR (including its modifications – quantitative and multi-target) has shown promising results, but there is insufficient evidence regarding its role in clinical practice.

Differential Diagnosis

The key to diagnosis of ocular tuberculosis in the current scenario lies in exclusion of other disease entities (infectious and noninfectious), found in a given geographic region that can mimic ocular tuberculosis. Therefore, the list of differential diagnosis depends on the specific clinical presentation and geographic location. Since tuberculosis can affect virtually every ocular tissue, the differential diagnosis can include nearly every ocular inflammatory condition except morphologically distinct entities like toxoplasma retinochoroiditis or viral retinitis.

Treatment

Treatment of ocular tuberculosis requires a combination of antimicrobial/antituberculosis therapy (ATT) and anti-inflammatory therapy (usually corticosteroids). In a large series of 360 patients, those treated with ATT had a significantly reduced rate of recurrent inflammation (15.74 %) compared to those treated only with corticosteroids (46.53 %) ([22], EBM: C, 2+). ATT should be administered in consultation with a pulmonologist or infectious disease specialist. According to the Centers for Disease Control and Prevention (CDC) guidelines, ATT should be given for a minimum of 6 months in total – 2 months of four-drug therapy (isoniazid 5 mg/kg daily, rifampicin 450 mg daily, pyrazinamide 30 mg/kg daily, and ethambutol 15 mg/kg daily) followed by a 4-month continuation phase of isoniazid and rifampicin ([9], EBM: 1+, A). Many authors have suggested a longer duration for the continuation phase, citing slow response to the drug in intraocular tuberculosis [10, 29]. It was found that those receiving >9 months ATT were significantly less likely to develop recurrence compared to those not receiving ATT ($p = 0.027$). However, the reduction in recurrence compared to other ATT durations (<6 months, 6–9 months) was not statistically significant ([10], EBM: C, 2-). Patients on ATT need to be monitored for ocular and systemic side effects. Ocular side effects include optic neuritis (ethambutol, especially if used >15 mg/day for >2 months, and rarely, isoniazid) and anterior uveitis (rifabutin).

Concomitant corticosteroid therapy is vital to control the inflammatory tissue damage caused by delayed-type hypersensitivity to *M. tuberculosis*. The importance of corticosteroid therapy can be judged from its role in the management of continued progression or paradoxical worsening of ocular inflammation that is occasionally seen after initiation of ATT for intraocular tuberculosis [100]. Such paradoxical worsening usually occurs in the initial 4–6 weeks after initiation of ATT and needs to be differentiated from various causes of treatment failure like drug resistance, reinfection, or missed diagnosis [25]. The mode of corticosteroid therapy (topical, periocular, intraocular, or systemic) depends on the degree and primary site of inflammation.

Future Directions

1. Definitive diagnosis based on PCR: Various modifications of PCR including quantitative PCR and multi-target PCR (targeting multiple gene sequences) are being applied to address the key challenge of low sensitivity of this technique [22].

10.1.4.2 Syphilis

Definition

Syphilis is a sexually transmitted disease caused by the spirochete *Treponema pallidum*. In acquired syphilis, the bacterium enters the body through small abrasions on the skin or the mucous membranes, mainly the genitals and mouth. If the condition is left untreated, it will progress through four stages with harmful effects in the major organs such as the heart and brain. Vertical transmission through the placental route is also possible but much less frequent, giving rise to congenital syphilis if the fetus survives.

Clinical Signs and Symptoms

Acquired Syphilis: Systemic Signs Primary Syphilis

The main sign is the genital chancre which appears 3 weeks after infection (an ulcerated painless lesion) associated with regional lymphadenopathy.

Secondary Syphilis

It appears 6 weeks after the appearance of the chancre and is characterized by flu-like illness, by maculopapular skin rash (mainly on soles and palms), and rarely by symptomatic or asymptomatic meningitis.

Latent Stage

This stage is divided into early and late latent. During this stage, the clinical disease is not detectable.

Tertiary Syphilis

At this stage, syphilis may present with "gumma," a small, rubbery granuloma with a necrotic center often located in the liver but also in the brain, heart, skin, and other tissues, leading to cardiovascular syphilis (aortitis and aortic aneurysms) and/or as neurosyphilis. In the late phase, neurosyphilis results in parenchymal lesions leading to encephalitis, stroke, tabes dorsalis, and Argyll-Robertson pupil, among other clinical findings.

Congenital syphilis can present during childhood and is divided into an early phase characterized by mucocutaneous lesions and osteochondritis and a late phase with the classic triad of Hutchinson keratitis, Hutchinson incisors, and eight nerve deafness.

Stages	Clinical findings
Primary syphilis	The initial clinical manifestation is the primary chancre Usually painless, which distinguishes it from other causes of genital ulcers: herpes simplex (genital herpes) and *Haemophilus ducreyi* (chancroid) Often heals without treatment over a period of a few weeks
Secondary syphilis	Untreated disease, approximately 25 % of patients will go on to develop systemic symptoms: rash, fever, headache, malaise, diffuse lymphadenopathy, alopecia
Latent syphilis	Latent syphilis refers to patients without symptoms who have positive serologic testing for syphilis Early latent: <1 year Late latent: >1 year
Tertiary syphilis	Clinical manifestations that may occur 1–30 years after infection when the infection is not treated

Ocular Signs

Syphilitic Posterior Segment Involve ment

Ocular syphilis manifests itself in the secondary and tertiary stage of syphilis. It often affects the eye as anterior granulomatous uveitis (mutton-fat KPs at the corneal endothelium, iris nodules) but may involve any other ocular structure. Because of its very variable presentation, syphilis earned the label as "great mimicker." Posterior pole manifestations vary ([122], EBM: 4, C). Unlike other infectious agents, treponemas have an affinity for all ocular layers including the posterior pole.

Deep chorioretinitis is the most common manifestation, with lesions, that can be divided into focal or multifocal lesions often located at the posterior pole. Focal lesions are often associated with serous retinal detachment and a significant degree of vitreous inflammation. Fluorescein angiography (FA) shows early hypofluorescence followed by late staining of the lesions.

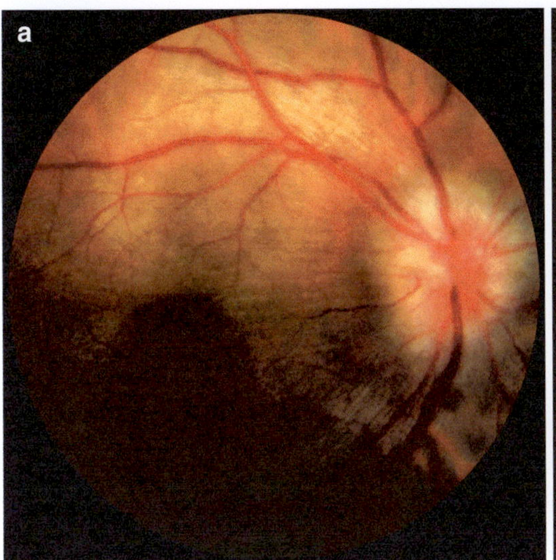
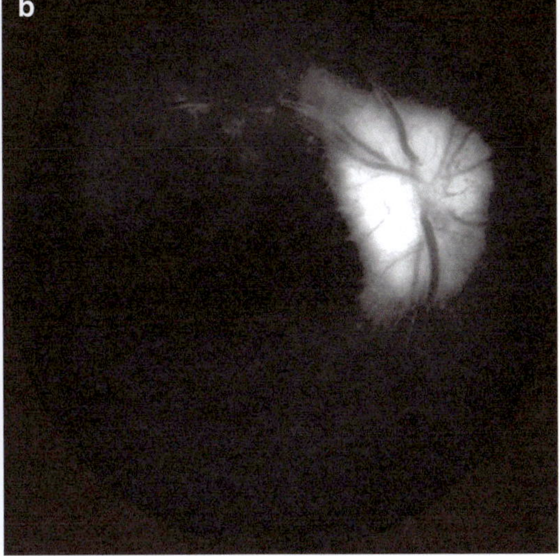

Fig. 10.7 Acute syphilitic posterior placoid chorioretinitis (ASPPC) characterized by placoid, yellowish subretinal lesions at the level of the RPE (**a**), associated with papillitis. Fluorescein angiography: note the corresponding staining of the dye at the late phases of the angiogram (**b**), with an evident hot disk

Acute syphilitic posterior placoid chorioretinitis (ASPPC, Fig. 10.7) is a specific, uncommon entity described by Gass, associated with placoid subretinal lesions at the level of the RPE and not infrequently associated with a retinal detachment in which macular pseudohypopyon can be observed ([77], EBM: 2++, B). FA shows typical leopard-spot pattern in the cicatricial phase of the lesions.

Syphilis may also manifest as a necrotizing retinitis, a severe condition associated with yellow-white patches of necrosis, retinal vasculitis, and vitritis, which can easily be confused with ARN.

Optic nerve involvement often occurs with minimal or no anterior segment inflammation. It often spills over into the retina being associated with either vasculitis, or focal areas of retinal edema. Untreated, it can lead to optic atrophy.

More peripheral involvement presenting as intermediate uveitis has been described, frequently associated with cystoid macular edema, vasculitis, and "hot disk." Pars plana exudates are characteristically absent.

The diagnostic approach offers the nonspecific tests which suffer a low level of sensitivity as compared to the high level of sensitivity and specificity offered by the specific tests.

Syphilis and HIV

The association between syphilis and HIV is quite common as both are sexually transmitted diseases. The frequency is sufficiently high that in the presence of one infection, one should always consider the presence of the other. However, the clinical presentation of syphilis does not appear to be altered by the presence of HIV and is not correlated with the severity of immune compromise. While the presentation may be similar to that in immunocompetent patients, relapses are more frequent, as is bilaterality. Patients with HIV infection may have a higher prevalence of posterior uveitis ([256], EBM: 2++ B), which may present in as a more severe and atypical form. Treatment will require more prolonged therapy with higher doses of antibiotics. Analysis of cerebrospinal fluid (CSF) should be performed in all patients with ocular syphilis due to a high prevalence of neurosyphilis and a poor sensitivity of systemic antibody titers in this patient population [144].

Treatment

In the presence of ocular involvement, all ocular manifestations of the infection should be treated as neurosyphilis. Intravenous penicillin G or procaine penicillin G 18–24 (MU) daily plus probenecid for 10–14 days should be given, followed by IM procaine penicillin G, 2.4 MU weekly for 3 weeks ([144] (EBM:1++, A), [50] (EBM: 2++, B)). For patients with tertiary stage ocular syphilis, a three-week course of benzathine penicillin should be added to the above regimen. In patients allergic to penicillin, ceftriaxone can be used instead.

Systemic corticosteroids can be used in combination with antibiotic therapy. If not used initially, vision and the severity of the inflammatory response need to be carefully monitored as a Jarisch-Herxheimer reaction can occur in severe enough cases where the use of steroids would be the preferred course of action ([130] (EBM:3, D), [254] (EBM:3, D)).

> **Core Message**
> - Syphilis is a sexually transmitted disease caused by the spirochete *Treponema pallidum.*
> - Ocular disease is characterized by a chronic granulomatous inflammation involving various ocular structures.
> - The most common eye manifestations are anterior uveitis, necrotizing retinitis, retinal vasculitis, panuveitis, and intermediate uveitis.
> - Because of its highly variable presentation and good treatment response, syphilis has always to be included in the differential diagnosis of any type of uveitis.
> - Syphilis is a treatable infection – especially in its primary and secondary stages – but is more difficult to manage in its tertiary stage.

10.1.4.3 Ocular Leptospirosis
Definition
Leptospirosis is a zoonosis caused by spirochetes of the genus *Leptospira*, whose natural reservoir is wild animals, mostly rodents and cattle. Initially, it was described by Adolf Weil in 1886 as a condition characterized by acute fever, malaise, and uveitis.

Etiology
Humans are accidental hosts, acquiring the disease by the contact with infected urine, tissues, or water. The disease can be considered occupational, infecting mostly farmers, veterinarians, and abattoir workers. It has the potential to occur both as epidemic outbreaks and as endemic disease, in tropical and temperate climates.

Clinical Symptoms and Signs
Leptospirosis is a multisystem disorder, characterized by a broad spectrum of illness ranging from subclinical illness to either a self-limited anicteric systemic illness (quasi 90 % of affected subjects) or a severe icteric septicemic illness associated with renal failure, liver failure, and pneumonitis with hemorrhagic diathesis. It is a biphasic disease with an initial septicemic phase followed by defervescence and the immune phase of illness. The most severe presentation that may develop after the initial leptospiremic phase is Weil's disease, which is associated with impaired liver and kidney function. Mortality rates in these patients range from 5 to 40 % ([192] (EBM:2+)).

Ocular manifestations are seen in both the acute leptospiremic and immune phases of the illness. In the former phase, the most prominent findings are conjunctival chemosis and scleral icterus, while in the latter phase, there is a myriad of ocular signs such as interstitial keratitis iritis, hypopyon, cataract, membranous vitreous opacities, and retinal vasculitis; meanwhile, the most important systemic features of this immune phase are meningitis and leptospiruria. In leptospiral uveitis, hypopyon is the primary expression of the intraocular inflammation. Nongranulomatous uveitis is the hallmark of leptospiral uveitis.

Differential Diagnosis
It includes Behcet's disease, HLA-B27-associated anterior uveitis, sarcoidosis, syphilis, toxoplasmosis, ARN, and endogenous endophthalmitis.

Treatment
Systemic leptospirosis has raised several controversies regarding antimicrobial treatment.

Despite a lack of evidence of the utility of antibiotic therapy for leptospirosis, penicillin, cephalosporins, and doxycycline are the commonly employed therapies in the management of leptospirosis. Despite its higher cost, interest in azithromycin against *Leptospira* spp. is increasing due to its broad activity against confounding pathogens, low mean inhibitory concentration (MIC), and fewer mild adverse events [286, 287].

For mild infection, doxycycline 100 mg po bid can be used for 7 days, amoxicillin 50 mg po q6 h for 7 days, and ampicillin 500–750 mg po q6 h for 7 days.

For moderate to severe infection, penicillin G 1.5 million UI IV q6 h can be used for 10 days, ampicillin 0.5–1 g q6 h for 10 days, and ceftriaxone 1 g IV qd for 10 days. For severe uveitis or neurological abnormalities or arthritis, ceftriaxone 2 g/day for 14–21 days ([78] (EBM:1+, B), [209] (EBM:2++, B), [42] (EBM:1-)) is given.

Corticosteroids are the mainstay of treatment for leptospiral uveitis. In unilateral panuveitis, sub-Tenon depot corticosteroids can be used, while in bilateral panuveitis, oral corticosteroids can be employed.

> **Core Message**
> - Leptospirosis is a zoonotic waterborne infection commonly classified as a tropical disease that mainly affects young and middle-aged men.
> - It has a wide-ranging clinical and public health impact, in particular, in developing countries with a broad variety of clinical manifestation and significant mortality rate.
> - MAT is considered as a gold standard diagnostic test.
> - The most important intraocular clinical manifestations are nongranulomatous panuveitis, papillitis, and vitritis. Despite the lack of evidence, utility of antibiotic therapy is common, whereas corticosteroids are the mainstay of treatment for ocular involvement.

10.1.4.4 Lyme Disease

Definition

Lyme borreliosis is a bacterial infection caused by *Borrelia burgdorferi*. The spirochete is transmitted through the bite of infected ticks. The diagnosis is based on clinical history and examination and can be supplemented by laboratory investigations.

Etiology

The disease was described in 1977 by Steere et al., who described a group of children presenting with inflammatory arthropathy similar to that in juvenile rheumatoid arthritis. This entity was labeled "Lyme disease" after the town of Lyme, Connecticut [35, 170]. A characteristic rash was associated with the disease, labeled as erythema chronicum migrans often associated with severe headaches. Erythema migrans is the most common clinical presentation. Ocular involvement is uncommon and occurs mainly in the second and late stages of the disease. The causative agent was later identified by Burgdorfer, who described the spirochete in the midgut of the Ixodes tick. The hosts (deer and small rodents) and the Ixodes tick often thrive in the climates of the endemic regions such as northern Asia, Europe, and North America.

Clinical Signs and Symptoms

The disease is divided into stages ([118] (EBM: A+)). During early infection, it can be identified as the first (local) stage which appears a few days after the tick bite and includes erythema migrans (bull's eye), fever, and arthralgias. However, 20–40 % of patients never develop a skin rash.

This is followed by the second (disseminated) stage during which the organism spreads to multiple organ systems. Particularly the skin, heart (associated with atrioventricular block), joints (associated with mono- or oligo-arthropathy), and nervous system are affected. Neurological involvement is frequently associated with palsies of the cranial nerves and meningitis. "Lymphocytoma benigna" is a bluish lesion occurring at the earlobes and nipple region.

The third or late (persistent) stage occurs after a disease-free period (months to years).

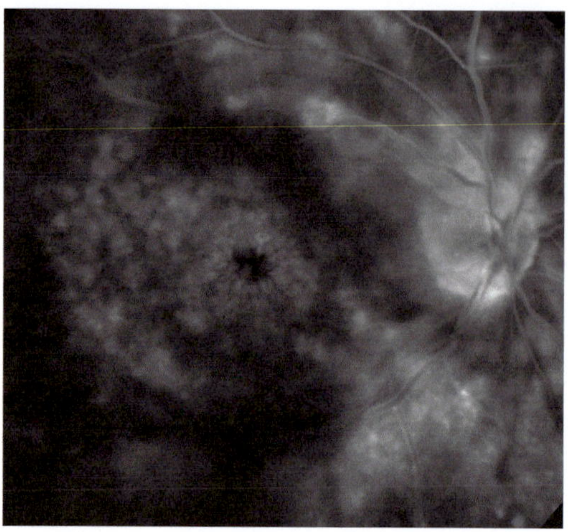

Fig. 10.8 Retinal vasculitis complicated by "honeycomb" cystoid macular edema in a patient with Lyme disease

Recurrent manifestations are the hallmark of this stage and include chronic relapsing arthritis mainly affecting the knee, acrodermatitis chronica atrophicans, chronic encephalopathy associated with cognitive dysfunction, and peripheral neuropathies.

Ocular Manifestations

Ocular manifestations are rare in patients with Lyme disease and can involve any of the ocular structures. Conjunctivitis is the most common finding, present in 11 % of patients with early disease. Episcleritis may occasionally be found with conjunctivitis during the local stage. Keratitis is one of the most common findings that appear during the late persistent stage.

Neuro-ophthalmic manifestations belong to the local and mainly disseminated stages, including optic neuritis, papillitis, papilledema, Bell's palsy which is the most common cranial neuropathy, and Horner's syndrome.

Intraocular inflammation has been reported to occur during the early and late stages of Lyme disease. Anterior uveitis, intermediate uveitis, posterior uveitis with choroiditis, and retinal vasculitis (Fig. 10.8) have been reported. Anterior uveitis associated with granulomatous KP-s and intermediate uveitis are the most common intraocular manifestations.

Differential Diagnosis

The most common infectious disorders are syphilis, TBC, viral keratitis, infectious arthritis, and viral encephalitis/meningitis. Noninfectious disorders that may have to be considered in the differential diagnosis from Lyme disease are sarcoidosis, VKH, multiple sclerosis, vasculitis, and collagen vascular disorders.

Treatment

Recommendations for the treatment of Lyme disease were reviewed by the Infectious Disease Society of America ([277] (EBM:1++, A)). In early infection, the adult doses are doxycycline 100 mg po bid for 14–21 days, amoxicillin 50 mg po tid for 14–21 days, and cefuroxime axetil 500 mg po bid for 14–21 days. In children, the doses are amoxicillin 50 mg/kg/day divided in three doses (maximum of 500 mg/dose) (Table 10.3).

In cases of severe ocular manifestations and neurological involvement, such as posterior uveitis, intravenous antibiotic therapy with ceftriaxone (2 g IV qd in adults for 2–4 weeks) is probably the treatment of choice ([277] (EBM:1++, A), [266] (EBM: 1+, A)). After systemic antibiotic treatment has been initiated, intraocular inflammation should be treated with topical corticosteroids and mydriatics. Systemic corticosteroids are proposed for severe posterior uveitis and neuro-ophthalmic involvement ([208] (EBM:4, D)). Attention should be directed at Jarisch-Herxheimer reaction after initiation of antibiotic therapy.

Core Message

- Lyme disease is characterized by a wide variety of changes including rather nonspecific flu-like symptoms associated with tiredness, headaches, arthralgia, and skin manifestations. The characteristic skin rash "erythema migrans" is the most common clinical presentation appearing about 3–30 days after a tick bite. Left untreated, later symptoms may involve the joints, heart, and central nervous system.

Table 10.3 Antibiotics frequently used in the treatment of *Lyme borreliosis* (EBM: 1A+))

Antibiotic	Route	Adult dose	Child dose	Duration
Erythema migrans	Doxycycline oral	200 mg daily	Not recommended	14 days
	Amoxicillin oral	500 mg/8 h	50 mg/kg/day in 3 divided doses	14 days
	Cefuroxime axetil oral	500 mg/12 h	30 mg/kg/day in 2 divided doses (Maximum 500 mg/dose)	14 days
Neurological Lyme borreliosis including uveitis	Doxycycline oral	200 mg daily (or 100 mg/12 h)	Not recommended	14 days
(Excluding encephalomyelitis or severe meningitis)	Ceftriaxone daily	IV 2 g 50–75 mg/kg (Maximum 2 g)	(Maximum 2 g) 50–75 mg/kg	14 days
Neurological Lyme borreliosis (Encephalomyelitis or severe meningitis)	Ceftriaxone daily	IV 2 g	50–75 mg/kg (Maximum 2 g)	14 days
Lyme arthritis or carditis or acrodermatitis chronica atrophicans	Doxycycline oral	200 mg daily	Not recommended	21 days
	Amoxicillin oral	500 mg/8 h	50 mg/kg/day in 3 divided doses	
	Ceftriaxone daily	IV 2 g	50–75 mg/kg (Maximum 2 g)	21 days

Based on Warshafsky et al. 2010 ([266]

- The ocular manifestations of Lyme borreliosis most commonly occur during the late stages of this tick-transmitted disease.
- A small proportion of patients who have had LB may go on to develop a post-infection syndrome resembling chronic fatigue syndrome or fibromyalgia, which has been termed "post-Lyme syndrome."
- Diagnostic strategies vary between early and late disease manifestations and usually include serologic methods. Erythema migrans is pathognomonic and does not require any further laboratory investigations. PCR has shown to be useful in the diagnosis of the disease, but serology should only be ordered in case of well-founded clinical suspicion for *Lyme borreliosis*, i.e., manifestations compatible with the diagnosis.
- Antibiotics are the mainstay of therapy, with corticosteroids associated during severe intraocular inflammation.

10.1.4.5 Cat Scratch Disease

Definition

Cat scratch disease (CSD) is a self-limited, systemic disease caused by a gram-negative bacillus, *Bartonella henselae* [64]. The disease manifests itself as a mild lymphadenitis involving the lymph nodes draining the dermal/conjunctival sites. CSD manifests a clinical spectrum ranging from a mild self-limiting disease with neuroretinitis and macular star formation to retinal vasculitis with subsequent severe vision loss.

Etiology

Within different species of *Bartonella*, there are four recognized as human pathogens: *B. bacilliformis* (Carrion's disease), *B. elizabethae* (endocarditis), *B. quintana* (trench fever), and *B. henselae* [271]. *Bartonella* species are gram-negative bacilli which have been associated with a clinical syndrome of self-limited lymphadenopathy associated with a transmission by cat scratch/bite. Human infections can be relatively asymptomatic or can produce symptoms such as fever, malaise, fatigue, and lymphadenopathy.

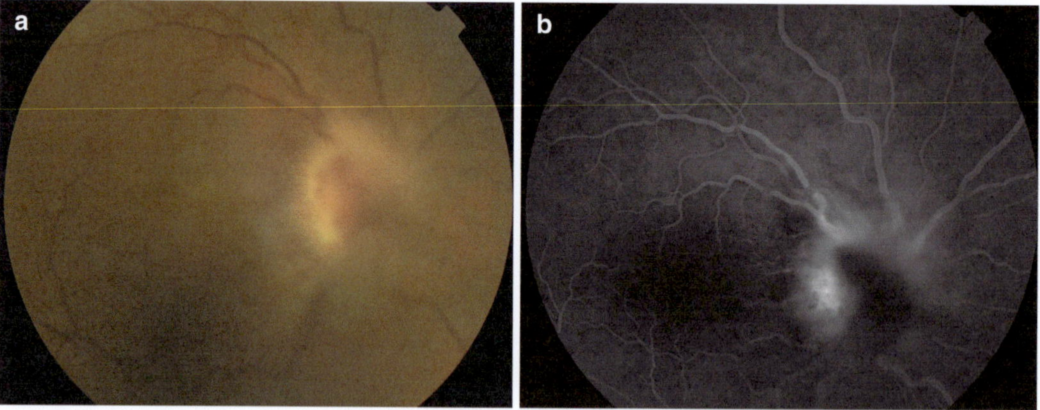

Fig. 10.9 (**a**) Color fundus photograph of the right eye of a patient with CSD shows a prominent optic disk edema associated with hemorrhage. (**b**) Fluorescein angiogram of the same eye shows optic disk leakage and masking effect by hemorrhages

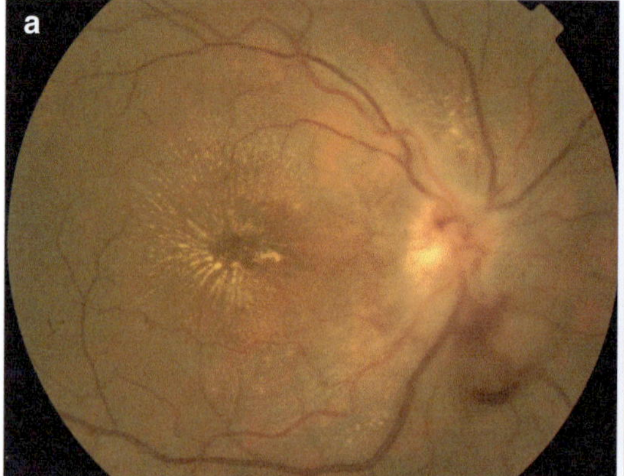

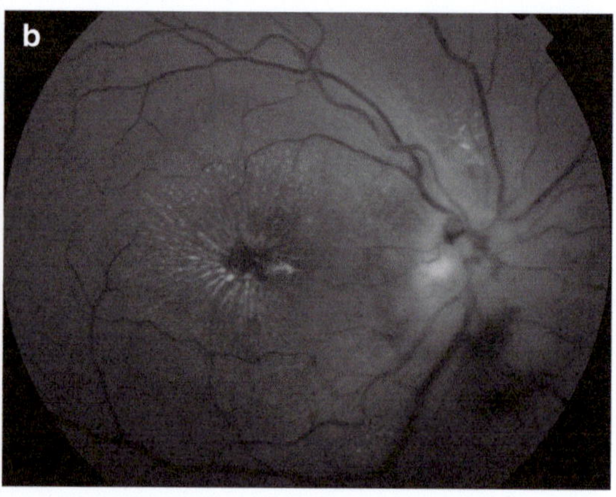

Fig. 10.10 (**a**) Photograph taken 15 days after initial presentation shows a complete macular star with partial resolution of optic disk edema. (**b**) Note the presence of optic disk telangiectatic vessels and associated preretinal hemorrhages

On the other hand, severe systemic involvement can occur, characterized by splenomegaly, encephalopathy, pneumonia, granulomatous hepatitis, and osteomyelitis. Cat fleas are the major vector for CSD.

The eye can be involved either with the primary inoculation complex resulting in Parinaud's oculoglandular syndrome, as is the most common presentation of *Bartonella* infection. The typical signs are unilateral granulomatous conjunctivitis and regional lymphadenopathy. Preauricular, submandibular, and cervical lymph nodes are typically affected. Vascular leakage from the optic nerve head (Fig. 10.9) ([56] (EBM:2, B)) and the "macular star" (Fig. 10.10) are the hallmark of the neuroretinitis, which may persist even after the resolution of posterior pole involvement. Typically, neuroretinitis is unilateral with a self-limited course.

Both multifocal retinitis and choroiditis are typically seen in conjunction with disk swelling. These lesions are typically juxtavascular. The inner white retinal infiltrates may look similar to cotton-wool spots, but their distribution is not necessarily associated with the distribution of arterioles as in the case of cotton-wool spots. Other clinical findings can be observed, such as branch retinal artery and vein occlusions, local serous retinal detachments, and intraretinal bleeding.

Differential Diagnosis

Etiologies that must be differentiated include other causes of optic nerve swelling such as optic neuritis and sarcoid papillitis. Pseudotumor cerebri can mimic the rare occurrence of the bilateral CSD. Syphilitic perineuritis, TBC, Lyme disease, leptospirosis, and, rarely, toxoplasmosis can produce similar clinical appearance. Other causes of macular star formation include systemic hypertension.

Other causes of conjunctivitis associated with regional lymphadenopathy include tularemia, sporotrichosis, TBC, syphilis, *lymphogranuloma venereum*, and leprosy.

Treatment

Usually, no treatment is recommended for mild to moderate forms of systemic CSD, since the disease runs a self-limited course. Treatment is recommended for severe ocular/systemic complications of *B. henselae* infection, both in immunocompetent and immunocompromised patients ([207] (EBM D 3)). Currently, no controlled clinical trial has demonstrated efficacy in immunocompetent patients. Doxycycline (100 mg twice daily) has good intraocular and CNS penetration. For pediatric patients (8–12 years), erythromycin is recommended. The duration of treatment lasts 2–4 weeks in immunocompetent patients and 4 months in immunocompromised patients. Azithromycin, intramuscular gentamicin, ciprofloxacin, and trimethoprim/sulfamethoxazole are alternative antibiotics ([207] (EBM:4, D)). The role of corticosteroids in atypical CSD is somewhat controversial.

> **Core Message**
> - *B. henselae* is a relatively common cause of neuroretinitis in CSD and probably underdiagnosed.
> - Mild to moderate forms of CSD run a self-limited course with no need for treatment. Patients with neuroretinitis, encephalopathy with or without hemiplegia, and acute solid organ transplant rejection have all been treated successfully with a combination of appropriate antibiotics and steroid therapy.
> - Patients with CSD have a good overall visual prognosis.
> - Good visual acuity at presentation was associated with a favorable visual outcome.

10.1.4.6 Rickettsial Diseases

Rickettsioses are worldwide distributed zoonoses due to obligate intracellular small gramnegative bacteria. Most of them are transmitted to humans by the bite of contaminated arthropods, such as ticks especially during spring or summer. Rickettsial agents are classified into three major categories: the spotted fever group, the typhus group, and the scrub typhus ([265] (EBM:2++, B)). The spotted fever group includes Mediterranean spotted fever (MSF), which is prevalent in Mediterranean countries and Central Asia; Rocky Mountain spotted fever, which is mainly encountered in the United States; and numerous other rickettsial agents.

Clinical Presentation

The initial clinical presentation includes high fever, myalgia, and headaches with a "tache noir" developing in the site of the bite. A maculopapular rash may be present at the time of presentation. Neurological signs ranging from small focal deficits to major neuropsychiatric disturbances have been reported.

Systemic Disease

The incubation period for rickettsial disease varies between 2 and 21 days. The initial presentation typically includes high fever with abrupt onset, headache, and myalgia. A maculopapular skin rash usually appears 3–5 days after the onset of fever. The skin rash, involving also the palms of the hands and the soles of the feet, is a hallmark of rickettsial infection. However, its absence should not rule out a possible rickettsial infection, especially during the first week of illness. A local skin lesion, termed tache noire (black spot), at the inoculating site may be seen in several rickettsial infections, including Mediterranean spotted fever, which is caused by *Rickettsia conorii*. Severe systemic complications may occur including interstitial pneumonitis, meningoencephalitic syndrome, acute renal failure, and disseminated intravascular coagulation [265].

Ocular Disease

Ocular involvement is common in patients with rickettsiosis, but since it is frequently asymptomatic and self-limited, it may be easily overlooked [265].

Bilateral or rarely unilateral non-necrotizing retinitis, with or without associated mild vitritis, is the most common ocular finding [265]. It typically presents in the form of white retinal lesions infiltrating the inner retinal layers (Fig. 10.11), located adjacent to retinal vessels, and varying in number, size, and location. Small retinal lesions in the posterior fundus may resemble cottonwool spots, and large retinal lesions are usually associated with macular edema and exudative retinal detachment, which are accurately detectable by OCT. FA usually shows early hypofluorescence and late staining of large retinal lesions (Fig. 10.12) and slight hypofluorescence or isofluorescence of small retinal lesions [265]. Retinal vascular lesions are a prominent feature of rickettsial disease. They may include focal or diffuse vascular sheathing, vascular leakage on fluorescein angiography (FA), retinal hemorrhages, and retinal vascular occlusions, which mainly involve small branch retinal arteries [133]. A subclinical choroidal involvement only detectable by FA or indocyanine green angiography (ICGA) is also common [265].

Other reported ocular manifestations of rickettsiosis include conjunctivitis, keratitis, nongranulomatous anterior uveitis, panuveitis, optic disk edema, optic disk staining, optic neuritis, neuroretinitis, anterior ischemic optic neuropathy, and endophthalmitis [265].

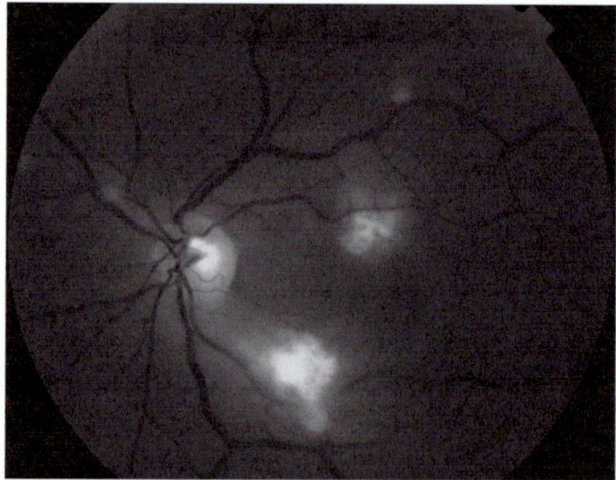

Fig. 10.11 Red-free fundus photograph of a patient with serologically proven rickettsial disease shows white retinal lesions of variable size, adjacent to retinal vessels

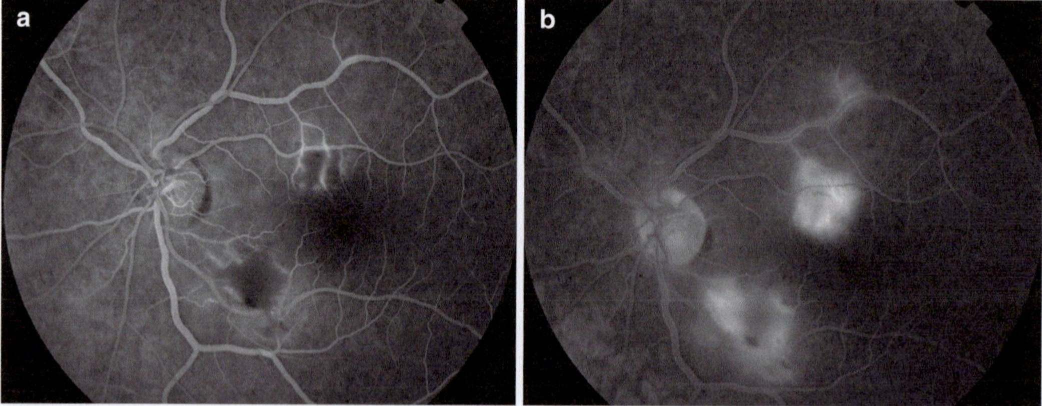

Fig. 10.12 Fluorescein angiography shows early hypofluorescence (**a**) and late staining of retinal lesions associated with focal retinal vascular leakage and optic disk hyperfluorescence (**b**)

Ophthalmic involvement associated with rickettsial diseases often has a self-limited course. Areas of retinitis usually completely disappear without causing scarring in 3–10 weeks. Causes of persistent visual impairment include residual retinal changes due to resolved retinitis, macular edema, exudative retinal detachment, branch retinal artery or vein occlusion, and optic neuropathy [265].

Laboratory Diagnosis

Early diagnosis of rickettsial infection, primarily based on clinical features and epidemiologic data, is of utmost importance for early initiation of antibiotic therapy. Confirmation of diagnosis usually relies on positive indirect immunofluorescent antibody test results. Positive serologic criteria usually include either initial high antibody titer or a fourfold rise of the titer in the convalescent serum. Case confirmation with serology might take 2–3 weeks. Other laboratory tests, such as serologic testing using Western blot or detection of rickettsiae in the blood or tissue using PCR, may be useful in selected cases [265].

Management

Early treatment is required for a better outcome. Oral tetracyclines, particularly doxycycline (100 mg, twice a day for 7–10 days), are effective in the treatment of systemic rickettsial disease [265]. Fluoroquinolones are also effective. Macrolides, including clarithromycin, azithromycin, and particularly josamycin, can be used as alternative therapy in children and pregnant women.

Specific ophthalmic therapy may be needed in patients with ocular involvement. It includes topical antibiotics for conjunctivitis and keratitis, topical corticosteroids and mydriatics for anterior uveitis, and systemic steroids in association with antibiotics in cases of severe ophthalmic involvement such as extensive retinitis threatening the macula or the optic disk, macular edema, exudative retinal detachment, severe vitritis, optic neuropathy, and retinal vascular occlusions [265]. Prevention of rickettsial disease includes personal protection against tick bites in endemic areas and improvement of sanitary conditions.

> **Core Message**
> - Ocular involvement in rickettsiosis is common but frequently asymptomatic.
> - Retinitis is a typical finding associated with vitritis and vascular lesions.
> - In order to diagnose this disease, a high index of suspicion is needed especially when associated with the specific clinical systemic symptoms and patients living or returning from endemic areas.
> - FA and ICGA are essential in subclinical cases.
> - Doxycycline is the mainstay of treatment.

10.1.5 Parasitic Uveitis

10.1.5.1 Ocular Toxoplasmosis
Definition
Ocular toxoplasmosis (OT) is considered as the most frequent infectious posterior uveitis. It is caused by the protozoan parasite *Toxoplasma gondii*, which exists in multiple clonal subpopulations, and in three stages, human seroprevalence of toxoplasmosis is high across the globe, but with remarkable geographic variation. A potential correlation of parasite genotype with disease is an area of current interest [160]. Ocular toxoplasmosis is more common in South America, Central America, and the Caribbean and parts of tropical Africa as compared to Europe and Northern America. Ocular disease in South America is more severe than in other continents due to the presence of extremely virulent genotypes of the parasite [200].

Etiology
The mode of *T. gondii* infection as either congenital or postnatally acquired is considered to be important. Although congenital infection frequently results in chronic recrudescent retinochoroiditis, most cases of OT are acquired after birth [249].

Clinical Symptoms and Signs
Symptoms vary but usually consist of unilateral floaters or blurred vision when the disease becomes active. Inactive disease rarely causes visual symptoms unless scarring is near the central retina

or macula. Acute OT appears as a well-defined focus of retinal necrosis accompanied by a vitreous inflammatory reaction. In addition, there may be diffuse inflammation in the retina and choroid. OT typically runs a clinical course of 2–4 months of active intraocular inflammation followed by more or less long disease-free intervals, which may extend for several years. The reactivation of OT shows satellite lesions close to an old atrophic scar (Fig. 10.13). In the area surrounding the active retinitis, hemorrhage and vasculitis may be observed. Anterior uveitis may also be present. Atypical clinical findings may occur as well, such as vascular occlusive events and Kyrieleis's arteritis [55]. Imaging can offer more information [97]. Bilateral involvement or atypical presentation can be observed in immune-compromised patients and often in congenital OT (Fig. 10.14).

Differential Diagnosis

Necrotizing retinochoroiditis is considered as the typical presentation of OT and considered characteristic to such a degree that often further diagnostic workup is not needed. However, even when it is the most frequent manifestation of OT, there is considerable variation in the clinical features. Therefore, other necrotizing retinopathies, such as viral diseases, fungi, and other parasites, are important differential diagnoses. In such patients, analysis of intraocular antibody production and, therefore, Goldmann-Witmer coefficient plays a decisive role in the diagnosis of ocular toxoplasmosis, even more than PCR [48, 268] (Table 10.4).

Treatment

Despite the fact that OT continues to be a very common and sight-threatening cause of infectious posterior uveitis, treatment remains highly controversial (Fig. 10.15). This is related to a number of factors:

- In many patients, *T. gondii* infection is a self-limited (often asymptomatic) disease that has been considered to need no treatment.
- The parasites are able to form cysts that are impenetrable to medications and host enzymes; therefore, they cannot be eliminated from retinal tissue.
- The persistence of retinal cysts also results in a very successful strategy for its survival and

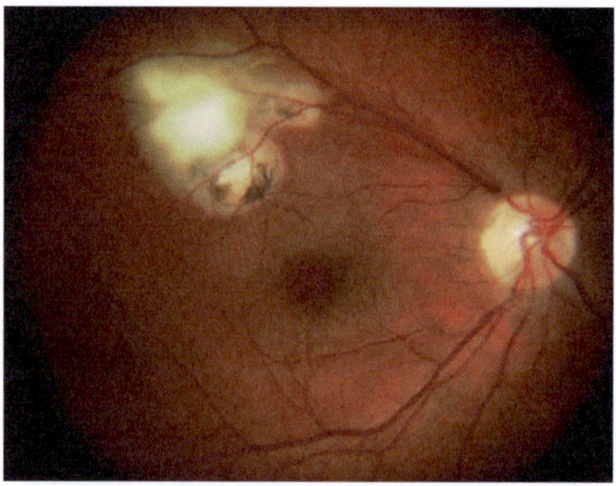

Fig. 10.13 Fundus photography of a 27-year-old patient presenting with recurrent paracentral retinochoroiditis caused by *T. gondii*. Aqueous humor analysis: Goldmann-Witmer coefficient >5

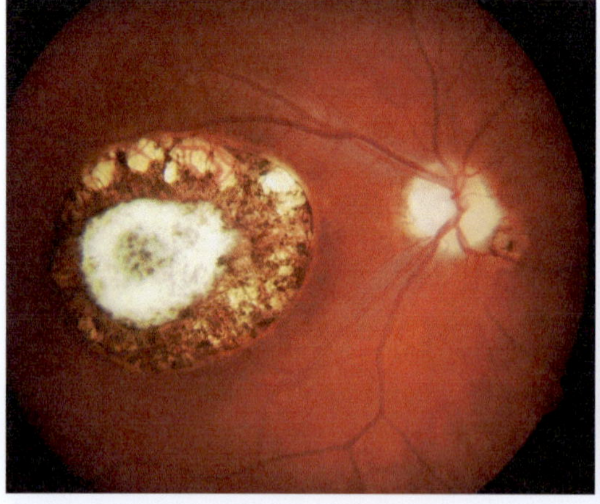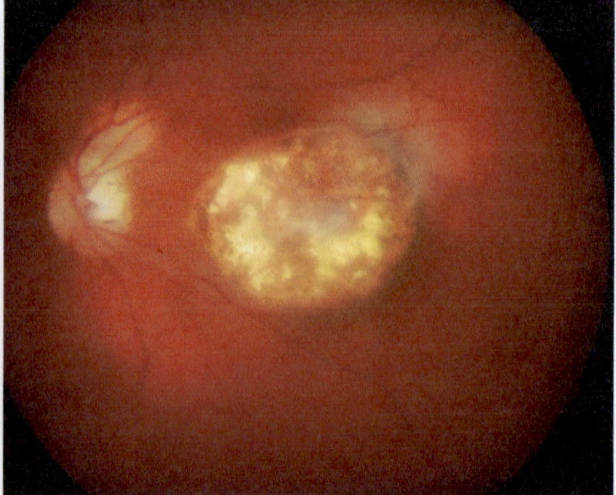

Fig. 10.14 Fundus photography of a 21-year-old patient affected by bilateral congenital ocular toxoplasmosis. The deep retinochoroidal lesion can be clearly seen

Table 10.4 Differential diagnosis of necrotizing retinopathies

Differential diagnosis	Clinical characteristics
Acute retina necrosis syndrome (herpes simplex virus, VZV CMV)	Acute onset; unilateral rapidly progressing necrotizing retinitis; initial: in peripheral retina; often anterior segment involvement
Tuberculosis	Symptoms depending on localization; often multiple choroidal infiltrates, hemorrhagic lesions; often no pulmonary involvement
Multifocal choroiditis	Often asymptomatic; initial: multiple, peripheral, (bilateral) choroidal lesions; progression with new lesions and increasing vitreous involvement occurs frequently
POHS ("histoplasmosis")	Often asymptomatic; multiple, sharply bordered, small lesions ("histo spots"); predominantly midperipheral retina; no vitreous involvement; frequently: choroidal neovascularization
PIC (punctate inner choroidopathy)	Often acute onset of symptoms (decreased vision, scotoma, photopsia; predominant in myopic females; small central lesions (100–300 um); often: choroidal neovascularization
Sarcoidosis	Multiple granulomatous changes in all ocular segments; bilateral active retina lesions; involvement of other organs (lung, skin, liver)

effectively avoids immunosurveillance by the host.

Despite the limited evidence of treatment effects, an increasing number of experienced ophthalmologists will treat patients with active OT [114].

Common clinical indications include:

- Lesions within the vascular arcades threatening central vision
- Active lesions in close proximity to the optic disk since substantial visual field defects may result
- Large lesions >2 optic disk diameter which are often associated with dense vitreous haze
- Immunosuppressed individuals because these patients very likely develop fulminant retinochoroiditis when left untreated

Several surveys of uveitis specialists indicate that even experts differ in their therapeutic approaches. Whereas some ophthalmologists will only care for sight-threatening lesions, others will treat all lesions independent on its location [28, 114, 255] (Fig. 10.16). Despite a lack of published evidence for effectiveness of current therapies, most ophthalmologists elect to treat patients with ocular toxoplasmosis that reduces or threatens visual acuity. Classic therapy consists of oral pyrimethamine and sulfadiazine, plus systemic corticosteroid. Substantial toxicity of this drug combination has spurred interest in alternative antimicrobials, as well as local forms of drug delivery ([217] [EBM C 3]). At this time, however, no therapeutic approach is curative of ocular toxoplasmosis.

In a Cochrane review, *Gilbert* et al. identified only three prospective, randomized, placebo-controlled clinical trials. Interestingly, two of these studies were conducted almost 40 years ago, using either eight weeks of pyrimethamine/trisulfapyrimidine vs. placebo or 4 weeks of pyrimethamine compared with placebo in acute OT [244] [EBM: B, 2++] [38] [EBM: 1+, B]. The third study determined the prophylactic effect of long-term (20 months) trimethoprim/sulfamethoxazole application vs. no treatment in patients with chronic relapsing OT [234] [EBM: B, 2++]. There was a lack of evidence in all three studies that antibiotics (short or long term) prevented vision loss. Only one study observing individuals infected with probably more aggressive South American strains of *T. gondii* demonstrated that long-term antibiotics (14 months) reduced the number of recurrences.

Because of toxicity and lack of effectivity, a number of alternative agents have been applied to OT patients. Clindamycin was a very promising substance when introduced in the 1980s [248] because it appeared to concentrate in ocular tissues and was considered to penetrate tissue cyst walls [248]. However, subsequent clinical experience showed no effect on disease recurrence [147] [EBM: C, 2+]. Recent treatment attempts focused on the use of clindamycin delivery as intravitreal injection [21, 140, 148] [EBM C 2+]. In a prospective randomized study comparing intravitreal clindamycin with 6 weeks of systemic clindamycin treatment, both

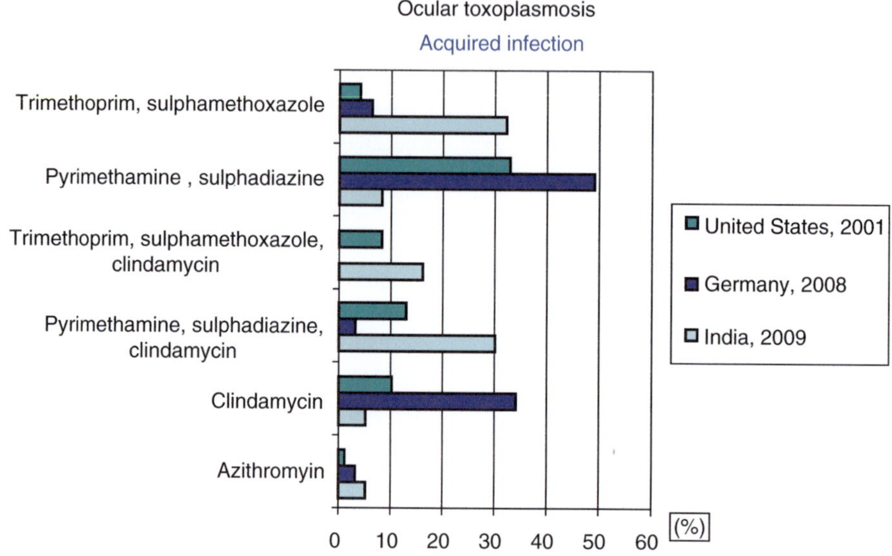

Fig. 10.15 Histogram illustrating the preferred practice pattern derived from three surveys focusing on treatment of acquired ocular toxoplasmosis (Adapted from Basu et al. [28])

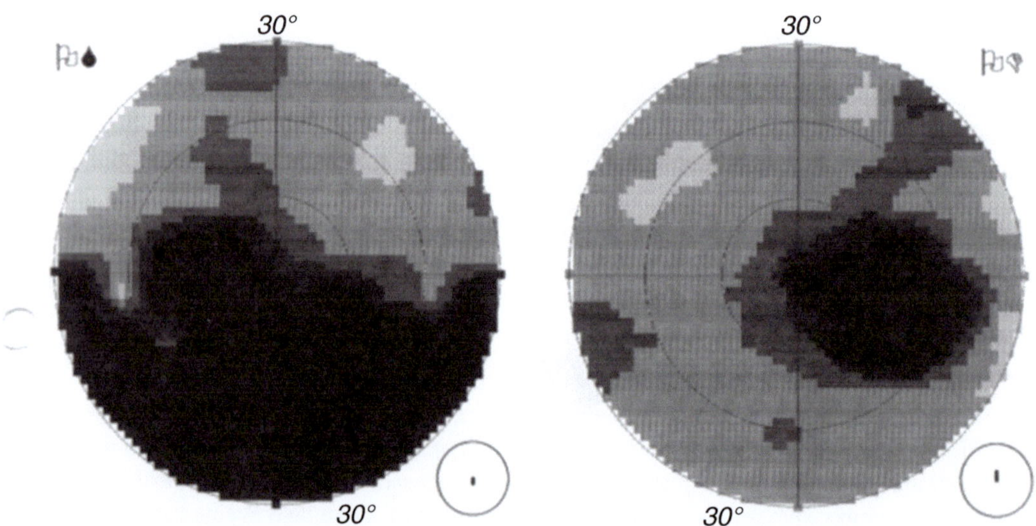

Fig. 10.16 Corresponding central scotoma of the patient of "Fig. 10.14" as findings in perimetry

appeared similarly effective [242] [EBM: B, 2++]. In a non-comparative, retrospective, multicentric interventional case series, 12 patients with active OT involving the posterior pole that were either intolerant to or contraindicated to oral medication received intravitreal injections of clindamycin (1.5 mg/0.1 ml) and dexamethasone (400 µg/0.1 ml) every 4 weeks (during pregnancy). During follow-up (24 months), reso-lution of OT was achieved in all cases and most eyes (83 %) improved, whereas two eyes (20 %) remained unchanged. No ocular or systemic adverse events were reported and furthermore no recurrences during 24 months of follow-up were observed [148] [EBM: C, 2+]. In particular, during pregnancy, sight-threatening lesions may be treated with intraocular injections of clindamycin and dexamethasone, combined with systemic

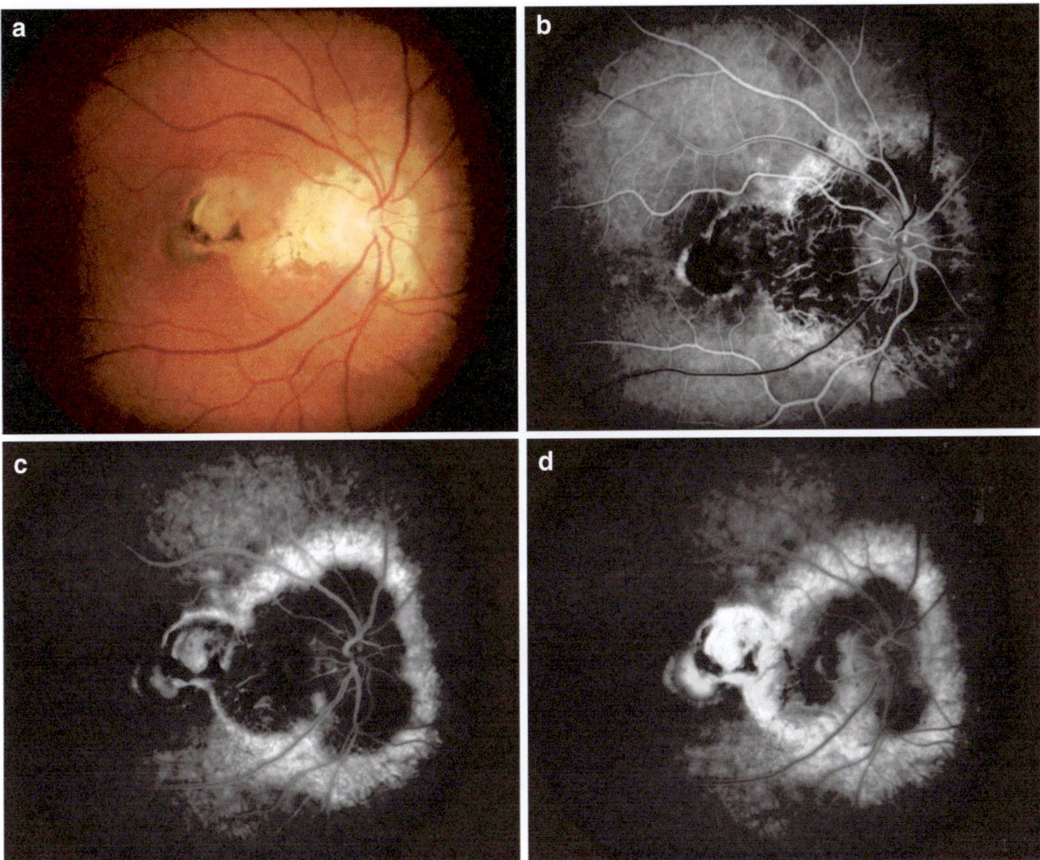

Fig. 10.17 Color picture (**a**) showing CNV in congenital ocular toxoplasmosis. Early (**b**), mid (**c**) and late (**d**) phases of FA showing an inactive CNV near the edge of an old, peripapillary toxoplasmic scar

sulfadiazine ([166] [EBM D 3]). Taken together, both studies demonstrated that IVI of clindamycin/dexamethasone might be an alternative to systemic treatment, offering a high drug availability and safer systemic adverse effect profile.

In addition, azithromycin [30] and atovaquone [197] were introduced into clinical use, but have not gained widespread acceptance (EBM: D, 3). There appears also an increasing use of the trimethoprim/sulfamethoxazole combination, offering a better option for compliance as does the standard combination of a dihydrofolate reductase inhibitor and sulphonamide. Small-scale uncontrolled studies showed apparently accelerated rates of resolution and improved acuities in patients on the combination [185] (EBM: D, 3). There remains, however, significant uncertainty with regard to proper medication by experts in the field. This is reflected by several surveys of uveitis specialists in the United States, Germany, and India, indicating that at least nine separate drugs in even more combinations are currently used in daily practice [28, 114, 255].

Management of Complications (CNV)

Several techniques have been proposed for CNV secondary to ocular toxoplasmosis (Fig. 10.17): PDT [EBM:C, 2+] [177], intravitreal anti-VEGF therapy [EBM: C, 2+] [164], and COMBO therapy [EBM: D, 3+] are the different therapeutic options [214].

Perioperative Prophylaxis

Perioperative prophylactic anti-toxoplasmic therapy may be warranted, in order to avoid reactivation of the disease [39] [EBM: C, 2+].

Management of Congenital Ocular Toxoplasmosis

Congenital OT is recognized as a major cause of child morbidity and mortality. Vertical transmission of toxoplasmosis occurs during primary infection in pregnant women, and generally, maternal disease goes unnoticed. Fetal infection occurs at up to 65–70 % and results in significant child morbidity with ocular lesions in up to 80 % of children as the most frequent manifestation [76, 169]. Therefore, prevention and treatment of congenital toxoplasmosis remains an important issue.

Worldwide remarkable differences exist regarding effective screening and treatment strategies. Reasons are related to the questionable benefit of early diagnosis and intervention since well-controlled studies are lacking and difficult to perform [83, 93, 94]. However, in most European centers, spiramycin remains the standard treatment and is immediately applied after diagnosis of maternal infection followed by pyrimethamine/sulphonamide as soon as a fetal infection is confirmed [93] [EBM: D, 2+]. Contrary, other treatment strategies rely initially on pyrimethamine/sulphonamide that will be changed to spiramycin if fetal diagnosis is negative [93] [EBM: C, 2+]. A meta-analysis investigating these different data in 2007 concluded that only weak evidence exists for an association between early treatment and reduced risk of congenital toxoplasmosis [252] [EBM: C, 2+]. However, it has been demonstrated by several studies that early treatment with spiramycin resulted in a significantly reduced rate (95 vs. 80 %) of placenta infection [61]. This led to a 50 % reduced incidence and lower severity of disease at birth of infected infants as compared to untreated individuals [135]. Recent observations confirm that it seems likely that more prompt diagnosis and treatment will result in better outcomes of congenital toxoplasmosis. New central chorioretinal lesions have been uncommon in children with congenital toxoplasmosis who are treated during their first year of life [201]. This contrasts markedly with previous observations for children left untreated or those treated for one month only ($\geq$82 % retinal lesions).

The Role of Corticosteroids

As in many other ocular infections, the host immune response may have detrimental effects. Therefore, early intervention, e.g., by the use of corticosteroids, is often beneficial to reduce tissue damage. Interestingly, histopathologic specimen of the eyes from immunocompromised patients with OT showed no inflammatory cells in the infected tissue. These observations suggest that parasite proliferation, rather than inflammation, is the major cause of tissue damage in these individuals. Therefore, corticosteroid therapy is probably not necessary to control OT in immune-compromised individuals. On the contrary, it is commonly agreed upon that corticosteroid therapy without concurrent use of antimicrobial agents can lead to severe retina destruction and large lesions. A recent Cochrane review did not find supportive evidence for steroid treatment in either immune-competent or immune-compromised OT patients [120] [EBM: B, 2+].

Alternative Treatment Options

Surgical Options

Since the effect of medical treatment is uncertain, surgical options have been considered for OT. Argon laser photocoagulation has been applied with the intention to directly disrupt the organism or to reduce recurrence by surrounding old OT lesions with laser spots [215, 243] [EBM: D, 1+]. Unfortunately, even when the parasite was confirmed to be heat sensitive, neither direct destruction of the organisms nor reduced reactivation of tissue cysts could be obtained. Laser treatment has now been abandoned. Since active intraocular inflammation always carries a risk of complications, also any other intraocular surgery is not advised.

Taken together, treatment practices in OT are highly diverse. There is still no consensus regarding the choice of antiparasitic agents for treatment regimens. Despite this uncertainty, uveitis specialists appear to be more likely to treat patients with OT as compared to a decade ago [114].

Core Message
- Ocular toxoplasmosis remains the most frequent infectious posterior uveitis in many parts of the world. Although congenital infection frequently results in retinochoroiditis, most ocular manifestations are acquired after birth (through nutrition).
- Atypical clinical findings can be observed mainly in immunocompromised individuals or elderly people.
- Although several treatment strategies have been proposed up to date, no therapeutic approach is curative of ocular toxoplasmosis.
- Steroids are frequently applied to decrease intraocular inflammation but need careful monitoring and concurrent antimicrobial treatment.

10.1.5.2 Ocular Toxocariasis

Definition

Toxocara canis and *Toxocara cati* are nematodes, which live and mature in the dog or cat intestines, respectively.

Etiology

As a mature adult, the organism releases eggs which are passed in the stool. Contact with infected materials leads to human infection.

Clinical Symptoms and Signs

Toxocariasis is a rare infection and typically is observed in children. Toxocara infection can present fever; pulmonary symptoms such as a dry, hacking cough or asthma-like attacks; splenomegaly and hepatomegaly; skin lesions; neurological symptoms such as convulsions; and meningeal symptoms [129]. Ocular symptoms comprehend decreased vision, pain, photophobia, and floaters.

The most common eye manifestation is a granuloma, either in the posterior pole or in the periphery of the retina, with massive vitritis.

Differential Diagnosis

Differential diagnosis comprehends retinoblastoma, Coats' disease, persistent fetal vasculature, retinopathy of prematurity, familial exudative vitreoretinopathy, idiopathic peripheral uveoretinitis, and toxoplasmosis. Retinoblastoma can be ruled out on the basis of B-scan echography, which typically finds calcifications, which are extremely uncommon in ocular toxocariasis. Non-inflamed eyes without cataract are also suggestive of retinoblastoma.

Laboratory tests are used to diagnose the disease: eosinophilia, hyperglobulinemia [232], and ELISA, even though a false-positive ELISA test can occur [161].

Treatment

The association of systemic prednisone (40 mg/day) and thiabendazole (2 g daily for 5 days) has been proposed ([220], EBM: D, 3). Albendazole (800 mg twice daily for adults or 400 mg twice daily for children, for 10 days to 2 weeks) can be considered as an alternative treatment option ([27], EBM: C, 2+).

Core Message
- Ocular toxocariasis should be differentiated from several ocular diseases, particularly retinoblastoma.
- Although different antihelminthic agents have been proposed, the role of such agents still remains unclear.

10.2 Noninfectious Posterior Uveitis

10.2.1 Multifocal Choroiditis (MFC)

MFC is part of the primary inflammatory choriocapillaropathies characterized by minimal signs of panuveitis mostly limited to cells in the posterior vitreous. ICGA made it clear that MFC typically involves primarily the choriocapillaris ([60, 238] (EBM:1+, A)) that shows inflammatory involvement even beyond the choriocapillaris in the choroidal stroma ([75] (EBM:3, D)). These findings may suggest an explanation for the more severe course and the propensity to develop choroidal neovascularization (CNV).

10.2.1.1 Clinical Symptoms and Signs

The majority of patients have bilateral disease that ranges from 66 to 79 % ([74, 213] (EBM:2+, D)), albeit asymmetric with the involved fellow eye. The most common symptoms are decreased central vision, photopsias, and subjective scotomas which are protracted in time. Signs of mild anterior uveitis including nongranulomatous keratic precipitates, cells, and flare can be seen associated with mild vitreous cellular activity when the disease is active. When keratic precipitates are granulomatous sarcoidosis, syphilis and tuberculosis have to be ruled out. Fundus examination reveals multiple round to oval, yellow-gray lesions, ranging in number from several to more than 100 scattered throughout the posterior pole and midperiphery. A distinct propensity for a peripapillary, nasal midperipheral, and peripheral distribution has been observed [213]. The active lesions evolve into round, atrophic chorioretinal scars with a punched-out appearance and varying degrees of hyperpigmentation. MFC shows a distinct peculiarity, that is, the high proportion of choroidal neovascular membranes complicating the disease, and typically, these almost always type II neovascular membranes seem to arise from atrophic scars or yellow nodular subretinal lesions frequently in association with active inflammation. Peripapillary atrophy similar to that seen in POHS is frequently seen on follow-up examination. Cystoid macular edema (CME) occurs in a range from 14 [74] to 41 % as reported by Nussenblatt et al. ([182] (EBM:4, D)). ICGA shows hypofluorescent areas during all the phases of the examination which are more numerous and involve a more extensive area than those appreciated on FA or clinical examination during the active stage of the disease. While during the active phase FA may show faint late hyperfluorescence reflecting the hypofluorescent lesion observed in ICGA, choroidal scars present a hyperfluorescent edge with a hypofluorescent center without leakage (Fig. 10.18). In a recent

paper from Vance SK et al. ([257] (EBM:2++, B)) regarding the characteristic findings of MFC in SD-OCT, the authors concluded that the acute lesions of MFC include the presence of sub-RPE material, choroidal hyper-reflectivity below the lesions, and overlying vitreous cells in comparison to the findings of myopic degeneration. Visual field testing can show small scotomas corresponding to the chorioretinal scars. In the active phases, scotomas are larger reflecting the choriocapillaris non-perfusion. ERG suggests that MFC is a diffuse process with the degree of dysfunction relating to the severity and extent of chorioretinal involvement. MFC is a chronic disease that may persist for many years with the majority of patients experiencing multiple inflammatory recurrences in one or both eyes and the pathology affects predominantly young, healthy adults in their mid-30s with women predominantly affected [74, 213]. Inflammatory reactivation may manifest with swelling of the choroidal scars with surrounding subretinal fluid.

10.2.1.2 Differential Diagnosis

ICGA is useful in ruling out the infectious causes such as West Nile virus choroiditis, Candida choroiditis, bacterial emboli, etc. However, in some instances, tuberculous choroiditis can also present with the same ICGA patterns as MFC. MFC exhibits anterior chamber and vitreous cells and a female predilection in contradistinction to POHS. MEWDS like MFC may present in young women with acute blind spot enlargement and vitreous inflammation; however, it is predominantly a unilateral disease. Although it has been suggested that SFU represents the terminal stage of MFC because of the multifocal lesions and the recurrent inflammatory episodes, SFU is limited to the posterior pole and eventuates in severe subretinal scarring. PIC is mostly related to MFC, with the high propensity in developing CNVM and its tendency towards bilaterality, but by definition, PIC is not associated with vitreous inflammation and the lesions tend to be smaller as compared to MFC. Other noninfectious entities to be considered in the differential diagnosis of MFC include sarcoidosis, APMPPE, and intraocular large cell lymphoma.

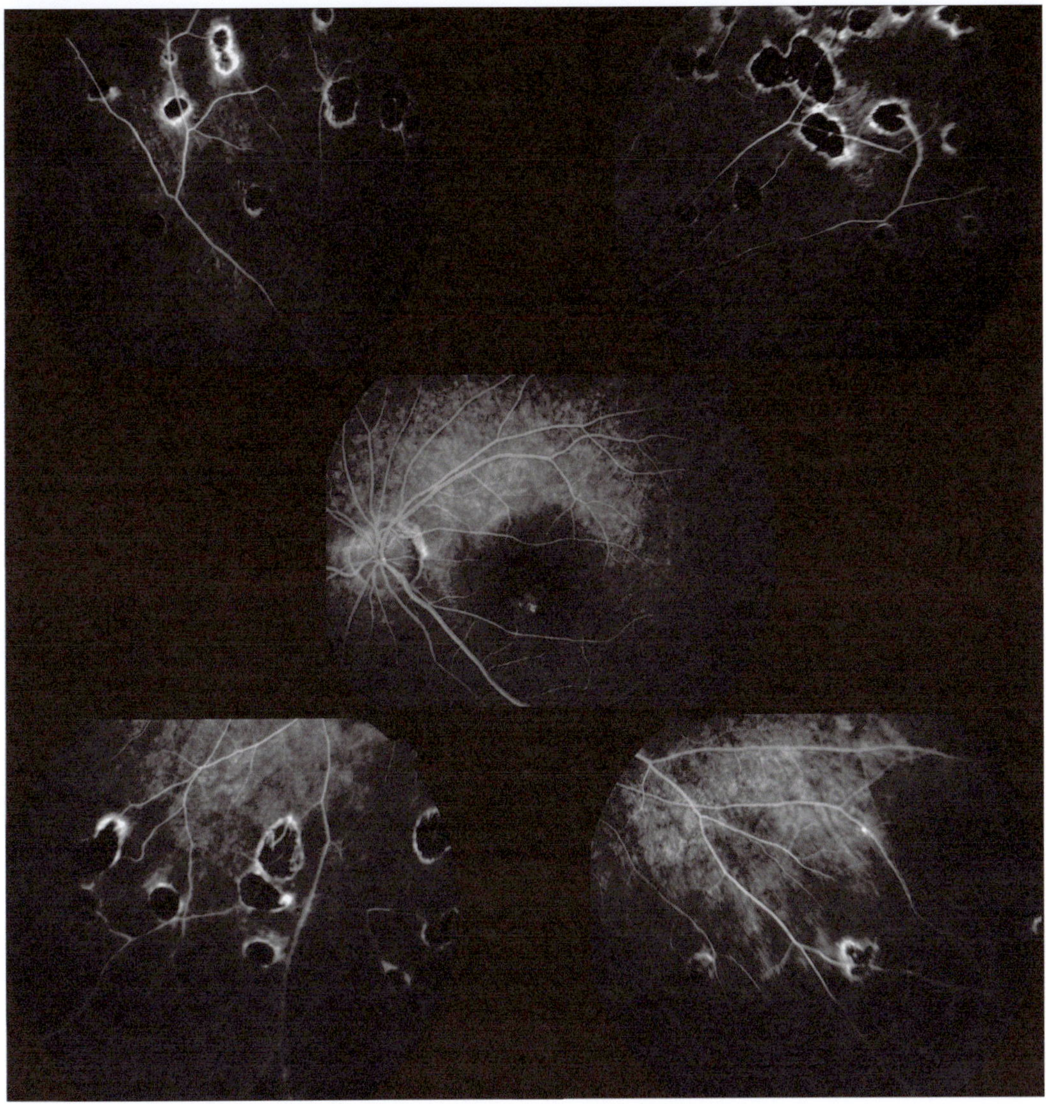

Fig. 10.18 FA showing multiple spots of a MFC associated with a juxtafoveal CNV

10.2.1.3 Treatment

Management, as for other entities under this group, is empirical. Although there are no controlled studies, clinical experience is probably sufficient to recommend corticosteroid therapy in cases with active disease; this can usually be diagnosed when patients complain of photopsia and is further evidenced by ICGA. If corticosteroids are insufficient, immunosuppressive agents may be added. The best follow-up parameter is ICGA which can show resolution of hypofluorescent areas. If inflammatory subretinal CNV is present, corticosteroids (sub-Tenon injections if the reactivation is unilateral or systemic if the reactivation is bilateral) should be tried first with concomitant or subsequent intravitreal anti-vascular endothelial growth factor (VEGF) therapy ([111] (EBM:4, D)). A recent paper published by Julian et al. reported the long-term results of 15 eyes (7 eyes with MFC) treated with intravitreal bevacizumab (IVB) as the first local treatment for CNV secondary to uveitis ([124] (EBM: 2++, C)). The intravitreal injections showed transient improvement in BCVA and CFT, in eyes under controlled inflammation, but further injections were needed in most cases with a mean number of 4.25 injections in 16 months. The peculiarity of this paper as compared to other works is the concomitant use of IVB in nine patients under systemic immunosuppression (corticosteroids and steroid-sparing agents). Another paper by Rouvas et al. ([219] (EBM:2+, C)) (three eyes) showed that ranibizumab resulted as a promising drug in maintaining stability or improving VA and OCT and FA findings in inflammatory choroidal neovascularization.

> **Core Message**
> - MFC is part of the primary inflammatory choriocapillaropathies.
> - It is characterized by recurrent episodes of chorioretinal inflammation: photopsias, scotomata, and visual loss.
> - Vitreous cells during the active stage.
> - ICGA: active disease shows hypofluorescent zones.
> - Choroidal inflammatory neovascularization is a frequent sequela.
> - Therapy: the association of corticosteroids and immunosuppressive therapy has shown to be useful in the light of multiple recurrences, with associated anti-VEGFs in cases of inflammatory CNVM.

10.2.2 Punctate Inner Choroidopathy

Punctate inner choroidopathy (PIC) is a subset of MFC (primary inflammatory choriocapillaropathy) characterized by a similar clinical picture as far as symptoms, fundus signs, and neovascular complications are concerned, except that the lesions are smaller. PIC affects predominantly young myopic women. Although PIC in the majority of cases is a self-limited disease with good visual prognosis, permanent and severe visual loss can occur as a result of the development of choroidal neovascular membranes.

10.2.2.1 Clinical Symptoms and Signs

The predominant symptoms at presentation are scotomatas, followed by blurred vision, floaters, photophobia, and metamorphopsia, and these visual disturbances are usually unilateral ([92] (EBM:1+, B)). An analysis of refractive errors in inflammatory choriocapillaropathies revealed that PIC patients had the highest refractive errors. There is lack of inflammatory reaction in the anterior chamber and vitreous. Fundus examination reveals multiple, small, gray or yellow, round lesions concentrated in the posterior pole in a random or linear pattern that sometimes can be associated with serous detachment of the overlying neuroepithelium. They usually evolve into atrophic scars, and after 2–3 months, they may resemble old punched-out lesions seen in POHS. The scars involve the RPE and the choriocapillaris sparing the rest of the choroid. The fundus abnormalities are usually bilateral in 80 % ([46] (EBM:2+, D)) of cases. The most harmful clinical sequela of PIC is the formation of CNVM, and it is estimated that 17–40 % [46] of the eyes with PIC will develop it. The most frequent visual field defect is enlargement of the blind spot. During the active phases, ICGA shows hypofluorescent areas during all the phases of the examination which gradually resolve or remain hypofluorescent in case of scarring. FA shows early hypofluorescence followed by late hyperfluorescence and staining of the lesions (Fig. 10.19). While most PIC CNVs begin as multiple, yellow-green lesions, over time a tendency towards coalescence is seen to form larger CNVMs with bridging networks. FA of these membranes shows early hyperfluorescence followed by late leakage.

10.2.2.2 Differential Diagnosis

PIC can be differentiated from POHS by the lack of peripapillary atrophic changes and peripheral retinal lesions. MEWDS lesions are also concentrated in the posterior pole as in PIC, but these lesions have a less distinct border and do not have an associated serous detachment. In contrast to PIC lesions, APMPPE lesions are typically placoid and often confluent. ICGA findings are useful in excluding the infectious causes [164].

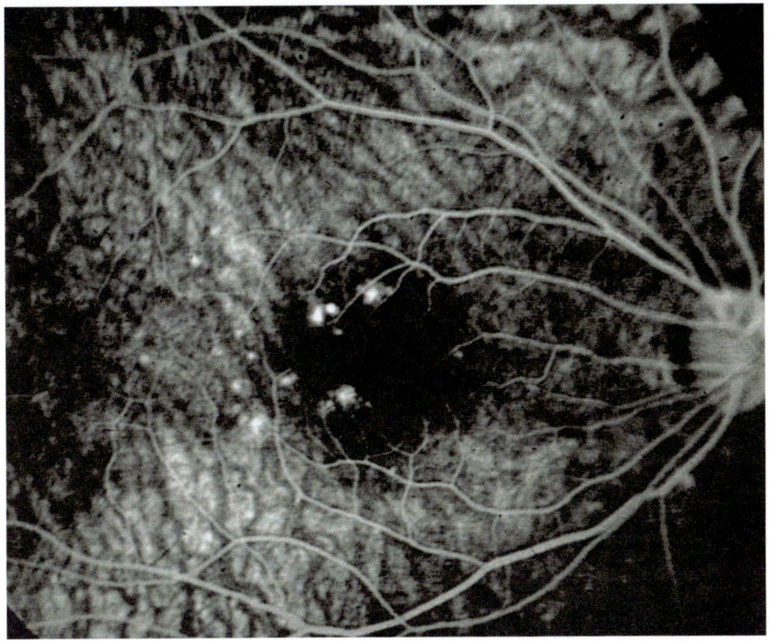

Fig. 10.19 FA showing multiple hyperfluorescent macular spots typically observed in PIC

10.2.2.3 Treatment

No treatment is advised for the majority of patients with PIC where there is no evidence of CNV as the visual prognosis is excellent. The only exception to this would be those patients with inflammatory lesions, but no CNV, very close to fixation in whom medical treatment can be considered ([8] (EBM:2++, B)). Like multifocal choroiditis, new lesions respond to systemic or sub-Tenon corticosteroids, and additional immunosuppressive therapy is not always necessary. Corticosteroids are also thought to have a beneficial effect on the neovascular membrane and are the first line of treatment ([111] (EBM:4, D)). Corticosteroids can limit the extent of RPE disturbance and of scar formation following the insult of the acute PIC lesions. The treatment of inflammatory CNV is still a challenge, since no guidelines are available. Laser photocoagulation [184], periocular and systemic steroids ([80] (EBM:2+, C)), PDT ([112] (EBM:2+, D), [154] (EBM:2+, D)), immune suppression ([70] (EBM:2+, D)), and surgical removal ([157] (EBM:2+, D)) have been employed for management of inflammatory CNV in the pre-anti-VEGF era. Steroid-sparing agents such as cyclosporine A can be used for immune modulation; mycophenolate mofetil offers a more favor-able safety and efficacy profile and is a promising drug for the long-term control of inflammatory CNV ([176] (EBM:2++, B)). Recent papers ([219] (EBM:2+, C), [14] (EBM:2++, C)) by Rouvas et al. (five eyes with PIC) and Arevalo et al.(eight eyes with PIC) showed that ranibizumab and bevacizumab, respectively, resulted as promising drugs in maintaining stability or improving VA and OCT and FA findings in inflammatory choroidal neovascularization [164].

> **Core Message**
> - Punctate inner choroidopathy (PIC) is a subset of MFC primary inflammatory choriocapillaropathy, predominantly seen in healthy young myopic women.
> - PIC is characterized by recurrent episodes of chorioretinal inflammation.
> - The symptoms are scotomatas, followed by blurred vision, floaters, photophobia, and metamorphopsia.
> - Multiple, small, gray or yellow, round lesions concentrated in the posterior pole, which are usually bilateral in 80 % of cases.

- ICGA: active disease shows hypofluorescent zones.
- FA: scars show early hypofluorescence followed by late hyperfluorescence.
- CNVM is estimated to occur in up to 40 % of eyes affected by PIC.
- Therapy: the association of corticosteroids and immunosuppressive therapy has shown to be useful in the light of multiple recurrences, with associated anti-VEGFs in cases of inflammatory choroidal neovascularization.

10.2.3 Serpiginous Choroiditis

10.2.3.1 Definition

Serpiginous choroiditis (SC) is a rare, chronic, progressive, and recurrent bilateral inflammatory disease involving the RPE, the choriocapillaris, and the choroid of unknown etiology [5, 19]. SC affects mainly healthy young to middle-aged adults with a higher prevalence in men and with no racial or familial predilection. Because of the rarity and the variable course of the disease, the long-term management of patients with SC remains a challenging issue in ocular immunology.

10.2.3.2 Clinical Symptoms and Signs

Patients present typically with a painless unilateral decrease in central vision, metamorphopsia, or bilateral scotoma. Scotomata may be absolute or relative depending on the inflammatory activity. Usually, the anterior segment and the anterior vitreous do not present inflammation. The disease is characterized acutely by irregular, gray-white, or creamy-yellow subretinal infiltrates at the level of the choriocapillaris and the RPE. The overlying retina is usually edematous and an associated neurosensory retinal detachment may occur. Around 80 % of cases with SC have the classic peripapillary geographic pattern. The peripapillary serpentine lesions in the fundus are a characteristic feature of this type. Classically, lesions develop first in the peripapillary area and tend to spread centrifugally in a pseudo-podial or serpentine fashion. Active lesions resolve spontaneously with or without treatment over 6–8 weeks leaving focal areas of atrophy. Recurrences usually, but not always, occur at the edges of previous atrophic scars, and they tend to be multiple at variable intervals ranging from months to years. Chronic cases are characterized by chorioretinal atrophy; subretinal fibrosis and extensive RPE clumping may be observed ([156] (EBM:2++, B)).

About two-thirds of patients with SC have scars in one or both eyes at the initial presentation 87 ([146] (EBM:2+, C)). Visual loss in one or both eyes with final VA of less than 20/200 is observed in up to 25 % of patients despite treatment ([59] (EBM:2+, C)). When SC begins in the macular area, it is termed "macular SC" [108]. Macular SC has a worse visual prognosis due to early foveal involvement and the higher risk of developing secondary choroidal neovascularization (CNV). This condition may be underdiagnosed. Occasionally, the lesions may occur in the periphery in an isolated or multifocal pattern termed "ampiginous choroiditis" [156] or "relentless placoid chorioretinitis" ([123] (EBM:4, D)). The evolution of APMPPE can mimic the clinical course of SC, with the difference that the multifocal nature of the lesions did not coincide to the extension of the old lesions. A paper by Gupta et al. reported that 20 out of 86 patients with SC presented with initially APMPPE which over time progressed to SC ([105] (EBM:1+, A)). Compared to patients with typical peripapillary SC, those with ampiginous choroiditis tend to have less central foveal involvement. ICGA findings are characterized by hypofluorescent areas during all the phases of the angiography. FA findings (Fig. 10.20) are the following: early serpiginous hypofluorescence followed by late diffuse staining and leakage at the edge of the retinal lesions ([40] (EBM:1+, A)). Visual field shows absolute scotomata associated with active lesions and relative ones associated with the resolution of the active lesions. ERG and EOG do not contribute to the evaluation of disease progression. The most common complication associated with SC is CNV, with a range from 13 to 35 % of patients [34, 59]. Other ocular conditions that may be

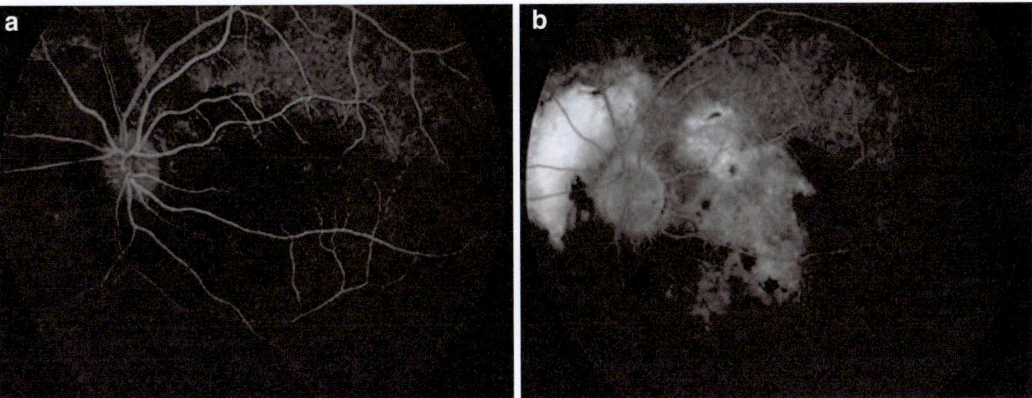

Fig. 10.20 Fluorescein angiography showing early hypofluorescence (**a**) and late hyperfluorescence with leakage at the edge of the retinal lesions (**b**) in a patient with noninfectious SC

considered as complications associated with SC are branch retinal vein occlusion (BRVO), periphlebitis, pigment epithelial detachment (PED), serous retinal detachment (SRD), cystoid macular edema (CME), optic disk neovascularization, and subretinal fibrosis.

10.2.3.3 Differential Diagnosis

The disease that most likely resembles the acute initial presentation of SC is APMPPE. The key difference is the clinical course where APMPPE lesions usually resolve spontaneously in two to three weeks, leaving a mottled RPE without significant choroidal involvement, and unlike SC, secondary CNV in APMPPE is rare and recurrence is uncommon. Patients with MFC differ from those with SC in that the latter do not show signs of vitreous inflammation and the lesions in MFC are smaller. Outer retinal toxoplasmosis may also mimic SC, but lesions do not coalesce and are virtually always unilateral. Tuberculosis infection, like SC, may affect the choroid and give rise to similar choroidal scars, but patients with ocular tuberculosis frequently present with vitritis, constitutional symptoms, and a positive tuberculin skin test. The angiographic features of choroidal ischemia and SC are similar, and conditions that result in occlusion of the posterior ciliary vessels, such as hypertension and systemic vasculitis, should be excluded. In older patients, metastatic tumors, non-Hodgkin's lymphoma, and choroidal osteoma may mimic the appearance of the acute unilateral lesion of SC.

10.2.3.4 Treatment

Untreated active lesions typically resolve over months with a gradual extension of the primary lesion characterized by a variable natural history. The frequent recurrences also increase the risk of secondary CNV. Fundus photography and angiography are necessary to document the non-progression of SC in order to evaluate treatment. The rapid control of the active lesions during recurrences and prevention of further recurrences seem to represent the mainstay of a successful therapy. Based on the different etiologies proposed, many different treatments have been proposed such as antibiotics ([1, 156] (EBM:2++, B)), antivirals [1, 59], and immunosuppressive therapy [146]. Systemic corticosteroids and retrobulbar steroidal injections were effective in controlling the active lesions and in shortening the duration of active disease, but not in preventing recurrences [267]. Intravitreal steroids will likely be effective in the treatment of acute lesions, but probably will not prevent recurrences if not administered on a continuous basis. Treatment of SC with cyclosporine A (CsA) as a monotherapy has produced mixed results. Christmas et al. [59] reported successful results in 4 out of 6 patients with SC treated with immunosuppressive drugs such as CsA, mycophenolate mofetil, or azathioprine in a period ranging from 2 to 40 months, in terms of discontinuation of therapy without recurrences. Triple-agent therapy consisting of CsA, azathioprine, and prednisolone was reported to show satisfying results in terms of inflammation control ([1, 116] (EBM:2+, C)). Because of the potentially serious side effects, alkylating agents should be limited to patients with sight-threatening lesions that are unresponsive to conventional immunosuppressives. Nowadays, better visual acuity results are achievable through VEGF inhibitor injections with or without PDT. This is proven by a few publications with greater numbers of patients because of the rarity of the diseases and several case reports in the literature. In addition to CNV treatment, the control of intraocular inflammation should never be forgotten because it forms the leading CNV trigger ([273] (EBM:4, D)). Recent reports from Julian et al. ([124] (EBM: 2++, C)) (one eye with SC and two eyes with ampiginous choroiditis) and Arevalo et al. ([14] (EBM:2++, C)) (six eyes with SC) showed that intravitreal bevacizumab resulted as a promising drug in maintaining stability or improving VA and OCT and FA findings in inflammatory choroidal neovascularization. Based on the studies reported so far, the rapid control of any active lesion with aggressive immunosuppression and the maintenance on appropriate immunosuppression for at least 6 months to prevent eventual recurrences can be considered the initial management of patients with SC. Subsequent treatment will depend on the severity of the disease.

> **Core Message**
> - SC is a rare, usually bilateral, chronic, progressive, recurrent inflammation of the choroid, RPE, and choriocapillaris.
> - SC can present into the peripapillary, macular, and ampiginous types.
> - SC is characterized by multiple recurrences.
> - Immunosuppressive treatment seems to be useful, but further clinical trials are required in order to achieve a gold standard of treatment.

10.2.4 Multiple Evanescent White Dot Syndrome (MEWDS) and Acute Idiopathic Blind Spot Enlargement (AIBSE)

10.2.4.1 Definition

MEWDS is a primary inflammatory choriocapillaritis of unknown etiology that results from inflammation at the level of the choriocapillaris causing areas of non-perfusion or hypoperfusion. The ischemic areas produce white lesions deep in the outer retina or at the level of the retinal pigment epithelium (RPE). AIBSE is most probably a variant of MEWDS ([72] (EBM:2+, C), [236] (EBM:2+, C)).

10.2.4.2 Clinical Symptoms and Signs

The majority of patients with MEWDS are within the younger age groups, and a definite female predominance is observed. In a large series, it was noted that a preceding flu-like episode or upper respiratory tract infection can occur in up to 50 % of patients ([36] (EBM:2++, B)). An autoimmune or immunologic mechanism is suspected after by reports of MEWDS developing after hepatitis B vaccination [20] or detection of HLA-B51 haplotype ([71] (EBM:2+, C)). Typically, patients with MEWDS present with unilateral visual impairment in the form of visual field defects including blind spot enlargement and central, cecocentral, and arcuate scotomas. Symptoms such as photopsias and scotomas are associated with ERG abnormalities in 80 % of cases and photoreceptor dysfunction. The lesions of MEWDS appear as multiple, small, round, yellow to white spots distributed over the posterior fundus especially at the perifoveal (around the vascular arcades) and peripapillary regions. Macular granularity is a uniform and distinguishing feature of MEWDS in the convalescent stage. Other common clinical features include anterior chamber cells, vitreous cells, an afferent papillary defect, and mild optic disk swelling. The disease usually hits once, and the evolution is spontaneously favorable with restoration of visual function within 6–12 weeks. Inflammation is usually moderate and limited to the vitreous, but the optic disk can be involved. Angiographic exams are essential in ascertaining the pathology. ICGA shows hypofluorescent dots and peripapillary hypofluorescence in the acute phases. FA is associated with early hypofluorescence and late hyperfluorescence (mild staining) and optic disk hyperfluorescence.

AIBSE manifests with peripapillary scotoma producing symptomatic enlargement of the blind spot that can be identified through visual field testing. ERG shows focal abnormalities around the optic disk. ICGA shows peripapillary hypofluorescence indicating choriocapillaris non-perfusion. AIBSE can be associated with several primary inflammatory choriocapillaropathies such as multifocal choroiditis and punctate inner choroidopathy.

10.2.4.3 Differential Diagnosis

The main differential diagnosis of MEWDS is retrobulbar optic neuritis, and the best way to ascertain the diagnosis is the performance of an ICGA.

10.2.4.4 Treatment

The lesions of MEWDS resolve spontaneously without treatment.

> **Core Message**
> - MEDWS is the result of primary inflammatory involvement of the choriocapillaris that in up to 50 % of cases is preceded by a viral flu-like syndrome.
> - Usually unilateral and unique episode.
> - The characteristics of the fundus are discrete discolorations in the midperiphery and granularity of the macula.
> - Photoreceptors dysfunction.
> - Visual field changes and blind spot enlargement.
> - ICGA hypofluorescent dots and peripapillary hypofluorescence resolving in two months.

10.2.5 Birdshot Retinochoroiditis

10.2.5.1 Definition

Birdshot retinochoroiditis (BC) is a form of posterior uveitis, characterized by multiple, distinctive, hypopigmented choroidal lesions, that is strongly associated with the human leukocyte antigen (HLA)-A29 [153]. The term "birdshot retinochoroidopathy" was first used in 1980, by Ryan and Maumenee [223], even though very recently the term is turning into "birdshot retinochoroiditis."

10.2.5.2 Etiology

The etiology of BC remains still receding. BC shows a strong association with the phenotype HLA-A29, which is present in 80–98 % of the white patients affected by this disease, compared to 7 % of controls [17, 18, 153]. The sensitivity (96 %) and specificity (93 %) of HLA-A29 phenotype can have a determining role in confirming the diagnosis [79]. BC has been diagnosed in 0.6–1.5 % of patients with uveitis who were referred to tertiary centers [168, 216]. BC is slightly predominant in females, with a mean age at onset of 53 years and with the majority of patients being Caucasians [229].

10.2.5.3 Clinical Symptoms and Signs

BC does not seem to be associated with systemic disorders, with the exception of a few studies showing associations with hypertension [206], hearing loss and cutaneous vitiligo [89], and loss of brightness and luster of colors. Involvement is always bilateral but can be asymmetric. The most common presentation of patients affected by BC is characterized by varying degrees of painless visual loss, blurred visual acuity, floaters, paracentral scotomas, photopsias, and nyctalopia [89, 126]. Visual acuity does not seem to be a specific marker for the disease severity [180]. The anterior segment usually remains quiet, but it can reveal a mild iritis associated with granulomatous keratic precipitates on the corneal endothelium in approximately 25 % of cases [142, 186]. Fundus examination reveals multiple, bilateral, ovoidal, cream-colored birdshot lesions, distributed throughout the post-equatorial retina. These spots can be best visualized in the inferotemporal quadrant [153]. Biomicroscopic examination points out that lesions are located at the level of the choroid and retinal pigment epithelium (RPE). The granulomatous nature of the inflammation in BC

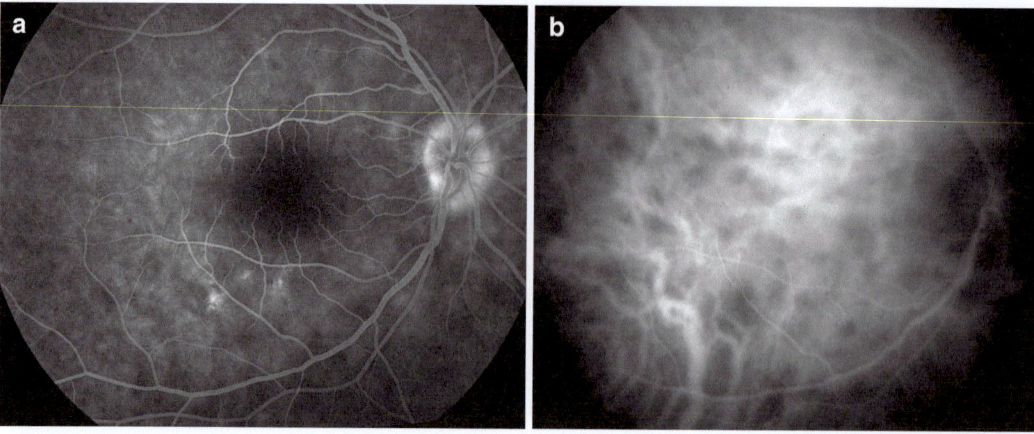

Fig. 10.21 Patient with Birdshot retinochoroiditis. Note the hot disk with few hyperfluorescent spots at the FA (**a**); a different clinical assessment can be done at the ICGA (**b**), where the distribution of the choroidal granulomata is better appreciated

has been verified histopathologically in a recent autopsy case [91]. At the onset of disease, fundus examination shows papillitis, periphlebitis, few cream-colored lesions, and vitreous infiltration which is usually present. Chronic cystoid macular edema (CME) is the most common complication of BC, occurring in up to 50 % of cases [206, 262]. The late findings of BC consist in epiretinal membranes [206], optic atrophy [49], macular and peripapillary choroidal neovascularization (CNV) in 6 % of cases [206], and RPE atrophy. The fundus fluoroangiographic (FFA) findings of the early and active phase show sectorial vasculitis mainly of the retinal veins, diffuse vasculitis of the retinal capillaries, pseudo-delay in arteriovenous circulation, optic disk hyperfluorescence, and CME, while the long-lasting cases "old lesions" show window defects of atrophic areas with early hypofluorescence and late hyperfluorescence and vessel attenuation [191]. The angiographic findings of indocyanine green angiography (ICGA) in the early and non-treated phase of the disease are numerous hypofluorescent dark dots corresponding to stromal granulomas (Fig. 10.21), regularly distributed along the posterior pole and midperiphery [190]. These dots may remain hypofluorescent or become isofluorescent in the late frames of ICGA; another characteristic angiographic sign pointed out by ICGA is the vasculitis of the larger choroidal vessels. Ocular coherence tomography (OCT) is

a complementary examination to FFA. It evaluates macular thickness in case of vascular leakage, the photoreceptors inner/outer segment junction in cases of blurred VA, abnormal color, etc. The fundus autofluorescence (FAF) examination reveals hypoautofluorescence due to RPE atrophy, nonuniform correspondence between hypoautofluorescent areas and birdshot lesions, linear hypoautofluorescent streaks along retinal blood vessels which correspond to the visible changes at the level of the RPE, placoid hypoautofluorescent area at the macula which is correlated to a best corrected VA $\leq 20/50$, macular RPE atrophy which predicts a low central VA, and non-correspondence of the RPE atrophic areas to hypopigmented lesions suggesting an independent affection of the RPE and choroid [143]. Visual field testing is a routine follow-up examination, and the occurrence or progression of visual field changes is considered an indication to introduce therapy [68]. Visual filed loss is much more indicative of the retinal dysfunction than VA alone. There are a variety of abnormalities despite normal best corrected VA such as multiple foci of scotomas, arcuate defects, and loss of the third highly reflective band on OCT that is associated with retinal damage. The introduction of immunomodulatory therapy (IMT) can reverse the visual field loss related to retinal dysfunction [253]. Full-field electroretinogram (ERG) becomes abnormal as the disease progresses, a fact that indicates relentless retinal deterioration. ERG shows decrease of the rod a- and b-wave amplitudes with an increase of their implicit times [85]. The most sensitive and prevalent abnormality is a delay of the cone system-derived 30 Hz flicker ERG [113].

10.2.5.4 Differential Diagnosis

The diagnosis of BC is mainly a clinical one, based on a careful ophthalmic examination and review of systems. The required diagnostic criteria are bilateral disease, birdshot lesions ≥3 inferior or nasal to optic nerve, low-grade anterior chamber inflammation, and low-grade vitreous inflammation. The supportive criteria are HLA-A29 positivity, retinal vasculitis, and CME. The exclusion criteria are posterior synechiae and other infectious, neoplastic, inflammatory entity [155]. Diagnosing birdshot retinochoroiditis is most challenging at the onset of disease, particularly if the typical birdshot lesions are subtle. The presence of the following signs such as mutton-fat keratic precipitates, hypopyon, or posterior synechiae in the early phase of the disease, in the majority of cases, is compatible with other pathologic entities such as Vogt-Koyanagi-Harada (VKH) disease, sarcoidosis, syphilis, and tuberculosis. The presence of concurrent systemic inflammatory disease suggests an alternative diagnosis, such as posterior scleritis, sarcoidosis, syphilis, tuberculosis, VKH disease, or intraocular lymphoma. The short and usually self-limited course of both acute posterior multifocal placoid pigment epitheliopathy (APMPPE) and multiple evanescent white dot syndrome (MEWDS) will distinguish these entities from the chronic and protracted course of birdshot retinochoroiditis. Pars planitis can almost always be distinguished from birdshot retinochoroiditis either by the presence of snowballs or snowbanking or by the absence of birdshot lesions in later phases of the disease. Sarcoidosis is the disease that is most difficult to distinguish from birdshot retinochoroiditis, because it shares a chronic course, and fundus lesions can occur in patients with sarcoidosis that mimics birdshot lesions [211, 264]. Patients with documented sarcoidosis who are HLA-A29-positive have been reported.

10.2.5.5 Treatment

The mainstay of treatment has been the employment of systemic and periocular corticosteroids (CS). CS are very important in the short-term management of vitritis and CME, but they show an inconsistent and transient efficacy in the long-term management because of the high maintenance dose of >15 mg/day to prevent CME and the severe adverse effects [85]. The use of regional CS is mainly adjunctive, employed in the inflammatory relapses in patients with systemic therapy or in asymmetrical disease. The early introduction of IMT shows an inherent anti-inflammatory effect and also a steroid-sparing effect of 10 mg/day of CS. The main treatment outcomes should include the reduction of inflammation and recurrences, preservation or reversal of a possible visual field loss, reduction of the risk of CME, and induction of long-term remission. The therapeutic modalities utilized in the treatment of BC include antimetabolites such as methotrexate (MTX), azathioprine, and mycophenolate mophetil (MMF); T-cell transduction inhibitors such as cyclosporine A (CSA), tacrolimus, and combination of MTX and MMF; biologics such as adalimumab, infliximab, and daclizumab; fluocinolone acetonide implant; emerging therapies such as voclosporin, anti-interleukin-17 monoclonal, and interferon α-2a; and intravenous immunoglobulins (IVIG). The indications for initiating therapy are symptomatic patients with photopsias, floaters and nyctalopia, vitritis, retinal vasculitis, CME, and peripheral retinal dysfunction revealed by visual field examination and ERG. A randomized, double-masked study comparing CSA to prednisolone in the treatment of endogenous uveitis by Nussenblatt RB et al. reported the efficacy of CSA in the treatment of two patients affected by BC at a dose of 10 mg/kg/day [179]. These findings were supported by Le Hoang et al., who treated 21 patients (42 eyes) affected by BC. There was a marked reduction of vitritis, improved visual acuity in 54.8 % of eyes, stabilization of VA in 26.2 % of eyes, and marked reduction of retinal vasculitis at the dose of 10 mg/kg/day of CSA [151]. This dose of CSA is now known to be associated with a high rate of nephrotoxic and hypertensive effects. Vitale et al. reported favorable outcomes in 19 patients (19 eyes) treated with CSA at a dosage of 2.5–5.0 mg/kg/day alone in 8 patients or in combination with AZA 1.5–2.0 mg/kg/day in 5 patients. The remaining patients were on systemic/periocular CS. Vitritis was controlled in 88.5 % of the cases; VA improved or stabilized in 83.8 % of the cases; there was a reduction of recurrences; and no nephrotoxic effects were observed [262]. Kiss et al. reported on a long-term follow-up of 81.2 months, in 28 patients affected by BC. All patients were treated with CS-sparing systemic IMT at some point during their follow-up: 92.9 % were treated with CSA, 67.9 % with MMF, 17.9 % with AZA, 10.7 % with oral MTX, and 7.1 % with daclizumab. VA remained stable or improved in 78.6 % OD, 89.3 % OS. The 30-Hz flicker implicit time was prolonged in 58.3 % of initial ERGs and in 62.5 % of final ERGs. The bright scotopic amplitude was abnormal in 45.5 % of initial and final ERGs [141]. Rothova et al. reported on the efficacy of low-dose MTX in 76 patients affected by BC, 46 of whom were followed for ≥ 5 years. The mean visual acuity underwent a statistically significant increase over time in the MTX-treated patients, remained unchanged in patients on systemic CS, and decreased in the patients without systemic treatment [218]. In a retrospective cohort study by Cervantes-Castaneda RA et al., there were 40 reported patients (80 eyes) affected by BC and treated with a combination therapy of CSA/MMF in a median time of 25.6 months with a median total patient follow-up of 52.6 months. At the 12-month point, a statistically significant reduction of vitritis and CME was achieved. Inflammatory control off systemic CS in 92.5 % of cases, long-term remission followed by absence of relapses in 64.9 % of cases, no reduction under 30 Hz of the amplitude/implicit times OD/OS, at least one relapse requiring change of IMT in 35.1 % of the cases, and a mean LogMAR VA not statistically different in both eyes were also reported [51]. In a report by Sorbin et al., there is satisfactory evidence of daclizumab employment in eight patients affected by BC and refractory to conventional IMT. The dose of daclizumab used was 1 mg/kg IV every 2 weeks with a mean follow-up of 25.6 months. Seven patients had either stabilization or improvement in visual acuity of both eyes and complete resolution of vitreous inflammation. Six patients had resolution of vasculitis on fluorescein angiography. The ERG 30-Hz implicit times and the bright scotopic amplitudes worsened in some patients despite abolition of clinically evident inflammation. Four patients were able to discontinue all other IMT and remain inflammation-free while receiving only daclizumab treatment. Two patients developed adverse effects that led to daclizumab treatment discontinuation [241], while Yeh et al. bring another modality of high doses of daclizumab in two patients with BC. They used 8 mg/kg at day 0 and 4 mg/kg at day 14. These treatment modality resulted in a mean visual acuity (10 eyes in 5 patients) that was 69.2 ETDRS letters and following treatment was 78.2 letters ($p < 0.12$). Anterior chamber cell, vitreous cell, and vitreous haze also improved in the majority of eyes. Adverse events were generally mild except for one episode of left-lower lobe pneumonia requiring hospitalization and treatment [283]. In a recent paper by Artornsombudh et al., there are reports on infliximab treatment of 22 patients with BC refractory to conventional IMT. The mean duration of the disease prior to infliximab was 58.62 months and the mean duration of infliximab therapy 13.55 months. All patients received 4–5 mg/kg infliximab at 4- to 8-week intervals. The main outcome measures were abolition of all evidence of active inflammation, visual acuity (VA), and presence of CME at 6 months and 1 year. Control of inflammation was achieved in 81.8 % at 6 months and in 88.9 % at the 1-year follow-up. The rate of CME decreased from 22.7 % at baseline to 13.9 % at 6 months and 6.7 % at 1 year after receiving the drug. Initial VA of 20/40 or better was found in 34 eyes (84.1 %). At 6 months and 1 year, 91.7 and 94.4 % of eyes, respectively, had VA of 20/40 or better. Three patients had active inflammation during therapy. Six patients developed adverse events requiring drug discontinuation [15]. Le Hoang et al. reported in a clinical study the tolerance and efficiency of IVIG treatment in 18 patients (36 eyes) with active BC with a mean follow-up of 39 months. IVIG was given as sole treatment at 1.6 g/kg every four weeks for six months, followed by injections of 1.2–1.6 g/kg at 6- to 8-week intervals. The results showed that the final VA of the 26 eyes with an initial VA of < or =20/30 was increased by two or more lines in 14 eyes (53.8 %) and decreased in two (7.7 %). When present, macular edema was improved in 17/23 eyes on fluorescein angiography and the visual field improved in 20/26 eyes. Benign side effects were observed in 12 patients: moderate transient arterial hypertension (7), headache (6), eczematous lesions (6), and hyperthermia (4) [152]. In a retrospective, multicenter, interventional case study, Rush et al., report on the outcomes in 22 patients (36 eyes) affected by BC and HLA-A29 positive following intravitreal implantation of a fluocinolone acetonide-containing drug delivery device. Nineteen of 22 patients (32 eyes) completed 12 months of follow-up with improvement in median visual acuity ($p=0.015$). Eyes with zero vitreous haze increased from 7 of 27 scored eyes (26 %) at baseline to 30 of 30 eyes (100 %) by 12 months ($p<0.001$). CME decreased from 13 of 36 eyes (36 %) at baseline to 2 of 32 eyes (6 %) at 12 months ($p=0.006$). Prior to implantation, 18 of 22 patients (82 %) received immunosuppressive therapy vs. 1 of 19 (5 %) by 12 months ($p<0.001$). Nineteen of twenty-two patients (32 eyes) completed 12 months of follow-up with improvement in median visual acuity ($p=0.015$). Nineteen patients underwent cataract surgery, and all of the 22 patients had ocular hypertension, while 33 % of the cases required glaucoma surgery or pressure-lowering therapy [222].

> **Core Message**
> - BC is a chronic progressive, sight-threatening disease.
> - Early and aggressive IMT limits ocular structural damage, preserves global visual function, and establishes long-term remission.
> - The treatment threshold is suggested by the markers of progressive disease such as the clinical indices of intraocular inflammation, visual field evaluation, ERG, and the various imaging modalities (Table 10.5).

Table 10.5 Treatment protocol for birdshot chorioretinopathy

Treatment protocol
A. Initial treatment with prednisone 1 mg/kg day
1. Up to 60 mg daily for 3–4 weeks
2. Taper CS off if possible, and if this seems not possible, try to achieve a maintenance dose of <10 mg/day
B. Initial treatment with antimetabolite
1. CellCept 1 g bid; maximum 1.5 g bid when there is evidence of failing prednisone tapering
2. MTX 15 mg/weekly with 1 mg folic acid daily; maximum 25 mg/weekly when there is evidence of failing prednisone tapering
3. Consider initial combined therapy consisting of CSA/MMF
C. Adjunctive periocular/intravitreal CS for CME
D. Add CSA (2.5–5.0 mg/kg/day) or tacrolimus (0.10–0.15 mg/kg/day) to the therapy with antimetabolites when there is evidence of significant inflammatory recurrence/failure prednisone tapering
E. Advance to TNF-α inhibitor (infliximab, adalimumab) when there is evidence of failing combined IMT, with significant inflammatory recurrence/failure prednisone tapering. Discontinue CSA/tacrolimus
F. Consider fluocinolone acetonide implant when there is evidence of systemic CS/IMT failure or intolerance

10.2.6 Acute Posterior Multifocal Placoid Pigment Epitheliopathy (APMPPE)

10.2.6.1 Definition

APMPPE is a primary inflammatory choriocapillaropathy characterized by sudden loss of vision caused by the sudden appearance of deep multiple yellow-white, flat inflammatory lesions.

10.2.6.2 Clinical Symptoms and Signs

APMPPE has a predilection for young adults with peak occurrence between the ages of 20 and 40 years and a range of 8–66 years [224] and both sexes are equally affected. APMPPE is most commonly bilateral and involvement may however be asymmetric and sequential in time. Patients present with sudden complaints of visual disturbance, photopsias, and scotomas without external evidence of ocular inflammation. During the active phase, fundus examination discloses multiple round, circumscribed, flat, yellow-white, subretinal lesions involving the RPE. The lesions may be multiple and confluent, forming large patches, and are localized mainly at the post-equatorial area. After several days to weeks, in the convalescent phase, the lesions begin to disappear leaving behind scattered areas of chorioretinal scars and mottling of the pigment epithelium in the zones of maximal involvement. Visual loss varies from minimal to severe and depends on the location of lesions. Visual field testing identifies the scotomas that are localized to the areas of fundus involvement. Other ocular findings include minimal anterior segment inflammation and cells in the vitreous and serous retinal detachment that can be seen in severe and hyperacute cases. Most of the patients with APMPPE have a history of a preceding flu-like syndrome before the onset of ocular symptoms ([16, 60] (EBM: 2++, C)) and even preceding infectious episodes such as mumps and streptococcal group A infection ([37] (EBM:3, D), [158] (EBM:3, D)). Most commonly, the disease has occurred once, but in rare instances, it may recur. ICGA shows geographic hypofluorescent areas during all the course of the exam, while FA shows early hypofluorescence followed by late hyperfluorescence that has a geographic aspect. Electroretinography shows moderate and transient abnormalities in APMPPE ([195] (EBM:4, D)). In general, the visual prognosis in patients with APMPPE is good, and the time between the onset of visual loss and improvement may take as long as 6 months.

10.2.6.3 Differential Diagnosis

The most important disease to exclude is the early stage of serpiginous choroiditis which can mimic APMPPE in the beginning. In the case of strong suspects of serpiginous choroiditis, the tubercular etiology must be ruled out. Vogt-Koyanagi-Harada is another pathology to be excluded in the hyperacute forms of APMPPE, and ICGA is essential.

10.2.6.4 Treatment

Corticosteroids and/or immunosuppressive therapy has not been proved to be useful in APMPPE. If the tubercular etiology has been ruled out, a systemic corticosteroid therapy can be considered in patients with macular involvement given the vasculitic component in APMPPE ([198] (EBM:4, D)).

> **Core Message**
> - Primary inflammatory choriocapillaropathy.
> - APMPPE usually has self-limiting course and is characterized by bilateral discolorations at the posterior pole.
> - The main symptoms are visual loss, scotomas, and photopsias.
> - FA: early hypofluorescence late hyperfluorescence.
> - ICGA: hypofluorescent areas.
> - ERG shows no abnormalities.
> - Most patients do not require therapy, but in cases of macular involvement, systemic steroid therapy can be considered because of the inflammatory etiology.

10.2.7 Vogt-Koyanagi-Harada (VKH) Disease

10.2.7.1 Definition

VKH disease is a severe granulomatous bilateral panuveitis and multisystem disorder affecting the eyes, auditory system, meninges, and skin [173, 239].

10.2.7.2 Etiology

Although the exact etiology of VKH remains unknown, the underlying immunopathological mechanism in VKH disease is believed to involve a T-cell-mediated autoimmune reaction against a melanocyte-related antigen, which is a member of the tyrosinase family of proteins [281]. VKH has been linked to human leukocyte antigen DR4 (HLA-DR4) and HLA-Dw53 [66], with the strongest associated risk for HLA-DRB1*0405 haplotype [233]. In the United States, Nussenblatt et al. reported that 44 % of the patients in their series were blacks [181]. VKH is a common cause of endogenous uveitis in Japan, with at least 8 % of the total cases

[247]. Most patients develop VKH in the second to fifth decades of life, showing a slight female predominance [173, 247].

10.2.7.3 Clinical Symptoms and Signs

The clinical course of VKH has been divided into four clinical stages [247]. The prodromal stage which mimics a systemic viral infection whose symptoms include fever, headache, nausea, vertigo, orbital pain, meningismus, and tinnitus that represents a typical clinical symptom. The symptoms of prodromal stage normally last for a few days and are followed by the acute uveitis phase that lasts for several weeks. Patients in this stage present with acute blurring of vision and bilateral uveitis in both eyes in up to 70 % of patients [247], while the remaining 30 % may show a delay of 1–3 days regarding the involvement of the second eye. The early findings of the posterior segment consist in thickening of the posterior choroid, manifested as an elevation of the peripapillary retinochoroidal complex, and swelling of the optic nerve head [98]. Subsequent retinal pigment epithelium (RPE) breakdown causes multifocal exudative non-rhegmatogenous retinal detachment which can give rise to frank bullous exudative retinal detachment. The swelling of the optic nerve head is a marker of severe inflammation and is noted in 87 % of the patients with evolving disease [183]. The uveitis in the anterior segment initially may manifest as a nongranulomatous nature, which transforms into granulomatous at the later stages, causing mutton-fat keratic precipitates (KP) and iris nodules. In the early stages, the anterior chamber may be shallow [138] because of ciliary edema, serous detachment of the ciliary body [96], and forward displacement of the lens-iris diaphragm. These findings may cause a rise of the intraocular pressure (IOP) and acute angle closure glaucoma [139]. Harada's disease represents the condition in which posterior uveitis, serous retinal detachment, and cerebrospinal fluid (CSF) pleocytosis are the only manifestations of VKH disease, while the Vogt-Koyanagi disease represents the form associated with bilateral iridocyclitis, vitiligo, poliosis, and auditory problems. The convalescent stage that follows may last for several months and is associated with depigmentation of the skin and uveal tract. Sugiura's sign is a typical finding of early perilimbal depigmentation highly occurring in Japanese patients [84, 183]. The sunset glow fundus or depigmentation of the choroid typically occurs 2–3 months after the uveitic phase [98]. Dalen-Fuchs-like nodules, similar to those described in sympathetic ophthalmia, are frequently found in the midperiphery. The chronic recurrent phase, which abruptly interrupts the convalescent stage, is characterized by smoldering panuveitis with exacerbations of, typically, acute episodes of granulomatous anterior uveitis that are often resistant to systemic steroid therapy. Iris nodules are a characteristic finding of these recurrent episodes of disease. Being that VKH is a systemic disease, the presence of extraocular manifestations has an important role regarding the diagnosis. In the integumentary system, poliosis and vitiligo usually occur during the convalescent stage. Headache is the most common neurological complaint [30]. CSF pleocytosis has been found in 80 % of VKH patients [247]. Hearing loss usually involves the high frequencies, but all the frequencies can be affected in the early stage [117]. In the acute stage of the VKH, fundus fluorescein angiography (FFA) shows multiple punctate hyperfluorescent dots at the RPE level, which gradually enlarge and pool in the subretinal fluid underlying areas of exudative retinal detachment [90]. Optic nerve leakage is usually seen. In the chronic stage, FFA shows multiple window defects of the RPE or blocked fluorescence corresponding to damage of RPE. In some eyes, choroidal neovascularization (CNV) and subretinal fibrosis can occur as late complications [279]. The indocyanine green angiography (ICGA) findings in the acute phase are represented by filling delay of larger choroidal artery, fewer choroidal vessels in the posterior and peripheral fundus, patchy filling delay of choriocapillaris, ICG dye leakage, and multiple hypofluorescent spots, while in the convalescent phase, ICGA shows improvement of all the signs mentioned superiorly. The main ICGA signs for the evaluation of the inflammation and follow-up are hypofluorescent dark dots (Fig. 10.22), early hyperfluorescent choroidal vessels, fuzzy

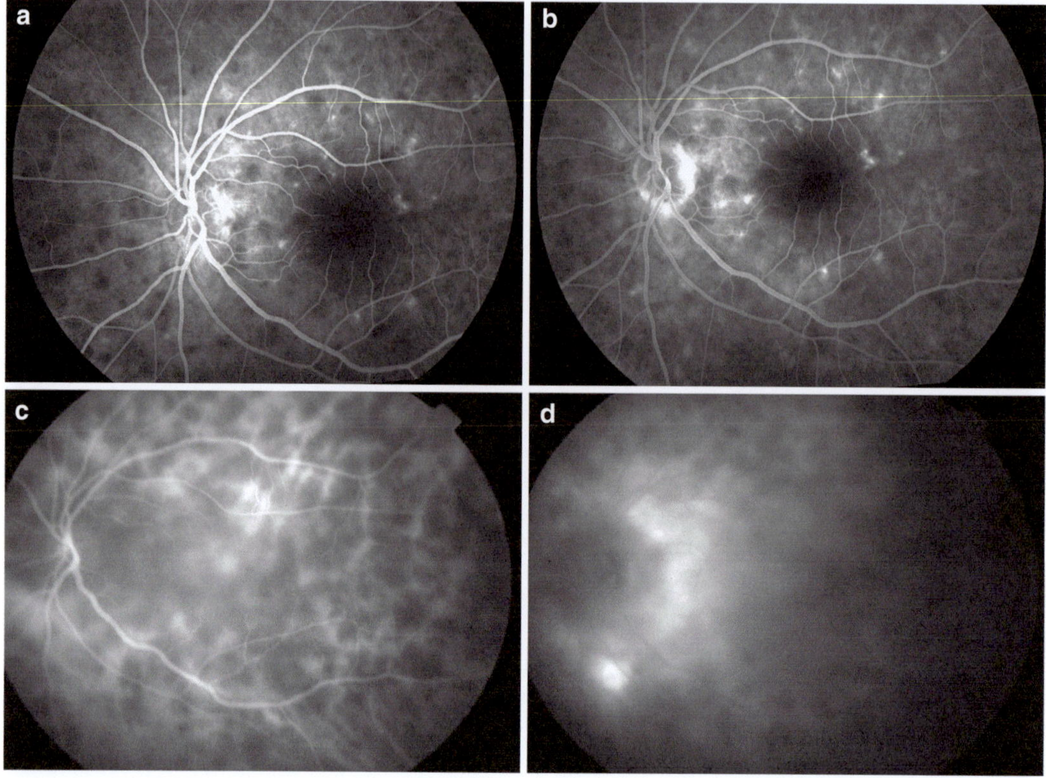

Fig. 10.22 FA of a patient with VKH disease. Note the widespread hypofluorescent spots at the early phase (**a**), followed by the hyperfluorescent spots at the late phase (**b**). Early (**c**) and late (**d**) phases of ICGA show a more extended involvement compromising the retina

choroidal stromal vessels, and ICGA optic disk hyperfluorescence [40, 41]. Recently, optical coherence tomography (OCT) has shown its importance in evaluating and monitoring serous retinal detachment during the acute and chronic phases of VKH disease [167, 193]. OCT can discover small serous detachments, otherwise not detectable by slit-lamp biomicroscopy [193]. Ultrasonography (USG) has shown its utility as a diagnostic tool in the presence of obscured fundus view or in atypical presentations of VKH [81]. Regarding the diagnosis of VKH disease, new criteria, taking into account the multisystem nature of Vogt-Koyanagi-Harada disease, with allowance for the different ocular findings present in the early and late stages of the disease, were formulated and agreed at the First International Workshop on VKH Disease on October 19–21, 1999, at the University of California, Los Angeles, Conference Center [210].

10.2.7.4 Differential Diagnosis

The differential diagnosis of VKH disease includes other causes that manifest with granulomatous inflammation, exudative retinal detachment, and white dot syndromes such as sympathetic ophthalmia, Lyme disease with ocular involvement, multiple evanescent white dot syndrome (MEWDS), posterior scleritis, acute posterior multifocal placoid pigment epitheliopathy (APMPPE), and uveal effusion syndrome.

10.2.7.5 Treatment

The typical treatment for VKH disease is high-dose corticosteroids (CS) in the range of 1–2 mg/kg/day followed by a slow tapering of the drug for at least 3–6 months in order to prevent further recurrence. Sasamoto et al. evaluated the significance of corticosteroid therapy on 47 new patients with VKH disease in a follow-up period of 6 months. Eighteen patients received systemic

CS as pulse therapy, 20 patients received high-dose CS starting with prednisolone 200 mg, 2 patients received conventional-dose CS, and 7 patients received no systemic CS therapy. After 6 months, anterior chamber inflammation was significantly less in patients with pulse and high-dose CS therapy than in those without systemic corticosteroid therapy, final visual acuity was significantly better in patients with pulse and high-dose CS than in those without them, while there was no significant difference between patients with pulse therapy and those with high-dose CS therapy [228]. In a paper of Rubsamen et al., we can find a review of 26 patients (44 eyes) affected by VKH disease treated with systemic CS, for a median period of 6 months, that was prolonged (48 months) in patients who developed chronic uveitis. The disease recurred in nine (43 %) of 21 patients in the first 3 months, usually in association with a rapid tapering of steroid dosage, and a final visual acuity of better than 20/30 in 29 (66 %) of 44 eyes and of worse than 20/400 in only 3 (7 %) of 44 eyes [221]. Yamanaka et al. evaluated through OCT the rapid effects of pulse CS therapy on the serous retinal detachment found at the acute phase of VKH disease on nine Japanese patients. OCT images showed a marked decrease in the retinal detachment immediately after the first intravenous injection of CS and subsequent resolution [282]. A multicenter study has shown an equal efficacy between the intravenous pulse steroid therapy and oral therapy with CS in improving the visual outcome [212]. Jaffe et al. investigated the safety and efficacy of a fluocinolone acetonide intravitreal implant in the treatment of 32 patients with a history of recurrent noninfectious posterior uveitis. None of these eyes experienced a recurrence for the first 2 years after implantation. There was a reduction in systemic and local therapy used in the device-implanted eyes. Inflammation was effectively controlled over the follow-up period. The posterior sub-Tenon capsule injection rate significantly decreased from a mean of 2.2 injections per eye per year to 0.07 injections per eye per year. Mean baseline visual acuity for the device-implanted eyes improved significantly from +1.1 logarithm of the minimum angle of resolution

(logMAR) units to +0.81 logMAR units (20/125) at 30 months. The most common adverse event was intraocular pressure (IOP) rise [119]. In a case report by Perente et al., sub-Tenon triamcinolone acetonide injection is recommended in addition to systemic CS and cyclosporine (CSA) treatments if systemic medications fail to stop the progression of the VKH disease activity [199]. Despite proper treatment with CS, several studies reported the development of chronic recurrent granulomatous inflammation and sunset glow fundus with peripapillary atrophy and depigmented small atrophic lesions at the level of RPE [3, 7, 194]. In the article of Paredes et al., the main focus was on the use of immunomodulatory therapy (IMT) in a group of patients with VKH disease and to compare the outcomes with those of another group of patients with VKH who were treated for prolonged periods with CS. Their results suggest that IMT as first-line therapy for VKH is associated with a superior visual outcome when compared to CS as monotherapy or with delayed addition of IMT [194]. Recently, several studies suggested that the use of nonsteroid immunomodulatory therapy with CSA, azathioprine (AZA), methotrexate (MTX), and mycophenolate mofetil (MMF) as first-line therapy in addition to corticosteroids is associated with good clinical results. In a retrospective chart review by Sachdev et al., the clinical profile, management with AZA in association with CS, and outcome in seven patients with posterior segment recurrence in Vogt-Koyanagi-Harada (VKH) disease were reported. All the recurrent episodes of VKH were bilateral and were characterized by vitritis (8 eyes), papillitis (14 eyes), multiple yellow-white oval subretinal lesions6 eyes), and exudative retinal detachment (10 eyes). The first episodes of recurrence were managed with oral CS (1.0–1.5 mg/day) and AZA (2.0–2.5 mg/day). Three patients experienced a second episode of posterior segment recurrence, which also responded to the CS-AZA combination [225]. In a recent retrospective analysis of 87 patients, of whom 53 have initial-onset acute VKH disease and 34 have chronic recurrent VKH disease, Abu El-Asrar et al. recommend the use of CSA and MMF as first-line therapy. The results pointed out that this treatment modality significantly reduced the development of complications in the whole study group and in the initial-onset acute group, while the visual outcomes improved in the whole study group and in the chronic recurrent group [2]. A recent paper by Cuchacovich et al. reported a prospective comparison between 2 immunosuppressive regimens in patients with active VKH disease in spite of systemic glucocorticoid treatment, in 44 patients. Twenty-one patients developed chronic intraocular inflammation in spite of glucocorticoid treatment and were randomized to receive either prednisone and AZA ($n=12$) or prednisone and CSA ($n=9$). The results suggested that both regimens showed a good clinical efficacy, but CSA seemed to be a better glucocorticoid-sparing agent than AZA [63]. Another prospective study by Abu El-Asrar et al. deals with the effectiveness of MMF as first-line therapy combined with systemic CS in 19 patients with acute uveitis related to VKH disease, with mean follow-up period of 27.0 ± 11.1 months. The results showed a statistically significant reduction of recurrent inflammation ($p=0.0383$) in the CS+MMF group (3 %) as compared to CS group (18 %). Development of all complications was significantly higher in the CS group (43 %) compared with the CS+MMF group (8 %) ($p<0.001$). None of the eyes in the CS+MMF group developed sunset glow fundus [3]. A case report by Dolz-Marco et al. reports the employment of rituximab in a patient with chronic recurrent VKH, refractory to conventional IMT treatment [73]. Wu et al. reported in their paper the usefulness of intravitreal bevacizumab in two patients who had developed subfoveal and extrafoveal CNV due to VKH disease.

> **Core Message**
> - VKH is a multisystem autoimmune disorder selectively targeting tissues containing melanocytes.
> - Ocular symptoms are preceded by headache, dysacousia, or tinnitus.
> - The ocular findings in the acute stage include bilateral and multifocal serous retinal detachment and swelling of the optic disk, while in the convalescent phase, the main findings are sunset glow fundus and irregular and linear pigmentation, which may result long after the onset of the disease.
> - The main FFA findings of the acute phase include multiple punctate hyperfluorescent dots at the RPE level, pooling in the subretinal fluid, and optic nerve leakage. The convalescent stage results in window defects due to RPE damage. The ICGA findings of the acute stage consist in by filling delay of larger choroidal artery, fewer choroidal vessels in the posterior and peripheral fundus, patchy filling delay of choriocapillaris, ICG dye leakage, and multiple hypofluorescent spots, while in the convalescent phase ICGA shows improvement of all the signs mentioned superiorly.
> - Though ocular inflammation responds to CS therapy, there is progressive depigmentation of the fundus. The damage to melanocyte-containing tissues goes on resulting in vitiligo, alopecia, and poliosis.
> - The principles of therapy in VKH disease are directed towards the suppression of the initial intraocular inflammation in the acute posterior uveitis stage with early and high-dose systemic CS followed by slow tapering, but despite proper treatment with corticosteroids, several studies have reported the development of chronic recurrent granulomatous inflammation and sunset glow fundus with peripapillary atrophy and depigmented small atrophic lesions at the level of retinal pigment epithelium. Recently published evidence is suggesting that the employment of non-steroid immunomodulatory therapy with CSA, AZA, MTX, and MMF as first-line therapy in addition to CS is associated with good clinical results.

10.2.8 Sympathetic Ophthalmia (SO)

10.2.8.1 Definition

SO is a bilateral diffuse granulomatous panuveitis occurring either after surgery or penetrating trauma to one eye. The eye responsible for initiation of the inflammation is called exciting eye while the noninjured eye is known as the sympathizing eye. Penetrating or surgical injury to the exciting eye leads to an inflammatory response in both the exciting and the sympathizing eye [6].

10.2.8.2 Etiology

Trauma was considered as the most common precipitating event [6], while the recent papers tend to consider ocular surgery as a major risk factor, particularly vitreoretinal surgery [88, 136, 204]. Kilmartin et al. [136] calculated the risk of developing SO in retinal surgical procedures, which resulted to be higher more than twice the risk of developing endophthalmitis after vitrectomy. Continuous advances in the management of traumatized eyes associated with less invasive microsurgical techniques may be held responsible for the observed etiologic and epidemiologic changes from penetrating injuries to surgical traumas. Other etiologic factors involved with the development of SO are laser and surgical procedures such as glaucoma filtration surgery, peripheral iridectomy, cataract surgery, scleral buckling, evisceration, Nd-YAG laser cyclotherapy, and cyclocryotherapy [95, 99, 109, 163, 230, 235].

10.2.8.3 Clinical Symptoms and Signs

SO is a bilateral granulomatous uveitis occurring either after intentional or unintentional penetrating trauma to one eye. The latent period is usually between 2 weeks and 3 months; however, there are reports of cases presenting as early as 5 days and as late as 66 years after the incident [261, 285]. Approximately 80 % of cases present within the first 3 months and 90 % of cases present by 1 year of the penetrating trauma [159]. The inflammatory response in the anterior chamber is a granulomatous one, with mutton-fat keratic precipitates (KPs) on the corneal endothelium and the typical findings of acute anterior uveitis such as ciliary flush, pain, and photophobia in the sympathizing eye. Iritis may manifest with posterior synechiae. In the early stages, the inflammation may be nongranulomatous, associated with cells in the retrolental space. Intraocular pressure (IOP) may be high or low as a result of inflammatory cells crowding the trabecular meshwork or ciliary shutdown, respectively. The posterior segment findings typically consist of moderate to severe vitritis associated with papillitis and multiple peripheral white to yellow choroidal lesions, which later show a tendency towards confluency. These represent the clinical appearance of Dalen-Fuchs nodules. Papillitis is an important marker of disease activity and progression. The clinical appearance of SO varies within a mild to severe range. In a long-term study of Gupta et al., the most important posterior segment manifestations were exudative retinal detachment in the majority of patients, Dalen-Fuchs nodules, papillitis, and vasculitis as secondary events [103]. The complications of chronic inflammation include secondary glaucoma, cataract, and chronic maculopathy. Misdiagnosis and inappropriate treatment of this condition may result in severe inflammatory sequela such as retinal and optic atrophy, inflammatory choroidal neovascularization (CNV), choroidal atrophy, and phthisis bulbi [103]. Rarely, SO may be associated with the typical extraocular findings accompanying Vogt-Koyanagi-Harada syndrome, such as alopecia, vitiligo, cells in the cerebrospinal fluid, and dysacousia. In the acute phase of SO, fundus fluorescein angiography (FFA) shows multiple hyperfluorescent sites of leakage at the retinal pigment epithelium (RPE) in the transit stage, while in the late phase, FFA shows late leakage. In severe cases, the sites of leakage may coalesce, with pooling of dye and consequent exudative neurosensory detachment. Late staining of the optic nerve head may sometimes be seen. Dalen-Fuchs lesions may appear hyper- or hypofluorescent, depending on the RPE condition [231]. During the intermediate phase of indocyanine green angiography (ICGA), the examiner observes hypofluorescent areas [31]. During the late phase of ICGA, the hypofluorescent areas seen in the intermediate phase may persist or may fade to isofluorescent ones, reflecting the behavior of full-thickness and partial-thickness choroidal granulomas, respectively. Late atrophic lesions of SO appear as hypofluorescent areas, not changing their behavior in ICGA even in the presence of systemic corticosteroids (CS).

10.2.8.4 Differential Diagnosis

SO represents a clinical diagnosis, relying essentially on a history of ocular trauma or surgery, which evolves in a bilateral granulomatous uveitis. The clinical findings of SO may be difficult to distinguish from those of VKH [98]. Patients with VKH do not have history of trauma. They typically show bilateral localized exudative neurosensory detachments, a sign which is absent in SO patients. VKH patients frequently present with auditory, integumentary, and meningeal signs, which are very rare in SO patients. VKH has a predilection for darkly pigmented races such as blacks and Asians, and most patients are affected during the 2nd–5th decades of life, while SO is not associated with these epidemiologic factors. VKH shows a tendency to involve choriocapillaris during its course, while SO does not. Other important differential diagnoses include granulomatous conditions such as tuberculosis, sarcoidosis, infective endophthalmitis, intraocular lymphoma, and lens-induced uveitis.

10.2.8.5 Treatment

Management of SO patients includes surgical and medical treatment. Enucleation of the injured eye is generally recommended within 14 days after ocular injury [159]. Because of the decreasing incidence of injured eyes developing SO, this approach is no longer advised. Nowadays, a lot of controversy exists regarding the value of enucleation once the inflammatory process has begun, as the exciting eye may actually present with better visual acuity (VA) than the sympathizing one. Lubin et al. reported that early enucleation of the exciting eye after onset of symptoms in the fellow eye was found to improve visual prognosis ([32] EBM C 2 +), while in another review of Winter, there are reports that show no benefits from enucleation of the exciting eye ([272] EBM D 4). Corticosteroids have served as the mainstay of treatment following onset ([52] EBM B

2+), which are used as intravenous, oral, topical, or regional injections ([54] EBM D 3, [110] EBM C3, [187] EBM D3). Nussenblatt et al. are recommending 3 months of high daily dose of 1–2 mg/kg CS, tapering in three to six months and considering uveitis quiescent with a maintenance dose of ≤15 mg of CS ([178] EBM D 4). In severe cases of SO, short courses of intravenous CS may be considered [110]. In cases that seem to be refractory to corticosteroids and in patients who show significant systemic side effects, steroid-sparing therapy that combines systemic corticosteroids and other immunosuppressive agents such as cyclosporine or azathioprine can improve prognosis, particularly in patients that have initial response to steroid but exhibit rebound activity when steroid is tapered to lower doses. Combining CS with other steroid-sparing agents such as cyclosporine A (CSA) and azathioprine (AZA) has shown benefits in patients that are refractory to the association of CS with a single immunosuppressive agent ([106] EBM C 3, [263] EBM C3). Nussenblatt suggests the employment of triple immunosuppressive therapy in patients where SO is difficult to control, such as CS, CSA, immunosuppressive agents, and biologics ([178] EBM C 4). Being that in attendance to recent studies, evidence suggests that sympathetic ophthalmia represents an autoimmune inflammatory response against choroidal melanocytes mediated by T cells ([65] EBM C 3, [203]); CSA represents the steroid-sparing agent of choice in CS refractory SO. Therapies including immunosuppressive agents such as mycophenolate mofetil (MMF) and chlorambucil have shown efficacy in patients refractory to "conventional" treatment ([149] EBM D3, [251] EBM D 3). Disruption of leukocyte recruitment by targeting gelatinase B (matrix metalloproteinase-9), CCL2, and CXCL12 may hold promise for future treatments ([4] EBM D 3). Furusato et al. reported that M1 macrophages, IL-23, CCL19, CXCL11, and IL-17 predominate within the granulomatous infiltrates of SO, findings which suggest the targeting of M1 macrophages and their cytokines and chemokines, Th17, or Th1 lymphocytes ([86] EBM D 3). Treatment with anti-TNFα agents has been used for uveitis suggesting potential benefit for sympathetic ophthalmia ([259] EBM D 3). Mahajan et al. examined the results of fluocinolone acetonide implantation (Retisert) in eight patients with active SO reporting satisfactory control of inflammation and a decrease in the dependence on systemic immunosuppression ([162] EBM D 3).

> **Key Points**
> 1. SO is a bilateral, diffuse granulomatous panuveitis that occurs after eye injury (trauma or surgery).
> 2. Other etiologic factors involved with the development of SO are laser and surgical procedures.
> 3. Histopathologic findings include granulomatous inflammation of the uvea, sparing the choriocapillaris.
> 4. The most common clinical findings include mutton-fat KPs, papillitis, Dalen-Fuchs nodules, and vitritis.
> 5. Chronic inflammation develops sequelae such as chronic maculopathy, CNV, optic atrophy, and secondary glaucoma.
> 6. The most important diagnostic tools include FFA and ICGA.
> 7. Management involves long-term CS, CSA, and other immunosuppressive agents, while enucleation is controversial.

References

1. Abrez H, Biswas J, Sudharshan S. Clinical profile, treatment, and visual outcome of serpiginous choroiditis. Ocul Immunol Inflamm. 2007;15(4):325–35.
2. Abu El-Asrar AM, Al Tamimi M, Hemachandran S, Al-Mezaine HS, Al-Muammar A, Kangave D. Prognostic factors for clinical outcomes in patients with Vogt-Koyanagi-Harada disease treated with high-dose corticosteroids. Acta Ophthalmol. 2013;91(6):e486–93.
3. Abu El-Asrar AM, Hemachandran S, Al-Mezaine HS, Kangave D, Al-Muammar AM. The outcomes of mycophenolate mofetil therapy combined with systemic corticosteroids in acute uveitis associated with Vogt-Koyanagi-Harada disease. Acta Ophthalmol. 2012;90(8):e603–8.
4. Abu El-Asrar AM, Struyf S, Van den Broeck C, Van Damme J, Opdenakker G, Geboes K, Kestelyn P. Expression of chemokines and gelatinase B in sympathetic ophthalmia. Eye (Lond). 2007;21(5):649–57 [3 D].
5. Abu el-Asrar AM. Serpiginous (geographical) choroiditis. Int Ophthalmol Clin. 1995;35:87–91.
6. Albert DM, Diaz-Rohena R. A historical review of sympathetic ophthalmia and its epidemiology. Surv Ophthalmol. 1989;34(1):1–14.
7. Al-Kharashi AS, Aldibhi H, Al-Fraykh H, Kangave D, Abu El-Asrar AM. Prognostic factors in Vogt-Koyanagi-Harada disease. Int Ophthalmol. 2007;27(2–3):201–10.
8. Amer R, Lois N. Punctate inner choroidopathy. Surv Ophthalmol. 2011;56(1):36–53.
9. American Thoracic Society. Targeted tuberculin testing and treatment of latent tuberculosis infection. MMWR Recomm Rep. 2000;49:1e51 (A).
10. Ang M, Hedayatfar A, Wong W, Chee SP. Duration of anti-tubercular therapy in uveitis associated with latent tuberculosis: a case-control study. Br J Ophthalmol. 2012;96(3):332–6 (C).
11. Ang M, Htoon HM, Chee SP. Diagnosis of tuberculous uveitis: clinical application of an interferon-gamma release assay. Ophthalmology. 2009;116(7):1391–6 (C).
12. Ang M, Wong WL, Li X, Chee SP. Interferon γ release assay for the diagnosis of uveitis associated with tuberculosis: a Bayesian evaluation in the absence of a gold standard. Br J Ophthalmol. 2013;97(8):1062–7. (C)s.
13. Anninger W, Lubow M. Visual loss with West Nile virus infection: a wider spectrum of a "new" disease. Clin Infect Dis. 2004;38:e55–6.
14. Arevalo JF, Adan A, Berrocal MH, Espinoza JV, Maia M, Wu L, Roca JA, Quiroz-Mercado H, Ruiz-Moreno JM, Serrano MA, Pan-American Collaborative Retina Study Group. Intravitreal bevacizumab for inflammatory choroidal neovascularization: results from the pan-American collaborative retina study group at 24 months. Retina. 2011;31(2):353–63.
15. Artornsombudh P, Gevorgyan O, Payal A, Siddique SS, Foster CS. Infliximab treatment of patients with birdshot retinochoroidopathy. Ophthalmology. 2013;120(3):588–92.
16. Azar P, Gohd RS, Waltman D, Gitter KA. Acute posterior multifocal placoid pigment epitheliopathy associated with an adenovirus type 5 infection. Am J Ophthalmol. 1975;80:1003–5.
17. Baarsma GS, Kijlstra A, Oosterhuis JA, et al. Association of birdshot retinochoroidopathy and HLA-A29 antigen. Doc Ophthalmol. 1986;61:267–9.
18. Baarsma GS, Priem HA, Kijlstra A. Association of birdshot retinochoroidopathy and HLA-A29 antigen. Curr Eye Res. 1990;9(Suppl):63–8.
19. Bacin F, Larmande J, Boulmier A, et al. Serpiginous choroiditis and placoid epitheliopathy. Bull Soc Ophthalmol Fr. 1983;83:1153–62.
20. Baglivo E, Safran AB, Borruat FX. Multiple evanescent white dot syndrome after hepatitis B vaccine. Am J Ophthalmol. 1996;122:431.

21. Baharivand N, Mahdavifard A, Fouladi RF. Intravitreal clindamycin plus dexamethasone versus classic oral therapy in toxoplasmic retinochoroiditis: a prospective randomized clinical trial. Int Ophthalmol. 2013;33(1):39–46.
22. Balne PK, Barik MR, Sharma S, Basu S. Development of a loop-mediated isothermal amplification assay targeting the mpb64 gene for diagnosis of intraocular tuberculosis. J Clin Microbiol. 2013;51(11):3839–40.
23. Banker A. Posterior segment manifestations of human immunodeficiency virus/acquired immune deficiency syndrome. Indian J Ophthalmol. 2008;56(5):377–83.
24. Bansal R, Gupta A, Gupta V, Dogra MR, Bambery P, Arora SK. Role of anti-tubercular therapy in uveitis associated with latent tuberculosis. Am J Ophthalmol. 2008;146(5):772–9. C.
25. Bansal R, Gupta A, Gupta V, Dogra MR, Sharma A, Bambery P. Tubercular serpiginous-like choroiditis presenting as multifocal serpiginoid choroiditis. Ophthalmology. 2012;119(11):2334–42.
26. Bansal R, Kulkarni P, Gupta A, Gupta V, Dogra MR. High-resolution spectral domain optical coherence tomography and fundus autofluorescence correlation in tubercular serpiginous-like choroiditis. J Ophthalmic Inflamm Infect. 2011;1(4):157–63.
27. Barisani-Asenbauer T, Maca SM, Hauff W, et al. Treatment of ocular toxocariasis with albendazole. J Ocul Pharmacol Ther. 2001;17:287–94.
28. Basu S, Biswas J, Pleyer U, Pathangay A, Manohar BB. An ophthalmologist survey-based study of the atypical presentations and current treatment practices of ocular toxoplasmosis in India. J Parasit Dis. 2011;35:148–54.
29. Basu S, Nayak S, Padhi TR, Das T. Progressive ocular inflammation following anti-tubercular therapy for presumed ocular tuberculosis in a high-endemic setting. Eye. 2013;27(5):657–62.
30. Beniz J, Forster DJ, Lean JS, Smith RE, Rao NA. Variations in clinical features of the Vogt-Koyanagi-Harada syndrome. Retina. 1991;11(3):275–80.
31. Bernasconi O, Auer C, Zografos L, Herbort CP. Indocyanine green angiographic findings in sympathetic ophthalmia. Graefes Arch Clin Exp Ophthalmol. 1998;236(8):635–8.
32. Bilyk JR. Enucleation, evisceration, and sympathetic ophthalmia. Curr Opin Ophthalmol. 2000;11(5):372–86 [2+ C].
33. Blacksell SD, Newton PN, Bell D, et al. The comparative accuracy of 8 commercial rapid immunochromatographic assays for the diagnosis of acute dengue virus infection. Clin Infect Dis. 2006;42:1127–34.
34. Blumenkranz MS, Gass JD, Clarkson JG. Atypical serpiginous choroiditis. Arch Ophthalmol. 1982;100:1773–5.
35. Bodaghi B. Ocular manifestations of Lyme disease. Med Mal Infect. 2007;37(7–8):518–22.
36. Borruat FX, Otheni-Girard P, Safran AB. Multiple evanescent white dot syndrome. Klin Monatsbl Augenheilkd. 1991;198:453–6.
37. Borruat FX, Piguet B, Herbort CP. Acute posterior multifocal placoid pigment epitheliopathy following mumps. Ocul Immunol Inflamm. 1998;6:189–93.
38. Bosch-Driessen LE, Berendschot TT, Ongkosuwito JV, Rothova A. Ocular toxoplasmosis: clinical features and prognosis of 154 patients. Ophthalmology. 2002;109:869–78.
39. Bosch-Driessen LH, Plaisier MB, Stilma JS, Van der Lelij A, Rothova A. Reactivations of ocular toxoplasmosis after cataract extraction. Ophthalmology. 2002;109:41–5.
40. Bouchenaki N, Cimino L, Auer C, et al. Assessment and classification of choroidal vasculitis in posterior uveitis using indocyanine green angiography. Klin Monatsbl Augenheilkd. 2002;219:243–9.
41. Bouchenaki N, Herbort CP. The contribution of indocyanine green angiography to the appraisal and management of Vogt-Koyanagi-Harada disease. Ophthalmology. 2001;108(1):54–64.
42. Brett-Major DM, Coldren R. Antibiotics for leptospirosis. Cochrane Database Syst Rev. 2012;2:CD008264. EbM 1-.
43. Brighton SW, Prozesky OW, de la Harpe AL. Chikungunya virus infection. A retrospective study of 107 cases. S Afr Med J. 1983;63:313–5.
44. Brighton SW. Chloroquine phosphate treatment of chronic Chikungunya arthritis. An open pilot study. S Afr Med J. 1984;66:217–8.
45. Briolant S, Garin D, Scaramizzino N, Jouan A, Crance JM. In vitro inhibition of Chikungunya and Semliki Forest viruses replication by antiviral compounds: synergistic effect of interferon-alpha and ribavirin combination. Antiviral Res. 2004;61:111–7.
46. Brown Jr J, Folk JC, Reddy CV, Kimura AE. Visual prognosis of multifocal choroiditis, punctate inner choroidopathy, and diffuse subretinal fibrosis syndrome. Ophthalmology. 1996;103:1100–5.
47. Burt FJ, Rolph MS, Rulli NE, Mahalingam S, Heise MT. Chikungunya: a re-emerging virus. Lancet. 2012;379(9816):662–7.
48. Butler NJ, Furtado JM, Winthrop KL, Smith JR. Ocular toxoplasmosis II: clinical features, pathology and management. Clin Experiment Ophthalmol. 2013;41:95–108.
49. Caballero-Presencia A, Diaz-Guia E, Lopez-Lopez JM. Acute anterior ischemic optic neuropathy in birdshot retinochoroidopathy. Ophthalmologica. 1988;196:87–91.
50. Centers for Disease Control and Prevention. Sexually transmitted diseases treatment guidelines, 2006. MMWR Morb Mortal Wkly Rep. 2006;55(No. RR-11):1–96.
51. Cervantes-Castaneda RA, Bhat P, Fortuna E, Acevedo S, Foster CS. Induction of durable remission in ocular inflammatory diseases. Eur J Ophthalmol. 2009;19(1):118–23.
52. Chan CC, Roberge RG, Whitcup SM, Nussenblatt RB. 32 cases of sympathetic ophthalmia. A retrospective study at the National Eye Institute, Bethesda, Md., from 1982 to 1992. Arch Ophthalmol. 1995;113(5):597–600.

53. Chan DP, Teoh SC, Tan CS, et al. Ophthalmic complications of dengue. Emerg Infect Dis. 2006;12:285–9.
54. Chan RV, Seiff BD, Lincoff HA, Coleman DJ. Rapid recovery of sympathetic ophthalmia with treatment augmented by intravitreal steroids. Retina. 2006;26(2):243–7 [3 D].
55. Chazalon E, Conrath J, Ridings B, Matonti F. Kyrieleis arteritis: report of two cases and literature review. J Fr Ophtalmol. 2013;36:191–6.
56. Chi SL, Stinnett S, Eggenberger E, Foroozan R, Golnik K, Lee MS, Bhatti MT. Clinical characteristics in 53 patients with cat scratch optic neuropathy. Ophthalmology. 2012;119(1):183–7. EbM 2b.
57. Chia A, Luu CD, Mathur R, Cheng B, Chee SP. Electrophysiological findings in patients with dengue-related maculopathy. Arch Ophthalmol. 2006;124(10):1421–6.
58. Chlebicki MP, Ang B, Barkham T, Lande A. Retinal hemorrhages in 4 patients with dengue fever. Emerg Infect Dis. 2005;11:770–1.
59. Christmas NJ, Oh KT, Oh DM, et al. Long-term follow up of patients with serpiginous choroiditis. Retina. 2002;22:550–6.
60. Cimino L, Auer C, Herbort CP. Sensitivity of indocyanine green angiography for the follow-up of active inflammatory choriocapillaropathies. Ocul Immunol Inflamm. 2000;8:275–83.
61. Couvreur J, Thulliez P, Daffos F, et al. In utero treatment of toxoplasmic fetopathy with the combination pyrimethamine-sulfadiazine. Fetal Diagn Ther. 1993;8:45–50.
62. Cruz-Villegas V, Berrocal AM, Davis JL. Bilateral choroidal effusions associated with dengue fever. Retina. 2003;23:576–8.
63. Cuchacovich M, Solanes F, Díaz G, Cermenati T, Avila S, Verdaguer J, Verdaguer JI, Carpentier C, Stopel J, Rojas B, Traipe L, Gallardo P, Sabugo F, Zanoli M, Merino G, Villarroel F. Comparison of the clinical efficacy of two different immunosuppressive regimens in patients with chronic Vogt-Koyanagi-Harada disease. Ocul Immunol Inflamm. 2010;18(3):200–7.
64. Cunningham ET, Koehler JE. Ocular bartonellosis. Am J Ophthalmol. 2000;130(3):340–9.
65. Damico FM, Kiss S, Young LH. Sympathetic ophthalmia. Semin Ophthalmol. 2005;20(3):191–7 [3C].
66. Davis JL, Mittal KK, Freidlin V, Mellow SR, Optican DC, Palestine AG, Nussenblatt RB. HLA associations and ancestry in Vogt-Koyanagi-Harada disease and sympathetic ophthalmia. Ophthalmology. 1990;97(9):1137–42.
67. De Amorim Garcia CA, Gomes AH, De Oliveira AG. Bilateral stellar neuroretinitis in a patient with dengue fever. Eye. 2006;20(12):1382–3.
68. De Courten C, Herbort CP. The potential role of computerized field testing for the appraisal and follow-up of birdshot chorioretinopathy. Arch Ophthalmol. 1998;116:1389–91.
69. De Lamballerie X, Boisson V, Reynier JC, et al. On chikungunya acute infection and chloroquine treatment. Vector Borne Zoonotic Dis. 2008;8:837–9.
70. Dees C, Arnold JJ, Forrester JV, Dick AD. Immunosuppressive treatment of choroidal neovascularization associated with endogenous posterior uveitis. Arch Ophthalmol. 1998;116:1456–61.
71. Desarnaulds AB, Borruat FX, Herbort CP, Spertini F. Multiple evanescent white dot syndrome: a genetic disorder? Klin Monatsbl Augenheilkd. 1996;208:301–2.
72. Dodwell DD, Jampol LM, Rosenberg M, et al. Optic nerve involvement associated with multiple evanescent white dot syndrome. Ophthalmology. 1990;97:862.
73. Dolz-Marco R, Gallego-Pinazo R, Díaz-Llopis M. Rituximab in refractory Vogt-Koyanagi-Harada disease. J Ophthalmic Inflamm Infect. 2011;1(4):177–80.
74. Dreyer RF, Gass JDM. Multifocal choroiditis and panuveitis: a syndrome that mimics ocular histoplasmosis. Arch Ophthalmol. 1984;102:1776.
75. Dunlop AA, Cree IA, Hagee S, Luthert PJ, Lightman S. Multifocal choroiditis, clinicopathologic correlation. Arch Ophthalmol. 1998;116:801–3.
76. Dunn D, Wallon M, Peyron F, Petersen E, et al. Mother-to-child transmission of toxoplasmosis: risk estimates for clinical counselling. Lancet. 1999;353:1829–33.
77. Eandi CM, Neri P, Adelman RA, Yannuzzi LA, Cunningham Jr ET, International Syphilis Study Group. Acute syphilitic posterior placoid chorioretinitis: report of a case series and comprehensive review of the literature. Retina. 2012;32(9):1915–41.
78. Faine S, Adler B, Bolin C, Perolat P. Leptospira and leptospirosis. 2nd ed. Melbourne: Med Sci; 1999. p. 1–230.
79. Feltkamp TE. Ophthalmological significance of HLA associated uveitis. Eye. 1990;4:839–44.
80. Flaxel CJ, Owens SL, Mulholland B, Schwartz SD, Gregor ZJ. The use of corticosteroids for choroidal neovascularization in young patients. Eye (Lond). 1998;12:266–72.
81. Forster DJ, Cano MR, Green RL, Rao NA. Echographic features of the Vogt-Koyanagi-Harada syndrome. Arch Ophthalmol. 1990;108(10):1421–6.
82. Forster DJ, Dugel PU, Frangieh GT, Liggett PE, Rao NA. Rapidly progressive outer retinal necrosis in the acquired immunodeficiency syndrome. Am J Ophthalmol. 1990;110(4):341–8.
83. Freeman K, Tan HK, Prusa A, Petersen E, et al. Predictors of retinochoroiditis in children with congenital toxoplasmosis: European, prospective cohort study. Pediatrics. 2008;121:e1215–22.
84. Friedman AH, Deutsch-Sokol RH. Sugiura's sign. Perilimbal vitiligo in the Vogt-Koyanagi-Harada syndrome. Ophthalmology. 1981;88(11):1159–65.
85. Fuerst DJ, Tessler HH, Fishman GA, et al. Birdshot retinochoroidopathy. Arch Ophthalmol. 1984;102:214–9.
86. Furusato E, Shen D, Cao X, Furusato B, Nussenblatt RB, Rushing EJ, Chan CC. Inflammatory cytokine and chemokine expression in sympathetic ophthalmia: a pilot study. Histol Histopathol. 2011;26(9):1145–51 [3 D].

87. Garg S, Jampol LM. Systemic and intraocular manifestations of West Nile virus infection. Surv Ophthalmol. 2005;50:3–13.

88. Gass JD. Sympathetic ophthalmia following vitrectomy. Am J Ophthalmol. 1982;93(5):552–8.

89. Gass JD. Vitiliginous chorioretinitis. Arch Ophthalmol. 1981;99:1778–87.

90. Gass JDM. Harada's disease. In: Gass JDM, editor. Stereoscopic atlas of macular disease. Diagnosis and treatment. St Louis: Mosby; 1987. p. 150–3.

91. Gaudio PA, Kaye DB, Brooks CJ. Histopathology of birdshot retinochoroidopathy. Br J Ophthalmol. 2002;86:1439–41.

92. Gerstenblith AT, Thorne JE, Sobrin I, et al. Punctate inner choroidopathy: a survey analysis of 77 persons. Ophthalmology. 2007;114:1201–4.

93. Gilber RE, Freeman K, Lago EG, Bahia-Oliveira LM, et al. Ocular sequelae of congenital toxoplasmosis in Brazil compared with Europe. PLoS Negl Trop Dis. 2008;2:e277.

94. Gilbert R, Dezateux C. Newborn screening for congenital toxoplasmosis: feasible, but benefits are not established. Arch Dis Child. 2006;91:629–31.

95. Glavici M. Sympathetic ophthalmia after a cataract operation. Oftalmologia. 1992;36(4):397–401.

96. Gohdo T, Tsukahara S. Ultrasound biomicroscopy of shallow anterior chamber in Vogt-Koyanagi-Harada syndrome. Am J Ophthalmol. 1996;122(1):112–4.

97. Goldenberg D, Goldstein M, Loewenstein A, Habot-Wilner Z. Vitreal, retinal, and choroidal findings in active and scarred toxoplasmosis lesions: a prospective study by spectral-domain optical coherence tomography. Graefes Arch Clin Exp Ophthalmol. 2013;251:2037–45.

98. Goto H, Rao NA. Sympathetic ophthalmia and Vogt-Koyanagi-Harada syndrome. Int Ophthalmol Clin. 1990;30(4):279–85.

99. Green WR, Maumenee AE, Sanders TE, Smith ME. Sympathetic uveitis following evisceration. Trans Am Acad Ophthalmol Otolaryngol. 1972;76(3):625–44.

100. Gupta A, Bansal R, Gupta V, Sharma A, Bambery P. Ocular signs predictive of tubercular uveitis. Am J Ophthalmol. 2010;149:562–70. C.

101. Gupta A, Bansal R, Gupta V, Sharma A. Fundus autofluorescence in serpiginous-like choroiditis. Retina. 2012;32(4):814–25.

102. Gupta V, Bansal R, Gupta A. Continued progression of tubercular serpiginous-like choroiditis after initiating antituberculosis treatment. Am J Ophthalmol. 2011;152:857–63.

103. Gupta V, Gupta A, Dogra MR. Posterior sympathetic ophthalmia: a single centre long-term study of 40 patients from North India. Eye (Lond). 2008;22(12):1459–64.

104. Gupta V, Gupta A, Rao NA. Intra-ocular tuberculosis – an update. Surv Ophthalmol. 2007;52:561–87.

105. Gupta V, Agarwal A, Gupta A, Bambery P, Narang S. Clinical characteristics of serpiginous choroidopathy in North India. Am J Ophthalmol. 2002;134(1):47–56.

106. Hakin KN, Pearson RV, Lightman SL. Sympathetic ophthalmia: visual results with modern immunosuppressive therapy. Eye (Lond). 1992;6(Pt 5):453–5 [3C].

107. Halstead SB. Dengue. Curr Opinion Infect Dis. 2002;15:471–6.

108. Hardy RA, Schatz H. Macular geographic helicoid choroidopathy. Arch Ophthalmol. 1987;105:1237–42.

109. Harrison TJ. Sympathetic ophthalmia after cyclocryotherapy of neovascular glaucoma without ocular penetration. Ophthalmic Surg. 1993;24(1):44–6.

110. Hebestreit H, Huppertz HI, Sold JE, Dämmrich J. Steroid-pulse therapy may suppress inflammation in severe sympathetic ophthalmia. J Pediatr Ophthalmol Strabismus. 1997;34(2):124–6 [3C].

111. Herbort CP, Papadia M, Neri P. Myopia and inflammation. J Ophthalmic Vis Res. 2011;6(4):270–83. EBM (4).

112. Hogan A, Behan U, Kilmartin DJ. Outcomes after combination photodynamic therapy and immunosuppression for inflammatory subfoveal choroidal neovascularization. Br J Ophthalmol. 2005;89:1109–11.

113. Holder GE, Ag R, Pavesio CP, Graham EM. Electrophysiological characterization and monitoring in the management of birdshot chorioretinopathy. Br J Ophthalmol. 2005;89:709–18.

114. Holland GN, Lewis KG. An update on current practices in the management of ocular toxoplasmosis. Am J Ophthalmol. 2002;134:102–14.

115. Holland GN. Standard diagnostic criteria for the acute retinal necrosis syndrome. Executive Committee of the American Uveitis Society. Am J Ophthalmol. 1994;117:663–7.

116. Hooper PL, Kaplan HJ. Triple agent immunosuppression in serpiginous choroiditis. Ophthalmology. 1991;98(6):944–51.

117. Hoshi H, Tamada Y, Murada Y, et al. Changes in audiogram in the course of Harada's disease. Jpn J Clin Ophthalmol. 1977;31:23–30.

118. Huppertz HI, Bartmann P, Heininger U, Fingerle V, Kinet M, Klein R, Korenke GC, Nentwich HJ, Committee for Infectious Diseases and Vaccinations of the German Academy for Pediatrics and Adolescent Health. Rational diagnostic strategies for Lyme borreliosis in children and adolescents: recommendations by the Committee for Infectious Diseases and Vaccinations of the German Academy for Pediatrics and Adolescent Health. Eur J Pediatr. 2012;171(11):1619–24.

119. Jaffe GJ, McCallum RM, Branchaud B, Skalak C, Butuner Z, Ashton P. Long-term follow-up results of a pilot trial of a fluocinolone acetonide implant to treat posterior uveitis. Ophthalmology. 2005;112(7):1192–8.

120. Jasper S, Vedula SS, John SS, Horo S, Sepah YJ, Nguyen QD. Corticosteroids for ocular toxoplasmosis. Cochrane Database Syst Rev. 2013;4:CD007417.

121. Jeon S, Kakizaki H, Lee WK, et al. Effect of prolonged oral acyclovir treatment in acute retinal necrosis. Ocul Immunol Inflamm. 2012;20(4):288–92.

122. John M, Samson CM, Foster CS. Syphilis. In: Foster CS, Vitale AT, editors. Diagnosis & treatment of uveitis. New Delhi: Jaypee Medical Publishers; 2013. p. 337–45.

123. Jones BE, Jampol LM, Yannuzzi LA, et al. Relentless placoid chorioretinitis: a new entity or an unusual variant of serpiginous choroiretinitis? Am J Ophthalmol. 2000;118:931–8.

124. Julián K, Terrada C, Fardeau C, Cassoux N, Français C, LeHoang P, Bodaghi B. Intravitreal bevacizumab as first local treatment for uveitis-related choroidal neovascularization: long-term results. Acta Ophthalmol. 2011;89(2):179–84.

125. Kanungo S, Shukla D, Kim R. Branch retinal artery occlusion secondary to dengue fever. Indian J Ophthalmol. 2008;56(1):73–4.

126. Kaplan HJ, Aaberg TM. Birdshot retinochoroidopathy. Am J Ophthalmol. 1980;90:773–82.

127. Kapoor HK, Bhai S, John M, Xavier J. Ocular manifestations of dengue fever in an East Indian epidemic. Can J Ophthalmol. 2006;41:741–6.

128. Kawaguchi T, Spencer DB, Mochizuki M. Therapy for acute retinal necrosis. Semin Ophthalmol. 2008;23(4):285–90.

129. Kennedy JJ, Defeo E. Ocular toxocariasis demonstrated by ultrasound. Ann Ophthalmol. 1981;13:1357–8.

130. Kent ME, Romanelli F. Reexamining syphilis: an update on epidemiology, clinical manifestations and management. Ann Pharmacother. 2008;42:226–36.

131. Khairallah M, Ben Yahia S, Attia S, Zaouali S, Ladjimi A, Messaoud R. Linear pattern of West Nile virus-associated chorioretinitis is related to retinal nerve fibres organization. Eye (Lond). 2007;21(7):952–5.

132. Khairallah M, Ben Yahia S, Ladjimi A, Zeghidi H, Ben Romdhane F, Besbes L, Zaouali S, Messaoud R. Chorioretinal involvement in patients with West Nile virus infection. Ophthalmology. 2004;111(11):2065–70.

133. Khairallah M, Kahloun R, Ben Yahia S, Jelliti B, Messaoud R. New infectious etiologies for posterior uveitis. Ophthalmic Res. 2013;49(2):66–72.

134. Khairallah M, Yahia SB, Letaief M, Attia S, Kahloun R, Jelliti B, Zaouali S, Messaoud R. A prospective evaluation of factors associated with chorioretinitis in patients with West Nile virus infection. Ocul Immunol Inflamm. 2007;15(6):435–9.

135. Kieffer F, Wallon M, Garcia P, Thulliez P, Peyron F, Franck J. Risk factors for retinochoroiditis during the first 2 years of life in infants with treated congenital toxoplasmosis. Pediatr Infect Dis J. 2008;27:27–32.

136. Kilmartin DJ, Dick AD, Forrester JV. Sympathetic ophthalmia risk following vitrectomy: should we counsel patients? Br J Ophthalmol. 2000; 84(5):448–9.

137. Kim SJ, Equi R, Belair ML, Fine HF, Dunn JP. Long-term preservation of vision in progressive outer retinal necrosis treated with combination antiviral drugs and highly active antiretroviral therapy. Ocul Immunol Inflamm. 2007;15:425–7.

138. Kimura R, Sakai M, Okabe H. Transient shallow anterior chamber as initial symptom in Harada's syndrome. Arch Ophthalmol. 1981;99(9):1604–6.

139. Kishi A, Nao-i N, Sawada A. Ultrasound biomicroscopic findings of acute angle-closure glaucoma in Vogt-Koyanagi-Harada syndrome. Am J Ophthalmol. 1996;122(5):735–7.

140. Kishore K, Conway MD, Peyman GA. Intravitreal clindamycin and dexamethasone for toxoplasmic retinochoroiditis. Ophthalmic Surg Lasers. 2001;32:183–92.

141. Kiss S, Ahmed M, Letko E, Foster CS. Long-term follow-up of patients with birdshot retinochoroidopathy treated with corticosteroid-sparing systemic immunomodulatory therapy. Ophthalmology. 2005;112(6):1066–71.

142. Knecht PB, Papadia M, Herbort CP. Granulomatous keratic precipitates in birdshot retinochoroiditis. Int Ophthalmol. 2013;33(2):133–7.

143. Koizumi H, Pozzoni MC, Spaide RF. Fundus autofluorescence in birdshot chorioretinopathy. Ophthalmology. 2008;115(5):e15–20.

144. Kunkel J, Schürmann D, Pleyer U, Rüther K, Kneifel C, Krause L, Reichert M, Ignatius R, Schneider T. Ocular syphilis-indicator of previously unknown HIV-infection. J Infect. 2009;58:32–6.

145. Kupperman BD, Petty JG, Richman DD, et al. Correlation between CD4+ counts and the prevalence of cytomegalovirus retinitis and human immunodeficiency virus-related noninfectious retinal vasculopathy in patients with acquired immunodeficiency syndrome. Am J Ophthalmol. 1993;115:575–82.

146. Laatikanen L, Erkkilä H. A follow-up study on serpiginous choroiditis. Acta Ophthalmol (Copenh). 1981;59:707–18.

147. Lakhanpal V, Schocket SS, Nirankari VS. Clindamycin in the treatment of toxoplasmic retinochoroiditis. Am J Ophthalmol. 1983;95:605–13.

148. Lasave AF, Diaz-Llopis M, Muccioli C, Belfort Jr R, Arevalo JF. Intravitreal clindamycin and dexamethasone for zone 1 toxoplasmic retinochoroiditis at twenty-four months. Ophthalmology. 2010;117:1831–8.

149. Lau CH, Comer M, Lightman S. Long-term efficacy of mycophenolate mofetil in the control of severe intraocular inflammation. Clin Exp Ophthalmol. 2003;31(6):487–91 [3 D].

150. Laurence B, Harold M, Thierry D. Ocular complications of dengue fever. Ophthalmology. 2008;115:1100–1.

151. Le Hoang P, Girard B, Deray G, Le Minh H, De Kozak Y, Thillaye B, Faure JP, Rousselie F. Cyclosporine in the treatment of birdshot retinochoroidopathy. Transplant Proc. 1988;20(3 Suppl 4):128–30.

152. LeHoang P, Cassoux N, George F, Kullmann N, Kazatchkine MD. Intravenous immunoglobulin (IVIg) for the treatment of birdshot retinochoroidopathy. Ocul Immunol Inflamm. 2000;8(1):49–57.

153. LeHoang P, Ryan SJ. Birdshot retinochoroidopathy. In: Pepose JS, Holland GN, Wilhelmus KR, editors.

Ocular infection & immunity. St. Louis: Mosby-Year Book Inc; 1996. p. 570–8.

154. Leslie T, Lois N, Christopoulou D, Olson JA, Forrester JV. Photodynamic therapy for inflammatory choroidal neovascularization unresponsive to immunosuppression. Br J Ophthalmol. 2005;89:147–50.

155. Levinson RD, Brezin A, Rothova A, Accorinti M, Holland GN. Research criteria for the diagnosis of birdshot chorioretinopathy: results of an international consensus conference. Am J Ophthalmol. 2006;141(1):185–7.

156. Lim WK, Buggage RR, Nussenblatt RB. Serpiginous choroiditis. Surv Ophthalmol. 2005;50(3):231–44.

157. Lit ES, Kim RY, Damico DJ. Surgical removal of subfoveal choroidal neovascularization without removal of posterior hyaloid: a consecutive series in younger patients. Retina. 2001;21:317–23.

158. Lowder CY, Foster RE, Gordon SM, Gutman FA. Acute posterior multifocal placoid pigment epitheliopathy after acute group A streptococcal infection. Am J Ophthalmol. 1996;122:115–7.

159. Lubin JR, Albert DM, Weinstein M. Sixty-five years of sympathetic ophthalmia. A clinicopathologic review of 105 cases (1913–1978). Ophthalmology. 1980;87(2):109–21.

160. Maenz M, Schlüter D, Liesenfeld O, Schares G, Gross U, Pleyer U. Ocular toxoplasmosis: past, present and new aspects of an old disease. Prog Retin Eye Res. 2014;39c:77–106.

161. Magnaval JF, Fabre R, Maurières P, et al. Application of the western blotting procedure for the immunodiagnosis of human toxocariasis. Parasitol Res. 1991;77:697–702.

162. Mahajan VB, Gehrs KM, Goldstein DA, Fischer DH, Lopez JS, Folk JC. Management of sympathetic ophthalmia with the fluocinolone acetonide implant. Ophthalmology. 2009;116(3):552–7 [3 D].

163. Maisel JM, Vorwerk PA. Sympathetic uveitis after giant tear repair. Retina. 1989;9(2):122–6.

164. Mansour AM, Arevalo JF, Fardeau C, Hrisomalos EN, et al. Three-year visual and anatomic results of administrating intravitreal bevacizumab in inflammatory ocular neovascularization. Can J Ophthalmol. 2012;47:269–74.

165. Martin DF, Sierra-Madero J, Walmsley S, Wolitz RA, Macey K, Georgiou P. A controlled trial of valganciclovir as induction therapy for cytomegalovirus retinitis. N Engl J Med. 2002;346:1119–26.

166. Martinez CE, Zhang D, Conway MD, et al. Successful management of ocular toxoplasmosis during pregnancy using combined intraocular clindamycin and dexamethasone with systemic sulfadiazine. Int Ophthalmol. 1999;22:85–8.

167. Maruyama Y, Kishi S. Tomographic features of serous retinal detachment in Vogt-Koyanagi-Harada syndrome. Ophthalmic Surg Lasers Imaging. 2004;35(3):239–42.

168. McCannel CA, Holland GN, Helm CJ, et al. Causes of uveitis in the general practice of ophthalmology. UCLA Community-Based Uveitis Study Group. Am J Ophthalmol. 1996;121:35–46.

169. Melamed J, Eckert GU, Spadoni VS, Lago EG, Uberti F. Ocular manifestations of congenital toxoplasmosis. Eye. 2010;24:528–34.

170. Mikkilä HO, Seppälä IJ, Viljanen MK, Peltomaa MP, Karma A. The expanding clinical spectrum of ocular lyme borreliosis. Ophthalmology. 2000;107(3):581–7.

171. Mittal A, Mittal S, Bharathi JM, Ramakrishnan R, Saravanan S, Sathe PS. Optic neuritis associated with chikungunya virus infection in South India. Arch Ophthalmol. 2007;125:1381–6.

172. Mittal A, Mittal S, Bharathi JM, Ramakrishnan R, Sathe PS. Uveitis during outbreak of chikungunya fever. Ophthalmology. 2007;114:1798.

173. Moorthy RS, Inomata H, Rao NA. Vogt-Koyanagi-Harada syndrome. Surv Ophthalmol. 1995;39:265–92.

174. Musch DC, Martin DF, Gordon JF, Davis MD, Kuppermann BD, Ganciclovir Implant Study Group. Treatment of cytomegalovirus retinitis with a sustained-release ganciclovir implant. N Engl J Med. 1997;337:83–90. 90.

175. Nazari Khanamiri H, Rao NA. Serpiginous choroiditis and infectious multifocal serpiginoid choroiditis. Surv Ophthalmol. 2013;58(3):203–32.

176. Neri P, Manoni M, Fortuna C, Lettieri M, Mariotti C, Giovannini A. Association of systemic steroids and mycophenolate mofetil as rescue therapy for uveitic choroidal neovascularization unresponsive to the traditional immunosuppressants: interventional case series. Int Ophthalmol. 2009;30:583–90.

177. Neri P, Mercanti L, Mariotti C, Salvolini S, Giovannini A. Long-term control of choroidal neovascularization in quiescent congenital toxoplasma retinochoroiditis with photodynamic therapy: 4-year results. Int Ophthalmol. 2010;30:51–6.

178. Nussenblatt R. Sympathetic ophthalmia. In: Nussenblatt RB SW, Whitcup SW, editors. Uveitis: fundamentals and clinical practice. 4th ed. St. Louis: Mosby Elsevier; 2010. p. 289–302 [4 D].

179. Nussenblatt RB, Palestine AG, Chan CC, Stevens Jr G, Mellow SD, Green SB. Randomized, double-masked study of cyclosporine compared to prednisolone in the treatment of endogenous uveitis. Am J Ophthalmol. 1991;112(2):138–46.

180. Nussenblatt RB, Whitcup SM, Palestine AG. Birdshot retinochoroidopathy. In: Nussenblatt RB, Whitcup SM, Palestine AG, editors. Uveitis: fundamentals and clinical practice. 2nd ed. St Louis: Mosby-Year Book; 1996. p. 325.

181. Nussenblatt RB, Whitcup SM, Palestine AG. Vogt-Koyanagi-Harada syndrome. In: Nussenblatt RB, Whitcup SM, Palestine AG, editors. Uveitis: fundamental and clinical practice. 2nd ed. St Louis: Mosby; 1996. p. 312–24.

182. Nussenblatt RB, Whitcup SM, Palestine AG. White dot syndromes. In: Nussenblatt RB, Whitcup SM, Palestine AG, editors. Fundamentals and clinical

practice. 2nd ed. St. Louis: Mosby-Year Book, Inc; 1996. p. 373.

183. Ohno S, Minakawa R, Matsuda H. Clinical studies of Vogt-Koyanagi-Harada's disease. Jpn J Ophthalmol. 1988;32(3):334–43.

184. Olk RJ, Burgess DB. Treatment of recurrent juxtafoveal subretinal neovascular membranes with krypton red laser photocoagulation. Ophthalmology. 1985;92:1035–46.

185. Opremcak EM, Scales DK, Sharpe MR. Trimethoprim-sulfamethoxazole therapy for ocular toxoplasmosis. Ophthalmology. 1992;99:920–5.

186. Opremcak EM. Birdshot retinochoroiditis. In: Albert DM, Jakobiec FA, editors. Principles and practice of ophthalmology, vol. 1. Philadelphia: W.B. Saunders; 1994. p. 475.

187. Ozdemir H, Karacorlu M, Karacorlu S. Intravitreal triamcinolone acetonide in sympathetic ophthalmia. Graefes Arch Clin Exp Ophthalmol. 2005;243(7):734–6 [3 D].

188. Palay D, Sternberg P, Davis J. Decrease in the risk of bilateral acute retinal necrosis by acyclovir therapy. Ophthalmology. 1991;112:250–5.

189. Palestine AG, Rodrigues MM, Macher AM, et al. Ophthalmic involvement in the acquired immune deficiency syndrome. Ophthalmology. 1984;91:1092–9.

190. Papadia M, Herbort CP. Indocyanine green angiography (ICGA) is essential for the early diagnosis of birdshot chorioretinopathy. Klin Monbl Augenheilkd. 2012;229(4):348–52.

191. Papadia M, Herbort CP. Reappraisal of birdshot retinochoroiditis (BRC): a global approach. Graefes Arch Clin Exp Ophthalmol. 2013;251(3):861–9.

192. Pappachan JM, Mathew S, Thomas B, Renjini K, Scaria CK, Shukla J. The incidence and clinical characteristics of the immune phase eye disease in treated cases of human leptospirosis. Indian J Med Sci. 2007;61(8):441–7. EbM 2+.

193. Parc C, Guenoun JM, Dhote R, Brézin A. Optical coherence tomography in the acute and chronic phases of Vogt-Koyanagi-Harada disease. Ocul Immunol Inflamm. 2005;13(2–3):225–7.

194. Paredes I, Ahmed M, Foster CS. Immunomodulatory therapy for Vogt-Koyanagi-Harada patients as first-line therapy. Ocul Immunol Inflamm. 2006;14(2):87–90.

195. Park D, Shatz H, McDonald R, Johnson RN. Indocyanine green angiography of acute posterior multifocal placoid pigment epitheliopathy. Ophthalmology. 1995;102:1877–83.

196. Park JJ, Pavesio C. Prophylactic laser photocoagulation for acute retinal necrosis: does it raise more questions than answers? Br J Ophthalmol. 2008;92(9):1161–2.

197. Pearson PA, Piracha AR, Sen HA, Jaffe GJ. Atovaquone for the treatment of toxoplasma retinochoroiditis in immunocompetent patients. Ophthalmology. 1999;106:148–53.

198. Pedroza Seres M. Acute posterior multifocal placoid pigment epitheliopathy. In: Foster CS, Vitale AT, editors. Diagnosis and treatments of uveatis. Philadelphia: W.B. Saunders Company; 2002. p. 772–7.

199. Perente I, Utine CA, Cakir H, Kaya V, Tutkun IT, Yilmaz OF. Management of ocular complications of Vogt-Koyanagi-Harada syndrome. Int Ophthalmol. 2009;29(1):33–7.

200. Petersen E, Kiilstra A, Stanford M. Epidemiology of ocular toxoplasmosis. Ocul Immunol Inflamm. 2012;20:68–75.

201. Phan L, Kasza K, Jalbrzikowski J, et al. Longitudinal study of new eye lesions in treated congenital toxoplasmosis. Ophthalmology. 2008;115:553–9. e558.

202. Pialoux G, Gaüzère BA, Jauréguiberry S, Strobel M. Chikungunya, an epidemic arbovirosis. Lancet Infect Dis. 2007;7:319–27.

203. Pleyer U, Dutescu M. Sympathetic ophthalmia. Ophthalmologe. 2009;106(2):167–75 [4C].

204. Pollack AL, McDonald HR, Ai E, Green WR, Halpern LS, Jampol LM, Leahy JM, Johnson RN, Spencer WH, Stern WH, Weinberg DV, Werner JC, Williams GA. Sympathetic ophthalmia associated with pars plana vitrectomy without antecedent penetrating trauma. Retina. 2001;21(2):146–54.

205. Powers AM, Brault AC, Tesh RB, Weaver SC. Re-emergence of chikungunya and O'nyong-nyong viruses: evidence for distinct geographical lineages and distant evolutionary relationships. J Gen Virol. 2000;81:471–9.

206. Priem HA, Oosterhuis JA. Birdshot chorioretinopathy: clinical characteristics and evolution. Br J Ophthalmol. 1988;72:646–59.

207. Prutsky G, Domecq JP, Mori L, Bebko S, Matzumura M, Sabouni A, Shahrour A, Erwin PJ, Boyce TG, Montori VM, Malaga G, Murad MH. Treatment outcomes of human bartonellosis: a systematic review and meta-analysis. Int J Infect Dis. 2013;17(10):e811–9. pii: S1201-9712(13)00107-0. (EbM 1-).

208. Rahn DW, Felz MW. Lyme disease: current approach to early, disseminated and late disease. Postgrad Med. 1998;103(5):51–4. 57–9: 63–4.

209. Rathinam SR, Ratnam S, Selvaraj S, et al. Uveitis associated with an epidemic outbreak of leptospirosis. Am J Ophthalmol. 1997;124:71–9.

210. Read RW, Holland GN, Rao NA, Tabbara KF, Ohno S, Arellanes-Garcia L, Pivetti-Pezzi P, Tessler HH, Usui M. Revised diagnostic criteria for Vogt-Koyanagi-Harada disease: report of an international committee on nomenclature. Am J Ophthalmol. 2001;131(5):647–52.

211. Read RW, Rao NA, Sharma OP. Sarcoid choroiditis initially diagnosed as birdshot choroidopathy. Sarcoidosis Vasc Diffuse Lung Dis. 2000;17:85–6.

212. Read RW, Yu F, Accorinti M, Bodaghi B, Chee SP, Fardeau C, Goto H, Holland GN, Kawashima H, Kojima E, Lehoang P, Lemaitre C, Okada AA, Pivetti-Pezzi P, Secchi A, See RF, Tabbara KF, Usui M, Rao NA. Evaluation of the effect on outcomes of the route of administration of corticosteroids in acute

Vogt-Koyanagi-Harada disease. Am J Ophthalmol. 2006;142(1):119–24.

213. Reddy CV, Brown J, Folk JC, et al. Enlarged blind spots in chorioretinal inflammatory disorders. Ophthalmology. 1996;103:606.

214. Rishi P, Venkataraman A, Rishi E. Combination photodynamic therapy and bevacizumab for choroidal neovascularization associated with toxoplasmosis. Indian J Ophthalmol. 2011;59:62–4.

215. Rodriguez A. Photocoagulation in toxoplasmic retinochoroiditis. Am J Ophthalmol. 1981;91:417–8.

216. Rodriguez A, Calonge M, Pedroza-Seres M, et al. Referral patterns of uveitis in a tertiary eye care center. Arch Ophthalmol. 1996;114:593–9.

217. Rothova A, Bosch-Driessen LE, van Loon NH, Treffers WF. Azithromycin for ocular toxoplasmosis. Br J Ophthalmol. 1998;82:1306–8.

218. Rothova A, Ossewaarde-van Norel A, Los LI, Berendschot TT. Efficacy of low-dose methotrexate treatment in birdshot chorioretinopathy. Retina. 2011;31(6):1150–5.

219. Rouvas A, Petrou P, Douvali M, Ntouraki A, Vergados I, Georgalas I, Markomichelakis N. Intravitreal ranibizumab for the treatment of inflammatory choroidal neovascularization. Retina. 2011;31(5):871–9.

220. Rubin ML, Kaufman HE, Tierney JP, et al. An intraretinal nematode. Trans Am Acad Ophthalmol Otolaryngol. 1968;72:855–66.

221. Rubsamen PE, Gass JD. Vogt-Koyanagi-Harada syndrome. Clinical course, therapy, and long-term visual outcome. Arch Ophthalmol. 1991;109(5):682–7.

222. Rush RB, Goldstein DA, Callanan DG, Meghpara B, Feuer WJ, Davis JL. Outcomes of birdshot chorioretinopathy treated with an intravitreal sustained-release fluocinolone acetonide-containing device. Am J Ophthalmol. 2011;151(4):630–6.

223. Ryan SJ, Maumenee AE. Birdshot retinochoroidopathy. Am J Ophthalmol. 1980;89:31–45.

224. Ryan SJ, Maumenee AE. Acute posterior multifocal placoid pigment epitheliopathy. Am J Ophthalmol. 1972;74:1066–74.

225. Sachdev N, Gupta V, Gupta A, Singh R. Posterior segment recurrences in Vogt-Koyanagi-Harada disease. Int Ophthalmol. 2008;28(5):339–45.

226. Samuel MA, Diamond MS. Alpha/beta interferon protects against lethal West Nile virus infection by restricting cellular tropism and enhancing neuronal survival. J Virol. 2005;79:13350–61.

227. Sanjay S, Wagle AM, Au Eong KG. Dengue optic neuropathy. Ophthalmology. 2009;116(1):170.

228. Sasamoto Y, Ohno S, Matsuda H. Studies on corticosteroid therapy in Vogt-Koyanagi-Harada disease. Ophthalmologica. 1990;201(3):162–7.

229. Shah KH, Levinson RD, Yu F, Goldhardt R, Gordon LK, Gonzales CR, Heckenlively JR, Kappel PJ, Holland GN. Birdshot chorioretinopathy. Surv Ophthalmol. 2005;50(6):519–41.

230. Shammas HF, Zubyk NA, Stanfield TF. Sympathetic uveitis following glaucoma surgery. Arch Ophthalmol. 1977;95(4):638–41.

231. Sharp DC, Bell RA, Patterson E, Pinkerton RM. Sympathetic ophthalmia. Histopathologic and fluorescein angiographic correlation. Arch Ophthalmol. 1984;102(2):232–5.

232. Shields JA. Ocular toxocariasis: a review. Surv Ophthalmol. 1984;28:361–81.

233. Shindo Y, Inoko H, Yamamoto T, Ohno S. HLA-DRB1 typing of Vogt-Koyanagi-Harada's disease by PCR-RFLP and the strong association with DRB1*0405 and DRB1*0410. Br J Ophthalmol. 1994;78(3):223–6.

234. Silveira C, Belfort Jr R, Muccioli C, et al. The effect of long-term intermittent trimethoprim/sulfamethoxazole treatment on recurrences of toxoplasmic retinochoroiditis. Am J Ophthalmol. 2002;134:41–6.

235. Singh G. Sympathetic ophthalmia after Nd:YAG cyclotherapy. Ophthalmology. 1993;100(6):798–9.

236. Singh K, de Frank MP, Shults WT, Watzke RC. Acute idiopathic blind spot enlargement. A spectrum of disease. Ophthalmology. 1991;98:497.

237. Siqueira RC, Vitral NP, Campos WR, Orefice F, de Moraes Figueiredo LT. Ocular manifestations in dengue fever. Ocul Immunol Inflamm. 2004;12:323–7.

238. Slakter JS, Giovannini A, Yannuzzi LA, et al. Indocyanine green angiography of multifocal choroiditis. Ophthalmology. 1997;104:1813.

239. Snyder DA, Tessler HH. Vogt-Koyanagi-Harada syndrome. Am J Ophthalmol. 1980;90(1):69–75.

240. Sobia S, Ashfaq UA. A brief review on dengue molecular virology, diagnosis, treatment and prevalence in Pakistan. Genet Vaccines Ther. 2012;10(1):6.

241. Sobrin L, Huang JJ, Christen W, Kafkala C, Choopong P, Foster CS. Daclizumab for treatment of birdshot chorioretinopathy. Arch Ophthalmol. 2008;126(2):186–91.

242. Soheilian M, Ramezani A, Azimzadeh A, et al. Randomized trial of intravitreal clindamycin and dexamethasone versus pyrimethamine, sulfadiazine, and prednisolone in treatment of ocular toxoplasmosis. Ophthalmology. 2011;118:134–41.

243. Spalter HF, Campbell CJ, Noyori KS, Rittler MC, Koester CJ. Prophylactic photocoagulation of recurrent toxoplasmic retinochoroiditis. A preliminary report. Arch Ophthalmol. 1966;75:21–31.

244. Stanford MR, See SE, Jones LV, et al. Antibiotics for toxoplasmic retinochoroiditis: an evidence-based systematic review. Ophthalmology. 2003;110:926–31.

245. Stewart JF, Croxson MC, Powell KF, Polkinghorne PJ. Identification of cytomegalovirus in vitreous using the polymerase chain reaction. Aust N Z J Ophthalmol. 1993;21(3):165–9.

246. Sudeep AB, Parashar D. Chikungunya: an overview. J Biosci. 2008;33:443–9.

247. Sugiura S. Vogt-Koyanagi-Harada disease. Jpn J Ophthalmol. 1978;22:9–35.

248. Tabbara KF, O'Connor GR. Treatment of ocular toxoplasmosis with clindamycin and sulfadiazine. Ophthalmology. 1980;87:129–34.

249. Talabani H, Mergey T, Yera H, Delair E, Brézin AP, Langsley G, Dupouy-Camet J. Factors of occurrence

of ocular toxoplasmosis. A review. Parasite. 2010; 17(3):177–82.

250. Taylor SRJ, Hamilton R, Hooper CY, et al. Valacyclovir in the treatment of acute retinal necrosis. BMC Ophthalmol. 2012;12:48.

251. Tessler HH, Jennings T. High-dose short-term chlorambucil for intractable sympathetic ophthalmia and Behçet's disease. Br J Ophthalmol. 1990;74(6):353–7 [3 D].

252. Thiébaut R, Leproust S, Chêne G, Gilbert R. Effectiveness of prenatal treatment for congenital toxoplasmosis: a meta-analysis of individual patients' data. Lancet. 2007;369:115–22.

253. Thorne JE, Jabs DA, Kedhar SR, Peters GB, Dunn JP. Loss of visual field among patients with birdshot chorioretinopathy. Am J Ophthalmol. 2008;145(1):23–8.

254. Tomsak RL, Lystad LD, Katirji MB, Brassel TC. Rapid response of syphilitic optic neuritis to posterior subtenon's steroid injection. J Clin Neuroophthalmol. 1992;12:6–7.

255. Torun N, Sherif Z, Garweg J, Pleyer U. Diagnosis and treatment of ocular toxoplasmosis: a survey of German-speaking ophthalmologists. Ophthalmologe. 2008;105:1023–8.

256. Tucker JD, Li JZ, Robbins GK, Davis BT, Lobo AM, Kunkel J, Papaliodis GN, Durand ML, Felsenstein D. Ocular syphilis among HIV-infected patients: a systematic analysis of the literature. Sex Transm Infect. 2011;87(1):4–8. doi:10.1136/sti.2010.043042. Epub 26 Aug 2010.

257. Vance SK, Khan S, Klancnik JM, Freund KB. Characteristic spectral-domain optical coherence tomography findings of multifocal choroiditis. Retina. 2011;31:717–23.

258. Vasconcelos-Santos DV, Rao PK, Davies JB, Sohn EH, Rao NA. Clinical features of tuberculous serpiginouslike choroiditis in contrast to classic serpiginous choroiditis. Arch Ophthalmol. 2010;128(7):853–8.

259. Vazquez-Cobian LB, Flynn T, Lehman TJ. Adalimumab therapy for childhood uveitis. J Pediatr. 2006;149(4):572–5 [3 D].

260. Venkatramani J, Lim WK. Bilateral vitreous haemorrhage associated with dengue fever. Eye. 2006;20(12):1405–6.

261. Verhoeff F. An effective treatment for sympathetic uveitis. Arch Ophthalmol. 1927;56:28.

262. Vitale AT, Rodriguez A, Foster CS. Low-dose cyclosporine therapy in the treatment of birdshot retinochoroidopathy. Ophthalmology. 1994;101:822–31.

263. Vote BJ, Hall A, Cairns J, Buttery R. Changing trends in sympathetic ophthalmia. Clin Experiment Ophthalmol. 2004;[3C](5):542–5 [3C].

264. Vrabec TR, Augsburger JJ, Fischer DH, et al. Taches de bougie. Ophthalmology. 1995;102:1712–21.

265. Walker DH, Raoult D. Rickettsia rickettsii and other spotted fever group rickettsiae (Rocky Mountain spotted fever and other spotted fevers). In: Mandell GL, Douglas JE, Bennett R, editors. Principles and practice of infectious disease. New York: Churchill Livingstone; 1995. p. 1721–7.

266. Warshafsky S, Lee DH, Francois LK, Nowakowski J, Nadelman RB, Wormser GP. Efficacy of antibiotic prophylaxis for the prevention of Lyme disease: an updated systematic review and meta-analysis. J Antimicrob Chemother. 2010;65(6):1137–44.

267. Weiss H, Annesley WH, Shields JA, et al. The clinical course of serpiginous choroidopathy. Am J Ophthalmol. 1979;87:133–42.

268. Westeneng AC, Rothova A, de Boer JH, et al. Infectious uveitis in immunocompromised patients and the diagnostic value of polymerase chain reaction and Goldmann-Witmer coefficient in aqueous analysis. Am J Ophthalmol. 2007;144:781–5.

269. Whitcup SM, Fortin E, Nussenblatt RB, et al. Therapeutic effect of combination antiretroviral therapy on cytomegalovirus retinitis. JAMA. 1997;277:1519–20.

270. Wichmann O, Lauschke A, Frank C, et al. Dengue antibody prevalence in German travelers. Emerg Infect Dis. 2005;11:762–5.

271. Windsor JJ. Cat scratch disease: epidemiology, etiology and treatment. Br J Biomed Sci. 2001;58:101–10.

272. Winter FC. Sympathetic uveitis; a clinical and pathologic study of the visual result. Am J Ophthalmol. 1955;39(3):340–7 [4 D].

273. Winterhalter S, Joussen AM, Pleyer U, Stübiger N. Inflammatory choroidal neovascularizations. Klin Monbl Augenheilkd. 2012;229(9):897–904.

274. Wong R, Pavesio CE, Laidlaw DAH, et al. The effects of intravitreal foscarnet and virus type on outcome. Ophthalmology. 2010;117(3):556–60.

275. Wong RW, Jumper JM, McDonald HR, Johnson RN, Fu A, Lujan BJ, Cunningham Jr ET. Emerging concepts in the management of acute retinal necrosis. Br J Ophthalmol. 2013;97(5):545–52. doi:10.1136/bjophthalmol-2012-301983. Epub 12 Dec 2012.

276. World Health Organization. Dengue hemorrhagic fever: diagnosis, treatment and control. 2nd ed. Geneva: WHO; 1997.

277. Wormser GP, Dattwyler RJ, Shapiro ED, Halperin JJ, Steere AC, Klempner MS, Krause PJ, Bakken JS, Strle F, Stanek G, Bockenstedt L, Fish D, Dumler JS, Nadelman RB. The clinical assessment, treatment, and prevention of lyme disease, human granulocytic anaplasmosis, and babesiosis: clinical practice guidelines by the Infectious Diseases Society of America. Clin Infect Dis. 2006;43(9):1089–134.

278. Wroblewski KJ, Hidayat AA, Neafie RC, Rao NA, Zapor M. Ocular tuberculosis: a clinicopathologic and molecular study. Ophthalmology. 2011;118:772–7.

279. Wu L, Evans T, Saravia M, Schlaen A, Couto C. Intravitreal bevacizumab for choroidal neovascularization secondary to Vogt-Koyanagi-Harada syndrome. Jpn J Ophthalmol. 2009;53(1):57–60.

280. Yahia SB, Khairallah M. Ocular manifestations of West Nile virus infection. Int J Med Sci. 2009;6(3):114–5.

281. Yamaki K, Gocho K, Hayakawa K, Kondo I, Sakuragi S. Tyrosinase family proteins are antigens specific to Vogt-Koyanagi-Harada disease. J Immunol. 2000;165:7323–9.

282. Yamanaka E, Ohguro N, Yamamoto S, Nakagawa Y, Imoto Y, Tano Y. Evaluation of pulse corticosteroid therapy for Vogt-Koyanagi-Harada disease assessed by optical coherence tomography. Am J Ophthalmol. 2002;134(3):454–6.

283. Yeh S, Wroblewski K, Buggage R, Li Z, Kurup SK, Sen HN, Dahr S, Sran P, Reed GF, Robinson R, Ragheb JA, Waldmann TA, Nussenblatt RB. High-dose humanized anti-IL-2 receptor alpha antibody (daclizumab) for the treatment of active, noninfectious uveitis. J Autoimmun. 2008;31(2):91–7.

284. Yin PD, Kurup SK, Fischer SH, Rhee HH, Byrnes GA, Levy-Clarke GA, Buggage RR, Nussenblatt RB, Mican JM, Wright ME. Progressive outer retinal necrosis in the era of highly active antiretroviral therapy: successful management with intravitreal injections and monitoring with quantitative PCR. J Clin Virol. 2007;38(3):254–9.

285. Zaharia MA, Lamarche J, Laurin M. Sympathetic uveitis 66 years after injury. Can J Ophthalmol. 1984;19(5):240–3.

286. Phimda K, Hoontrakul S, Suttinont C, Chareonwat S, Losuwanaluk K, Chueasuwanchai S, Chierakul W, Suwancharoen D, Silpasakorn S, Saisongkorh W, Peacock SJ, Day NP, Suputtamongkol Y. Doxycycline versus azithromycin for treatment of leptospirosis and scrub typhus. Antimicrob Agents Chemother. 2007;51(9):3259–63. Epub 2007 July 16.

287. Ressner RA, Griffith ME, Beckius ML, Pimentel G, Miller RS, Mende K, Fraser SL, Galloway RL, Hospenthal DR, Murray CK. Antimicrobial susceptibilities of geographically diverse clinical human isolates of Leptospira. Antimicrob Agents Chemother. 2008;52(8):2750–4. doi: 10.1128/AAC.00044-08. Epub 2008 Apr 14.

288. Holland GN, Lewis KG. An update on current practices in the management of ocular toxoplasmosis. Am J Ophthalmol. 2002;134(1):102–14.

Cystoid Macular Edema

11

Marc D. de Smet

Contents

M.D. de Smet, MDCM, PhD, FRCSC
MIOS sa, Av. Du Leman 32,
Lausanne 1005, Switzerland
e-mail: mddesmet1@mac.com,
doctors@retina-uveitis.eu

11.1   Introduction

Macular edema is a frequent long-term complication of chronic uveitis, confirmed by a number of epidemiological studies. Its prevalence among uveitis patients is estimated between 20 and 30 % and is a major cause of permanent vision loss [1–3]. About 35 % of uveitis patients with a vision less than 0.1 (6/60) have macular edema, though its prevalence as a cause of poor vision varies with the duration of uveitis. It is reported in 17 % of cases at year 1 and increases to 30 % by year 5 [4].

It develops typically in patients with posterior uveitis, but it can be seen in patients with isolated anterior segment inflammation, in particular HLA-B27-related uveitic syndromes [2]. Among the posterior pole entities with the highest prevalence of cystoid macular edema, birdshot retinochoroidopathy, sarcoidosis, and intermediate uveitis stand out, present in 60 % or more of patients with disease of more than 1 year duration [2, 5, 6]. Significant vision impairment due to macular edema is also reported in the presence of acute retinal necrosis or toxoplasmosis but at an incidence of less than 15 %. Chronic macular edema has a significant impact on the quality of life of patients: affecting their ability to read and their function in society and in comparison to other causes of macular edema, in a younger population, often between 30 and 50 years of age [7, 8].

U. Pleyer et al. (eds.), *Immune Modulation and Anti-Inflammatory Therapy in Ocular Disorders*,
DOI 10.1007/978-3-642-54350-0_11, © Springer-Verlag Berlin Heidelberg 2014

> **Core Message**
> - Macular edema is a major cause of severe vision loss in patients with uveitis [EBM: 2++, B].
> - Prevalence varies depending on the disease entity. It is particularly frequent in intermediate uveitis and birdshot retinochoroiditis [EBM: 2+, C].

11.2 Definition and Etiology

Macular edema is present whenever retinal thickening is caused by the presence of intraretinal cysts or lacunae. It is caused by an imbalance between fluid influx and fluid clearance. Edema develops by vascular leakage (vasogenic edema) and/or neuronal and glial cell swelling (cytotoxic edema) [9]. The oncotic pressure within the extracellular compartment is regulated by water transport across the blood-ocular barrier formed by tight junctions in retinal capillaries and between retinal pigment epithelial cells. Breakdown in either of these barriers can lead to leakage of fluid and protein into the interstitial space. Under normal physiologic conditions, IOP-driven bulk flow and choroidal osmotic pressure promote passive fluid reabsorption by the RPE, preventing the buildup of subretinal fluid [10]. Active RPE fluid transport is required to oppose oncotic water accumulation when the blood-retinal barrier is disrupted and proteins aberrantly enter the subretinal space [11]. However, in the retina, the plexiform layers constitute a high-resistance barrier against paracellular fluid movement [12]. To eliminate fluid accumulating in the inner retina, a transcellular water flux is required, which occurs through Mueller cells [13]. Aquaporins and chloride intracellular channels (AQP1 and 4, CLIC4) play an important role in this active transport process, particularly at the apices of RPE cells and along the footplates of Mueller cells [9, 14]. Silencing CLIC4 in RPE cells leads, for example, to the appearance of serous retinal detachments [14]. Modulation in the expression of these channels is influenced by inflammation as has recently been demonstrated [15, 16].

Severity and persistence of macular edema may be influenced by additional factors. Vasodilatation induced by inflammation results in increased vascular flow and intraluminal pressure. Hence, systemic diseases which alter hemodynamics or vascular wall plasticity such as hypertension, diabetes, and hypercholesterolemia may favor the development and persistence of macular edema as was shown in a retrospective study in 2004 [17]. Mechanical vitreous traction on the fovea or leakage from the optic nerve can enhance or favor the persistence of edema [18, 19]. Smoking also acts as an independent risk factor for both diabetic and uveitic macular edema [20–22]. Smoking has been shown to increase TNF-α activity in the peripheral blood of rheumatoid arthritis patients [23]. Both the cellular and humoral components of the immune system are affected [24]. While the role of smoking in initiating or aggravating immune mediated diseases is established, it is less clear if cessation can lead to an improved outcome. There are currently no articles published on this subject in the ophthalmic literature. A prospective trial in rheumatoid arthritis patients suggests that those who stop smoking for 6 or more months maintain the same severity disease scores as smokers, both of which are higher than for nonsmokers [25]. It may take several years, up to 20 years according to some authors, for severity scores to return back to those of nonsmokers [26].

> **Core Message**
> - Active fluid transport occurs through the RPE and Mueller cells in cases of fluid overload.
> - Aquaporin and chloride intracellular channels play an important role in the active transport process. Their expression is modulated by inflammation.
> - Smoking is an independent risk factor. Cessation has not been studied so far in uveitis. In other inflammatory diseases, it does not provide short-term benefits [EBM: 1+, A].

11.3 Clinical Symptoms and Signs

A decrease in vision is the main symptom of macular edema. This may be associated with metamorphopsia when associated with a macular traction syndrome. The vision decrease may be fluctuating based on the severity of the macular edema. In subtle cases, it may be more noticeable when reading rather than with distance vision [7].

Clinically on biomicroscopy, cystic spaces of various sizes, possibly associated with intraretinal hemorrhages, or wrinkling of the retinal surface is seen. When affecting the foveal region, particularly in very early stages, a yellow coloration to the cysts (due to the lutein located in the superficial retina) can be seen. This is absent with more prolonged involvement. With the advent of spectral OCT, the extent of retinal involvement can be precisely defined. OCT is required for adequate evaluation and follow-up of patients [27–31]. Its drawback is a focus limited to the macular area. Hence, biomicroscopy and fluorescein angiography remain useful to determine the overall severity of posterior pole involvement.

11.3.1 Fluorescein Angiography

Retinal vascular integrity in the retina and optic nerve can be determined by using fluorescein angiography. During the arteriovenous phase, the integrity of the perifoveal vascular network can be assessed as well as the location and severity of vascular leakage. Leakage can be present on the basis of localized ischemia or on the basis of inflammation (Fig.11.1) [32]. Inflammation generally causes a more diffuse microvascular leakage, though it may be patchy in nature. It will not be limited to the zone surrounding the foveal avascular zone or areas of non-perfusion [19]. The frames taken during the venous phase provide information on the extent and severity of diffuse microvascular leakage originating from either the retina or the RPE (Fig.11.2), as well as providing an indication of large vessel involvement. Optic disk leakage and hyperfluorescence can be assessed in late frames and is often present in chronic macular edema [18, 33, 34]. In cases of choroidal inflammation, ICG may provide additional information regarding the severity of disease and help orient the choice of immunosuppression [35].

11.3.2 OCT

Optical coherence tomography (OCT) provides reliable cross-sectional images of the retina and remains clinically useful in the presence of media opacity particularly when using high-definition systems [36]. Studies using time domain OCT were able to show a negative correlation between

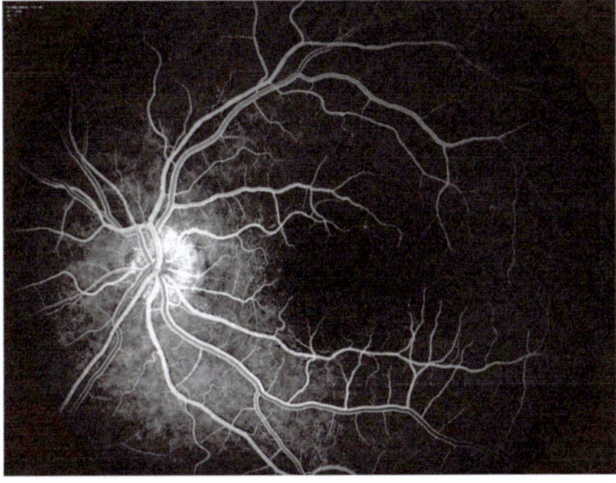
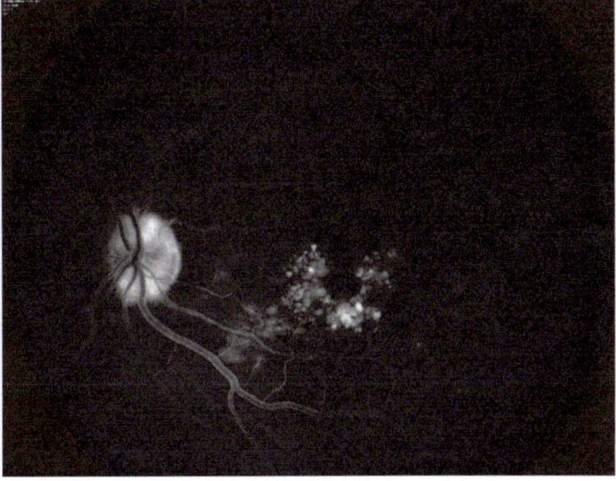

Fig. 11.1 Early midphase (*left*) and late (*right*) angiograpm of a patient with intermediate uveitis. The uveitis shows limited activity. The foveal avascular zone is increased in size with microvascular dilatation. The macular edema observed here is mainly due to loss of vascular channels and not due to inflammation response. Therapy is oriented towards the stabilization of the blood-ocular barrier

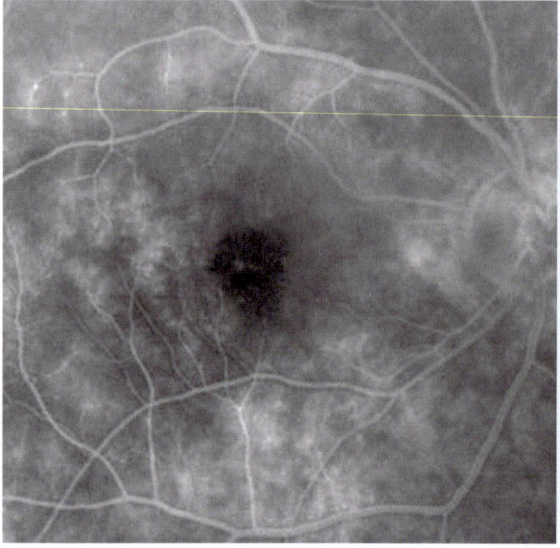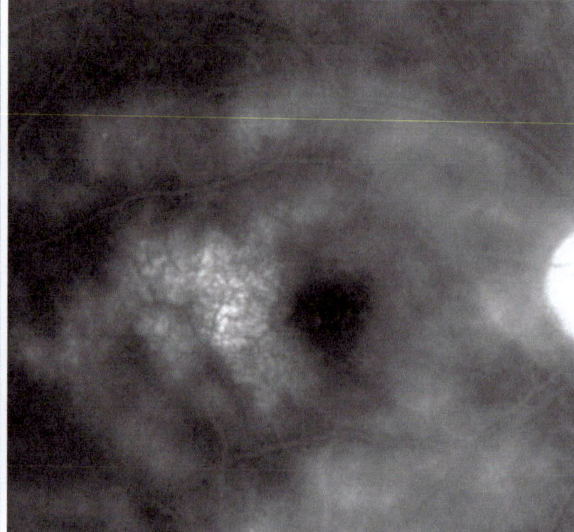

Fig. 11.2 Mid (*left*) and late (*right*) phase angiogram showing preservation of the foveal avascular zone, and diffuse microvascular leakage. Leakage is present both in the retinal vasculature and at the level of the RPE. Assessment of the level of leakage is facilitated by using stereo images. Note in the late image the lack of cystoid edema, but rather a diffuse leakage more prominent on the temporal side

visual acuity and central macular thickness but were poorly correlated with the likelihood of vision recovery [31, 37]. Certain structural correlates such as the presence of cystoid versus diffuse edema were shown to have prognostic significance, as the former is associated with a higher probability for vision improvement after treatment [31]. The presence of a partially intact junction between the inner and outer photoreceptor segments is also positively correlated with visual improvement [5, 38]. Foveal serous detachment presents in about 15 % of uveitis patients with macular edema and mostly during its acute phase [27, 39]. However, it does not impact on visual recovery [31]. In cases of diffuse edema, microperimetry may be an interesting adjunct to assess the potential for vision recovery [32, 40, 41].

There has been a recent effort to find a correlation between vision and retinal thickness and define a minimum significant change for clinical response. Correlations within aggregate data have been disappointing [29, 31]. Based on such correlations, a 20 % reduction in retinal thickness is associated with a balanced percentage of false-positives and false-negatives for a 10-letter change in visual acuity (77 % sensitivity and 75 % specificity) [29]. A better correlation between thickness and vision can be obtained by transforming retinal thickness to a logarithmic scale [42]. Such transformations tend to normalize measurements while maintaining their statistical integrity and achieve a certain degree of linearity [43]. However, wide variations in slopes are observed between patients indicating that the degree of vision recovery is not only dependent on thickness but intrinsic factors within the retina and duration of disease [29].

> **Core Message**
> - SD-OCT provides prognostic information with regard to vision improvement [EBM: 2++, B].
> - Cystoid edema is associated with vision improvement after treatment [EBM: 2++, B].
> - A partially intact inner-outer segment junction is correlated with potential vision improvement [EBM: 2+, C].
> - Foveal serous detachment is present early in 15 % of cases and does not appear to have prognostic significance [EBM 2+, C].

11.4 Differential Diagnosis

There is little diagnostic challenge in establishing the diagnosis of macular edema. The clinical signs as well as adjunctive imaging should confirm the diagnosis without much difficulty. Several factors which potentially can aggravate the disease have been mentioned in Sect. 11.2 including diabetes, vaso-occlusive disease, and vitreomacular traction.

Macular edema can also occur in what are best considered inflammatory masquerades [6]. It may be necessary to differentiate these from true inflammatory edema. Retinal detachments with its associated ischemia may lead to macular edema as well as an apparent inflammatory response. Not uncommonly, retinitis pigmentosa patients develop a mild vitritis and a clearly visible macular edema on OCT [44]. Vascular anomalies such as macular telangiectasis type I (Coat's disease) and IRVAN syndrome should also be considered [45, 46]. Both topical and systemically administered drugs may be to blame, including prostaglandin analogs [47, 48], epinephrine, nicotinic acid, tamoxifen, thiazolidinediones [49], and sphingosine-1-phosphate receptor modulators (fingolimod) [50].

Recently, the prevalence of macular edema was shown to be higher in both diabetes and central serous retinopathy in patients suffering from sleep apnea [51, 52]. Such an association has not yet been shown in uveitis but may be present. Treating the apnea has not so far modified the severity of macular edema.

11.5 Treatment

A systematic review was published in 2011 which reviewed the effectiveness of immunosuppressants and biological therapies in the treatment of macular edema due to noninfectious uveitis [53]. PubMed, MEDLINE, and EMBASE were searched from inception to October 2007 using terms to catch uveitis and CME. Of the 1,833 articles found on the treatment of CME, only 18 articles were retained based on their search criteria. Between 2007 and July 2012, an additional 292 articles were identified in MEDLINE using as search terms noninfectious uveitis and edema. Of these, 24 articles related to the pharmacological management of macular edema. All above articles were reviewed and complemented with additional articles mentioned in their reference list. The results of the review are summarized in Table 11.1.

No consensus has emerged for the management of inflammatory macular edema. Guidelines have been proposed on two recent occasions [54, 122]. A group of uveitis experts were polled for their preferred treatment in the presence of bilateral edema [28].

The management of a patient with uveitis and macular edema starts with the elimination of an infectious cause and the treatment of any underlying systemic inflammation. Acute disease is likely to respond to a course of systemic or periocular corticosteroids supplemented if needed with acetazolamide. If this treatment is insufficient or in the presence of chronic uveitis, the choice of secondary treatment will depend on whether one or both eyes are affected. In the case of unilateral disease, local treatment will be preferred. Periocular steroids (triamcinolone 40 mg) are generally effective with a primary success rate of about 50 % increasing to 80 % with a second injection [58]. A more rapid initial response can be obtained by direct intraocular injection (triamcinolone free of preservative 4 mg) (Table 11.1). RTC data for the fluocinolone implant suggests a rapid and sustained decrease in edema following implantation [76, 77]. A similar response is observed with the dexamethasone implant for up to 6 months [80–82]. Among newer intravitreal agents used to control macular edema, methotrexate (400 μg in a standard size eye) appears to provide a sustained effect for up to 4 months, but a reduced effect may be observed following repeated injections [111, 112]. Anti-VEGF antibodies (bevacizumab 1.25 mg) in combination with other modalities may be an interesting adjunct [59, 123].

In the presence of bilateral disease, a preference will be given to systemic immunomodulators in first instance. Bilateral implantation has been proposed and, from the MUST trial, appears to be equivalent to tight systemic control

Table 11.1 Treatment modalities of macular edema in the context of uveitis

Treatment	Mode of delivery	Recommendation	Evidence level (maximal)	Comment	References
Methylprednisolone/prednisone	Systemic (oral, IM, IV)	D	4	Expert opinion favors its use in first line for bilateral disease. Limited study data suggests 50 % response in either oral or deep IM dosing. IV may give a more rapid response based on expert opinion. First line if active inflammation present	[28, 54–57]
Corticosteroid	Subtenon or orbital floor	B	2++	Subtenon injection may be more effective than orbital floor according to some studies. Comparative prospective study shows no difference. Risk of glaucoma increases on repeated injection. Response in 50 % within 1 month, mean time to recurrence 20 weeks	[58–65]
Triamcinolone	Intravitreal	D	2	Response as compared to periocular is more rapidly visible. At 3 months, there is little difference between the two approaches. Side effects are more severe and pronounced than with external approaches	[61, 64, 66–75]
Fluocinolone	Sustained release	B	1++	Edema responds promptly. More intense reduction in the area of edema on FA compared to standard therapy. In the MUST trial, lower prevalence macular edema in the implanted group at 6 months, no difference between groups at 24 months. Many patients require cataract and glaucoma surgery	[76–79]
Dexamethasone	Sustained release	B	1+	Sustained effect seen up to 6 months postinjection compared to control. Transient IOP increase in 38.5 %, responsive to therapy. Data specifically on macular edema is limited though effect on vision in an RCT is statistically significant	[80–82]
Acetazolamide	Systemic (oral)	B	1+	When inflammation under control or when combined with concomitant immunosuppressive therapy, macular edema is responsive. Considered as early-line treatment before other immunosuppressants	[83–87]
INF-α2a	Systemic (SC)	B	2++	Effective in 80 % of patients resistant to first-line treatment. Allows taper of concomitant medications but in a fair proportion must be maintained for continued benefit. One study with INF-α2b shows similar results [88]. No RTCs	[89–94]

Treatment	Mode of delivery	Recommendation	Evidence level (maximal)	Comment	References
Cyclosporine	Systemic (oral)	B	1	Effective in half the population unresponsive to first-line treatment. More effective if given as an adjunct to systemic corticosteroids. No RTCs directed at the management of macular edema	[55, 95–97]
Mycophenolate mofetil	Systemic (oral)	C	2+	Short-term efficacy up to 1 year in one study. Relapses are frequent	[98, 99]
Anti-TNF (infliximab, adalimumab)	Systemic (IV, IM)	D	2	Rapid resolution of edema is seen particular in cases associated with vasculitis	[100–103]
Anti-TNF	Intravitreal	D	2	Improvement in visual acuity and macular edema 1 month after intravitreal injection. This effect is not sustained. Other studies are less supportive for macular edema	[104–107]
Octreotide	Systemic (SC)	C	2+	In 70 % of patients with chronic macular edema with nonactive uveitis, growth hormone analog will be effective. Recurrence occurs in many patients upon cessation of therapy	[108–110]
Methotrexate	Systemic	D	4	Survey of uveitis experts suggests its use in second line	[28]
Methotrexate	Intravitreal	C	2+	In patients unresponsive to first line, appeared effective in up to 16 weeks. Effective with repeated injection although long-term effectiveness is not established	[111–114]
Anti-VEGF	Intravitreal	C	1	Comparable to periocular steroids in patients failing primary therapy. Less effective than intravitreal steroids. Effective for up to 16 weeks. One RCT with small numbers	[59, 115–119]
Nonsteroidal anti-inflammatory drugs	Intravitreal	D	3	Transient improvement in edema and vision with no IOP rise at 8 weeks. Data limited to very few patients	[120, 121]

of inflammation [76]. Mounting evidence indicates that interferon 2a (various dosing regimens have been proposed) may be a particularly good choice for patients in whom more conventional systemic immunosuppression is not adequate. Other biologics such as the anti-TNF agents may also be of benefit, particularly in patients with Behçet's disease. Sustained release devices in patients with bilateral disease may be considered but are not readily available in many countries.

In macular edema present without evidence of active uveitis, certain alternatives have been proposed including the use of octreotide [108, 109], interferon 2a [89, 90], and intravitreal implants. Response to treatment in these cases depends on a prolonged and sustained effect as it may take several weeks to see any improvement. Cessation of therapy is often accompanied by recurrences over a number of weeks. In all cases, therapy should be tailored to the patient's needs and responses.

> **Core Message**
> - Rule out systemic and infectious causes, the treatment of which will lead in most cases to the resolution of edema or require only adjunctive local therapy.
> - Sustained release devices allow for a reduction in edema over several weeks, particularly in chronic cases [EBM 1+, A].
> - Interferon 2a and growth hormone analogs may be useful in the management of bilateral chronic edema unresponsive to other therapies [EBM2+, C].

11.6 Future Directions

Identifying patients at risk and determining which patients will benefit from therapy requires further elucidation. While the OCT has helped us to identify patients with macular edema, it is difficult based on the images currently available to predict who will benefit from therapy. A better understanding of the mechanisms underlying the development of macular edema may allow us to provide more specific therapy particularly in patients with more chronic inflammation. Currently, the levels of medications given to patient often reflect a need to control macular edema and exceed the levels required to prevent other manifestations of inflammation. Pharmacological agents with fewer side effects, which can be administered locally with a prolonged intraocular effect, require further development.

References

1. Rothova A, Suttorp- van Schulten MSA, Terffers WF, Kijlstra A. Causes and frequency of blindness in patients with intraocular inflammatory disease. Br J Ophthalmol. 1996;80:332–6.
2. Lardenoye CWTA, van Kooij B, Rothova A. Impact of macular edema on visual acuity in uveitis. Ophthalmology. 2006;113(8):1446–9.
3. Rothova A. Inflammatory cystoid macular edema. Curr Opin Ophthalmol. 2007;18:487–92.
4. Smith JA, Mackensen F, Sen HN, Leigh JF, Watkins AS, Pyatetsky D, et al. Epidemiology and course of disease in childhood uveitis. Ophthalmology. 2009; 116:1544–51.
5. Monnet D, Levinson RD, Holland GN, Haddad L, Yu F, Brézin AP. Longitudinal cohort study of patients with birdshot chorioretinopathy. III. Macular imaging at baseline. Am J Ophthalmol. 2007;144(6): 818–28.e2.
6. Johnson MW. Etiology and treatment of macular edema. Am J Ophthalmol. 2009;147(1):11–21.e1.
7. Kiss CG, Barisani-Asenbauer T, Maca S, Richter-Mueksch S, Radner W. Reading performance of patients with uveitis-associated cystoid macular edema. Am J Ophthalmol. 2006;142(4):620–4.e1.
8. Hazel A, Petre K, Armstrong RA. Visual function and subjective quality of life compared in subjects with acquired macular disease. Invest Ophthalmol Vis Sci. 2000;41:1309–15.
9. Bringmann A, Wiedemann P. Muller glial cells in retinal disease. Ophthalmologica. 2012;227(1):1–19. Epub 17 Sept 2011.
10. Marmor MF. Mechanisms of fluid accumulation in retinal edema. Doc Ophthalmol. 1999;97:239–49.
11. Verkman AS, Ruiz-Ederra J, Levin MH. Functions of aquaporins in the eye. Prog Retin Eye Res. 2008;27(4):420–33. Epub 27 May 2008.
12. Antcliff RJ, Marshall J. The pathogenesis of edema in diabetic maculopathy. Semin Ophthalmol. 1999;14: 223–32.
13. Bringmann A, Uckermann O, Pannicke T, Iandiev I, Reichenbach A, Wiedemann P. Neuronal versus glial cell swelling in the ischaemic retina. Acta Ophthalmol Scand. 2005;83(5):528–38. Epub 29 Sept 2005.
14. Chuang JZ, Chou SY, Sung CH. Chloride intracellular channel 4 is critical for the epithelial morphogenesis

of RPE cells and retinal attachment. Mol Biol Cell. 2010;21(17):3017–28. Epub 9 Jul 2010.

15. Motulsky E, Koch P, Janssens S, Liénart M, Vanbellinghen AM, Bolaky N, et al. Aquaporin expression in blood-retinal barrier cells during experimental autoimmune uveitis. Mol Vis. 2010;16:602–10.

16. Eberhardt C, Amann B, Feuchtinger A, Hauck SM, Deeg CA. Differential expression of inwardly rectifying K+ channels and aquaporins 4 and 5 in autoimmune uveitis indicates misbalance in Muller glial cell-dependent ion and water homeostasis. Glia. 2011;59(5):697–707. Epub 10 Feb 2011.

17. van Kooij B, Fijnheer R, Roest M, Rothova A. Trace microalbuminuria in inflammatory cystoid macular edema. Am J Ophthalmol. 2004;138:1010–5.

18. van Kooij B, Probst K, Fijnheer R, Roest M, de Loos W, Rothova A. Risk factors for cystoid macular oedema in patients with uveitis. Eye. 2008;22(2):256–60.

19. Forooghian F, Yeh S, Faia LJ, Nussenblatt RB. Uveitis foveal atrophy. Arch Ophthalmol. 2009;127:179–86.

20. Lin P, Loh AR, Margolis TP, Acharya NR. Cigarette smoking as a risk factor for uveitis. Ophthalmology. 2010;117(3):585–90.

21. Thorne JE, Daniel E, Jabs DA, Kedhar SR, Peters GB, Dunn JP. Smoking as a risk factor for cystoid macular edema complicating intermediate uveitis. Am J Ophthalmol. 2008;145:841–6.

22. Kaercher Kramer C, de Azevedo MJ, da Costa Rodrigues T, Canani LH, Esteves J. Smoking habit is associated with diabetic macular edema in type I diabetes mellitus patients. J Diabetes Complications. 2008;22:430.

23. Glossop JR, Dawes PT, Mattey DL. Association between cigarette smoking and release of tumor necrosis factor α and its soluble receptor by peripheral blood mononuclear cells in patients with rheumatoid arthritis. Rheumatology. 2006;45:1223–9.

24. Edwards D. Immunological effects of tobacco smoking in "healthy" smokers. COPD. 2009;6(1):48–58. Epub 21 Feb 2009.

25. Fisher MC, Hochberg MC, El-Taha M, Kremer JM, Peng C, Greenberg JD, et al. Smoking, smoking cessation, and disease activity in large cohort of patients with rheumatoid arthritis. J Rheumatol. 2012;39:904–9.

26. Costenbader KH, Feskanich D, Mandl LA, Karlson EW. Smoking intensity, duration, and cessation, and risk of rheumatoid arthritis in women. Am J Med. 2006;119:503–11.

27. Simmons-Rear A, Yeh S, Chan-Kai BT, Lauer AK, Flaxel CJ, Smith JR, et al. Characterization of serous retinal detachments in uveitis patients with optical coherence tomography. J Ophthal Inflamm Infect. 2012;2:191–7.

28. Sreekantam S, Denniston AK, Murray PI. Survey of expert practice and perceptions of the supporting clinical evidence for the management of uveitis-related cataract and cystoid macular oedema. Ocul Immunol Inflamm. 2011;19(5):353–7. Epub 10 Aug 2011.

29. Sugar EA, Jabs DA, Altaweel MM, Lightman S, Acharya N, Vitale AT, et al. Identifying a clinically meaningful threshold for change in uveitic macular

edema evaluated by optical coherence tomography. Am J Ophthalmol. 2011;152:1044–52.e1045.

30. Jittpoonkuson T, Garcia P, Rosen RB. Correlation between fluorescein angiography and spectral domain optical coherence tomography in the diagnosis of cystoid macular edema. Br J Ophthalmol. 2010;94: 1197–200.

31. Tran THC, de Smet MD, Bodaghi B, Fardeau C, Cassoux N, Lehoang P. Uveitic macular oedema: correlation between optical coherence tomography patterns with visual acuity and fluorescein angiography. Br J Ophthalmol. 2008;92(7):922–7.

32. de Smet MD, Okada AA. Cystoid macular edema in uveitis. Dev Ophthalmol. 2010;47:136–47.

33. Pruett R, Brockhurst RJ, Letts N. Fluorescein angiography of peripheral uveitis. Am J Ophthalmol. 1974;77:448–53.

34. Pelitli Gürlü V, Alimgil ML, Esgin H. Fluorescein angiographic findings in cases with intermediate uveitis in the inactive phase. Can J Ophthalmol. 2007;42:107–9.

35. Tugal-Tutkun I, Herbort CP, Kharairallah M, The Angiography Scoring for Uveitis Working Group (ASUWOG). Scoring of dual fluorescein and ICG inflammatory angiographic signs for the grading of posterior segment inflammation (dual fluorescein and ICG angiographic scoring system for uveitis). Int Ophthalmol. 2008;30:539–52.

36. Gupta V, Gupta P, Singh R, Dogra MR, Gupta A. Spectral-domain Cirrus high-definition optical coherence tomography is better than time-domain stratus optical coherence tomography for evaluation of macular pathologic features in uveitis. Am J Ophthalmol. 2008;145(6):1018–22.e2.

37. Markomichelakis NN, Halkiadais I, Pantelia E, Peponis V, Patelis A, Theodossiadis P, et al. Patterns of macular edema in patients with uveitis. Qualitative and quantitative assessment using optical coherence tomography. Ophthalmology. 2005;111:946–53.

38. Roesel M, Henschel A, Heinz C, Spital G, Heiligenhaus A. Time-domain and spectral-domain optical coherence tomography in uveitic macular edema. Am J Ophthalmol. 2008;146(4):626–7.

39. Ossewaarde-van Norel A, Berg EM, Sijssens KM, Rothova A. Subfoveal serous retinal detachment in patients with uveitis macular edema. Arch Ophthalmol. 2011;129:158–62.

40. Pilotto E, Vujosevic S, Grgic V, Sportiello P, Convento E, Secchi A, et al. Retinal function in patients with serpiginous choroiditis: a microperimetry study. Graefes Arch Clin Exp Ophthalmol. 2010;248(9): 1331–7.

41. Vujosevic S, Midena E, Pilotto E, Radin PP, Chiesa L, Cavarzeran F. Diabetic macular edema: correlation between microperimetry and optical coherence tomography findings. Invest Ophthalmol Vis Sci. 2006;47(7):3044–51.

42. Payne JF, Bruce BB, Lee LBK, Yeh S. Logarithmic transformation for spectral-domain optical coherence tomography data in uveitis-associated macular edema. Invest Ophthalmol Vis Sci. 2011;52:8939–43.

43. Ferris 3rd FL, Miller KM, Glassman AR, Beck RW. A proposed method of logarithmic transformation of optical coherence tomography data for use in clinical research. Ophthalmology. 2010;117(8):1512–6. Epub 7 Apr 2010.

44. Hajali M, Fishman GA, Anderson RJ. The prevalence of cystoid macular oedema in retinitis pigmentosa patients determined by optical coherence tomography. Br J Ophthalmol. 2008;92(8):1065–8. Epub 26 Jul 2008.

45. Samuel MA, Equi RA, Chang TS, Mieler WF, Jampol LM, Hay D, et al. Idiopathic retinitis, vasculitis, aneurysms, and neuroretinitis (IRVAN): new observations and a proposed staging system. Ophthalmology. 2007;114:1526–9.

46. Rothova A. Fuchs' heterochromic uveitis and Coat's disease. Ocul Immunol Inflamm. 1994;2:187–8.

47. Wand M, Shields BM. Cystoid macular edema in the era of ocular hypotensive lipids. Am J Ophthalmol. 2002;133:393–7.

48. Digiuni M, Fogagnolo P, Rossetti L. A review of the use of latanoprost for glaucoma since its launch. Expert Opin Pharmacother. 2012;13:723–45.

49. Idris I, Warren G, Donnelly R. Association between thiazolidinedione treatment and risk of macular edema among patients with type 2 diabetes. Arch Intern Med. 2012;172(13):1005–11. Epub 13 Jun 2012.

50. Gelfand JM, Nolan R, Schwartz DM, Graves J, Green AJ. Microcystic macular oedema in multiple sclerosis is associated with disease severity. Brain. 2012;135(Pt 6):1786–93. Epub 28 Apr 2012.

51. Kloos P, Laube I, Thoelen A. Obstructive sleep apnea in patients with central serous chorioretinopathy. Graefes Arch Clin Exp Ophthalmol. 2008;246(9):1225–8. Epub 12 Jun 2008.

52. Mason RH, West SD, Kiire CA, Groves DC, Lipinski HJ, Jaycock A, et al. High prevalence of sleep disordered breathing in patients with diabetic macular edema. Retina. 2012;32(9):1791–8.

53. Pato E, Munoz-Fernandez S, Francisco F, Abad MA, Maese J, Ortiz A, et al. Systematic review on the effectiveness of immunosuppressants and biological therapies in the treatment of autoimmune posterior uveitis. Semin Arthritis Rheum. 2011;40(4):314–23. Epub 27 Jul 2010.

54. Ossewaarde-van Norel A, Rothova A. Clinical review: update on treatment of inflammatory macular edema. Ocul Immunol Inflamm. 2011;19(1):75–83. Epub 3 Nov 2010.

55. Nussenblatt RB, Palestine AG, Chan CC, Stevens G, Mellow SD, Green SB. Randomized, doubled-masked study of cyclosporine compared to prednisolone in the treatment of endogenous uveitis. Am J Ophthalmol. 1991;112:138–46.

56. Tehrani NN, Saeed T, Murray PI. Deep intramuscular methylprednisolone for the treatment of cystoid macular oedema in uveitis. Eye. 2000;14:691–4.

57. Jabs DA, Rosenbaum JT, Foster CS, Holland GN, Jaffe GJ, Louie JS, et al. Guidelines for the use of immunosuppressive drugs in patients with ocular inflammatory disorders: recommendations of an expert panel. Am J Ophthalmol. 2000;130(4):492–513.

58. Leder HA, Jabs DA, Galor A, Dunn JP, Thorne JE. Periocular triamcinolone acetonide injections for cystoid macular edema complicating noninfectious uveitis. Am J Ophthalmol. 2011;152(3):441–8 e2. Epub 10 Jun 2011.

59. Bae JH, Lee CS, Lee SC. Efficacy and safety of intravitreal bevacizumab compared with intravitreal and posterior sub-tenon triamcinolone acetonide for treatment of uveitis cystoid macular edema. Retina. 2011;31:111–8.

60. Venkatesh P, Kumar CS, Abbas Z, Garg S. Comparison of the efficacy and safety of different methods of posterior subtenon injection. Ocul Immunol Inflamm. 2008;16(5):217–23.

61. Choudhry S, Ghosh S. Intravitreal and posterior subtenon triamcinolone acetonide in idiopathic bilateral uveitic macular oedema. Clin Experiment Ophthalmol. 2007;35(8):713–8. Epub 14 Nov 2007.

62. Habot-Wilner Z, Sallam A, Roufas A, Kabasele PM, Grigg JR, McCluskey P, et al. Periocular corticosteroid injection in the management of uveitis in children. Acta Ophthalmol. 2010;88(8):e299–304. Epub 1 Dec 2010.

63. Tanner V, Kanski JJ, Frith PA. Posterior sub-Tenon's triamcinolone injections in the treatment of uveitis. Eye. 1998;12:679–85.

64. Roesel M, Gutfleisch M, Heinz C, Heimes B, Zurek-Imhoff B, Heiligenhaus A. Intravitreal and orbital floor triamcinolone acetonide injections in noninfectious uveitis: a comparative study. Ophthalmic Res. 2009;42(2):81–6. Epub 30 May 2009.

65. Roesel M, Gutfleisch M, Heinz C, Heimes B, Zurek-Imhoff B, Heiligenhaus A. Orbital floor triamcinolone acetonide injections for the management of active non-infectious uveitis. Eye (Lond). 2009;23(4):910–4. Epub 10 May 2008.

66. Cunningham MA, Edelman JL, Kaushal S. Intravitreal steroids for macular edema: the past, the present, and the future. Surv Ophthalmol. 2008;53(2):139–49.

67. Atmaca L, Yalçindağ F, Özdemir Ö. Intravitreal triamcinolone acetonide in the management of cystoid macular edema in Behçet's disease. Graefes Arch Clin Exp Ophthalmol. 2007;245(3):451–6.

68. Park CH, Jaffe GJ, Fekrat S. Intravitreal triamcinolone acetonide in eyes with cystoid macular edema associated with central retinal vein occlusion. Am J Ophthalmol. 2003;136:419–25.

69. Martidis A, Duker JS, Puliafito CA. Intravitreal triamcinolone for refractor cystoid macular edema secondary to birdshot retinochoroidopathy. Arch Ophthalmol. 2001;119:1380–3.

70. Sallam A, Comer RM, Chang JH, Grigg JR, Andrews R, McCluskey PJ, et al. Short-term safety and efficacy of intravitreal triamcinolone acetonide for uveitic macular edema in children. Arch Ophthalmol. 2008;126(2):200–5.

71. Choi YJ, Oh IK, Oh JR, Huh K. Intravitreal versus posterior subtenon injection of triamcinolone acetonide for diabetic macular edema. Korean J Ophthalmol. 2006;20:205–9.

72. Kok H, Lau C, Maycock N, McCluskey P, Lightman S. Outcome of intravitreal triamcinolone in uveitis. Ophthalmology. 2005;112(11):1916.e1-.e7.

73. Maca SM, Abela-Formanek C, Kiss CG, Sacu SG, Benesch T, Barisani-Asenbauer T. Intravitreal triamcinolone for persistent cystoid macular edema in eyes with quiescent uveitis. Clin Exp Immunol. 2009;37(8): 389–96.

74. Tao Y, Jonas JB. Intravitreal triamcinolone. Ophthalmologica. 2011;225(1):1–20. Epub 10 Aug 2010.

75. Oueghlani E, Pavesio CE. Intravitreal triamcinolone injection for unresponsive cystoid macular oedema in probable Behçet's disease as additional therapy. Klin Monatsbl Augenheilkd. 2007;225:497–9.

76. Multicenter Uveitis Steroid Treatment (MUST) Trial Research Group, Kempen JH, Altaweel MM, Holbrook JT, Jabs DA, Louis TA, et al. Randomized comparison of systemic anti-inflammatory therapy versus fluocinolone acetonide implant for intermediate, posterior, and panuveitis: the multicenter uveitis steroid treatment trial. Ophthalmology. 2011;118(10): 1916–26. Epub 16 Aug 2011.

77. Pavesio C, Zierhut M, Bairi K, Comstock TL, Usner DW. Evaluation of an intravitreal fluocinolone acetonide implant versus standard systemic therapy in noninfectious posterior uveitis. Ophthalmology. 2010;117(3): 567–75.e1.

78. Callanan DG, Jaffe GJ, Martin DF, Pearson PA, Comstock TL. Treatment of posterior uveitis with a fluocinolone acetonide implant: three-year clinical trial results. Arch Ophthalmol. 2008;126(9):1191–201.

79. Jaffe GJ, Martin D, Callanan D, Pearson PA, Levy B, Comstock T. Fluocinolone acetonide implant (Retisert) for noninfectious posterior uveitis: thirty-four-week results of a multicenter randomized clinical study. Ophthalmology. 2006;113(6):1020–7.

80. Lowder C, Belfort Jr R, Lightman S, Foster CS, Robinson MR, Schiffman RM, et al. Dexamethasone intravitreal implant for noninfectious intermediate or posterior uveitis. Arch Ophthalmol. 2011;129(5): 545–53. Epub 12 Jan 2011.

81. Williams GA, Haller JA, Kuppermann BD, Blumenkranz MS, Weinberg DV, Chou C, et al. Dexamethasone posterior-segment drug delivery system in the treatment of macular edema resulting from uveitis or Irvine–Gass syndrome. Am J Ophthalmol. 2009;147(6):1048–54.e2.

82. Kuppermann BD, Blumenkranz MS, Haller JA, Williams GA, Weinberg DV, Chou C, et al. Randomized controlled study of an intravitreous dexamethasone drug delivery system in patients with persistent macular edema. Arch Ophthalmol. 2007;125(3):309–17.

83. Zierhut M, Thiel HJ, Schlote T. Treatment of uveitic macular edema with acetazolamide. Doc Ophthalmol. 1999;97:409–13.

84. Cox SN, Hay E, Bird AC. Treatment of chronic macular edema with acetazolamide. Arch Ophthalmol. 1988;106:1190–5.

85. Farber MD, Lam S, Tessler HH, Jennings TJ, Cross A, Rusin MM. Reduction of macular oedema by acetazolamide in patients with chronic iridocyclitis: a randomised prospective crossover study. Br J Ophthalmol. 1994;78:4–7.

86. Whitcup SM, Csaky KG, Podgor MJ, Chew EY, Perry CH, Nussenblatt RB. A randomized, masked, crossover trial of acetazolamide for cystoid macular edema in patients with uveitis. Ophthalmology. 1996;103: 1054–62.

87. Lashay AR, Rahimi A, Chams H, Davatchi F, Shahram F, Hatmi ZN, et al. Evaluation of the effect of acetazolamide on cystoid macular oedema in patients with Behçet's disease. Eye. 2003;17(6):762–6.

88. Butler NJ, Suhler EB, Rosenbaum JT. Interferon alpha 2b in the treatment of uveitic cystoid macular edema. Ocul Immunol Inflamm. 2012;20(2):86–90. Epub 14 Mar 2012.

89. Deuter CM, Kotter I, Gunaydin I, Stubiger N, Doycheva DG, Zierhut M. Efficacy and tolerability of interferon alpha treatment in patients with chronic cystoid macular oedema due to non-infectious uveitis. Br J Ophthalmol. 2009;93(7):906–13. Epub 27 Mar 2009.

90. Paire V, Lebreton O, Weber M. Effectiveness of interferon alpha in the treatment of uveitis macular edema refractory to corticosteroid and/or immunosuppressive treatment. J Fr Ophtalmol. 2010;33: 152–63.

91. Bodaghi B, Gendron G, Wechsler B, Terrada C, Cassoux N, Thi Huong DL, et al. Efficacy of interferon alpha in the treatment of refractory and sight threatening uveitis: a retrospective monocentric study of 45 patients. Br J Ophthalmol. 2007;91(3): 335–9.

92. Deuter CME, Koetter I, Ouenaydin I, Stuebiger N, Zierhut M. Interferon alfa-2A: a new treatment option for long lasting refractory cystoid macular edema in uveitis? Retina. 2006;26:786–91.

93. Plskova J, Greiner K, Forrester JV. Interferon-[alpha] as an effective treatment for noninfectious posterior uveitis and panuveitis. Am J Ophthalmol. 2007;144(1):55–61.e2.

94. Kötter I, Eckstein AK, Stübiger N, Zierhut M. Treatment of ocular symptoms of Behçet's disease with interferon α_{2a}: a pilot study. Br J Ophthalmol. 1998;82:488–94.

95. Nussenblatt RB, de Smet MD, Rubin B, Freidlin V, Whitcup SM, Davis J, et al. A masked, randomized, dose-response study between cyclosporine A and G in the treatment of sight-threatening uveitis of noninfectious origin. Am J Ophthalmol. 1993; 115:583–91.

96. Whitcup SM, Salvo Jr EC, Nussenblatt RB. Combined cyclosporine and corticosteroid therapy for sight-threatening uveitis in Behçet's disease. Am J Ophthalmol. 1994;118:39–45.

97. Vitale AT, Rodriguez A, Foster CS. Low-dose cyclosporine therapy in the treatment of birdshot retinochoroidopathy. Ophthalmology. 1994;101:822–31.

98. Neri P, Mariotti C, Cimino L, Mercanti L, Giovannini A. Long-term control of cystoid macular oedema in noninfectious uveitis with Mycophenolate Mofetil. Int Ophthalmol. 2009;29(3):127–33. Epub 26 Feb 2008.

99. Doycheva D, Zierhut M, Blumenstock G, Stuebiger N, Deuter C. Mycophenolate mofetil in the therapy of uveitic macular edema – long-term results. Ocul Immunol Inflamm. 2012;20(3):203–11. Epub 12 Apr 2012.

100. Abu El-Asrar AM, Abboud EB, Aldibhi H, Al-Arfaj A. Long-term safety and efficacy of infliximab therapy in refractory uveitis due to Behcet's disease. Int Ophthalmol. 2005;26(3):83–92. Epub 13 Oct 2006.

101. Cantini F, Niccoli L, Nannini C, Kaloudi O, Cassara E, Susini M, et al. Efficacy of infliximab in refractory Behcet's disease-associated and idiopathic posterior segment uveitis: a prospective, follow-up study of 50 patients. Biologics. 2012;6:5–12. Epub 1 Feb 2012.

102. Markomichelakis NN, Theodossiadis PG, Pantalia E, Papaefthimiou S, Theodossiadis GP, Sfikakis PP. Infliximab for chronic cystoid macular edema associated with uveitis. Am J Ophthalmol. 2004;138:648–50.

103. Erckens RJ, Mostard RL, Wijnen PA, Schouten JS, Drent M. Adalimumab successful in sarcoidosis patients with refractory chronic non-infectious uveitis. Graefes Arch Clin Exp Ophthalmol. 2012;250(5):713–20. Epub 29 Nov 2011.

104. Farvardin M, Afarid M, Mehryar M, Hosseini H. Intravitreal infliximab for the treatment of sight-threatening chronic noninfectious uveitis. Retina. 2010;30:1530–5.

105. Farvardin M, Afarid M, Shahrzad S. Long-term effects of intravitreal infliximab for treatment of sight-threatening chronic noninfectious uveitis. J Ocul Pharmacol Ther. 2012;28:628–31.

106. Markomichelakis N, Delicha E, Masselos S, Sfikakis PP. Intravitreal infliximab for sight-threatening relapsing uveitis in Behcet disease: a pilot study in 15 patients. Am J Ophthalmol. 2012;154:534–41.

107. Androudi S, Tsironi E, Kalogeropoulos C, Theodoridou A, Brazitikos P. Intravitreal adalimumab for refractory uveitis-related macular edema. Ophthalmology. 2010;117(8):1612–6. Epub 10 Apr 2010.

108. Kafkala C, Choi JY, Choopong P, Foster CS. Octreotide as a treatment for uveitic cystoid macular edema. Arch Ophthalmol. 2006;124:1353–5.

109. Missotten T, van Laar JAM, van der Loos TL, van Daele PLA, Kuijpers RWAM, Baarsma GS, et al. Octreotide long-acting repeatable for the treatment of chronic macular edema in uveitis. Am J Ophthalmol. 2007;144(6):838–43.

110. Papadaki T, Zacharopoulos I, Iaccheri B, Fiore T, Foster CS. Somatostatin for uveitic cystoid macular edema (CME). Ocul Immunol Inflamm. 2005;13(6):469–70.

111. Taylor SR, Habot-Wilner Z, Pacheco P, Lightman S. Intravitreal methotrexate in uveitis. Ophthalmology. 2012;119(4):878–9. Epub 5 Apr 2012.

112. Taylor SRJ, Habot-Wilner Z, Pacheco P, Lightman SL. Intraocular methotrexate in the treatment of uveitis and uveitic cystoid macular edema. Ophthalmology. 2009;116(4):797–801.

113. Bae JH, Lee SC. Effect of intravitreal methotrexate and aqueous humor cytokine levels in refractory retinal vasculitis in Behcet disease. Retina. 2012;32:1395–1402.

114. Hardwig PW, Pulido JS, Erie JC, Baratz KH, Buettner H. Intraocular methotrexate in ocular diseases other than primary central nervous system lymphoma. Am J Ophthalmol. 2006;142:883–5.

115. Mirshahi A, Namavari A, Djalilian A, Moharamzad Y, Chams H. Intravitreal bevacizumab (avastin) for the treatment of cystoid macular edema in Behcet disease. Ocul Immunol Inflamm. 2009;17(1):59–64. Epub 19 Mar 2009.

116. Soheilian M, Rabbanikhah Z, Ramezani A, Kiavash V, Yaseri M, Peyman GA. Intravitreal bevacizumab versus triamcinolone acetonide for refractory uveitic cystoid macular edema: a randomized pilot study. J Ocul Pharmacol Ther. 2010;26(2):199–206. Epub 24 Mar 2010.

117. Lasave AF, Zeballos DG, El-Haig WM, Diaz-Llopis M, Salom D, Arevalo JF. Short-term results of a single intravitreal bevacizumab (avastin) injection versus a single intravitreal triamcinolone acetonide (kenacort) injection for the management of refractory noninfectious uveitic cystoid macular edema. Ocul Immunol Inflamm. 2009;17(6):423–30. Epub 17 Dec 2009.

118. Cervantes-Castañeda RA, Giuliari GP, Gallagher MJ, Yilmaz T, MacDonell RE, Quinones K, et al. Intravitreal bevacizumab in refractory uveitic macular edema: one-year follow-up. Eur J Ophthalmol. 2009;19:622–9.

119. Weiss K, Steinbrugger I, Weger M, Ardjomand N, Maier R, Wegscheider BJ, et al. Intravitreal VEGF levels in uveitis patients and treatment of uveitic macular edema with intravitreal bevacizumab. Eye. 2009;23:1812–8.

120. Soheilian M, Karimi S, Ramezani A, Peyman GA. Pilot study of intravitreal injection of diclofenac for treatment of macular edema of various etiologies. Retina. 2010;30:509–15.

121. Kim SJ, Doherty TJ, Cherney EF. Intravitreal ketorolac for chronic uveitis and macular edema. Arch Ophthalmol. 2012;130:456–60.

122. Pleyer U, Roider J, Heiligenhaus A, Sauer S, Bertram B, Thurau S, et al. Stellungnahme der Deutschen Ophthalmologischen Gesellschaft, der Retinologischen Gesellschaft und des berufsverbandes der Augenärzte Deutschlands sur intravitrealen therapie des makula"dems bei uveitis. Ophthalmologe. 2012;109:93–9.

123. Acharya NR, Hong KC, Lee SM. Ranibizumab for refractory uveitis-related macular edema. Am J Ophthalmol. 2009;148(2):303–9.e2.

Safety of Immunosuppressive Therapy for Eye Diseases

12

Dana M. Hornbeak and John H. Kempen

Contents

Ocular inflammation is a significant cause of ocular morbidity and visual impairment. Topical, periocular, intraocular, and systemic corticosteroids all are highly effective for treating appropriate forms of ocular inflammation, but use of corticosteroids is constrained by a high risk of local and/or systemic side effects, especially if long-term therapy is required. As a result, drawing upon the discipline of rheumatology, immunosuppressive agents increasingly have been used to manage ocular inflammation alongside or in place of corticosteroids. The four major categories of immunosuppressive drugs currently used for ocular inflammatory diseases include antimetabolites, T-cell inhibitors, alkylating agents, and "biologics" (Table 12.1).

The antimetabolites most commonly used to treat ocular inflammatory diseases are

Financial Support This study was supported primarily by National Eye Institute Grant EY014943 (JHK). Additional support was provided by Research to Prevent Blindness and the Paul and Evanina Mackall Foundation.

Financial Disclosure(s) The author(s) have made the following disclosure(s): John H. Kempen consultant of Lux Biosciences, Allergan, Alcon, Sanofi-Pasteur, Harbor BioSciences, and Xoma and recipient of grant from the National Eye Institute, Food and Drug Administration, and EyeGate Pharma.

Contributions Design and conduct of the study (DMH, JHK); collection, management, analysis, and interpretation of the data (DMH, JHK); preparation, review, or approval of the manuscript (DMH, JHK)

Institutional Review Board Approval Not Applicable

D.M. Hornbeak, MD, MPH
Department of Ophthalmology, The Scheie Eye Institute, The University of Pennsylvania, 51 N. 39th Street, Philadelphia, PA 19104, USA
e-mail: dana.hornbeak@gmail.com, dana.hornbeak@uphs.upenn.edu

J.H. Kempen, MD, MPH, MHS, PhD (✉)
Department of Ophthalmology, Biostatistics and Epidemiology, The Scheie Eye Institute, The University of Pennsylvania Perelman School of Medicine, 3535 Market Street, Suite 700, Philadelphia, PA 19104, USA
e-mail: john.kempen@uphs.upenn.edu

U. Pleyer et al. (eds.), *Immune Modulation and Anti-Inflammatory Therapy in Ocular Disorders*, DOI 10.1007/978-3-642-54350-0_12, © Springer-Verlag Berlin Heidelberg 2014

Table 12.1 Four major classes of immunosuppressive drugs used in ocular inflammation

Immunosuppressive class
Agent
Antimetabolites
Methotrexate
Mycophenolate mofetil
Azathioprine
Mycophenolic acid[a]
T-cell inhibitors
Cyclosporine
Tacrolimus
Sirolimus[a]
Alkylating agents
Cyclophosphamide
Chlorambucil
Biologics
TNF inhibitors (infliximab, adalimumab, golimumab, certolizumab pegol, etanercept)
Interferons[a]
Rituximab[a]

[a]Promising but not currently in widespread use

methotrexate [1], mycophenolate mofetil [2], and azathioprine [3], although mycophenolic acid [4] has been suggested as potentially useful as well. With the exception of mycophenolic acid, all of these agents are available in generic form, and for methotrexate and azathioprine, decades of experience with use in other fields are available. Among T-cell inhibitors, cyclosporine [5] (also available as a generic) has been most widely used for ocular inflammatory diseases, although use of tacrolimus [6] is on the increase, and sirolimus has been suggested as potentially useful [7] but is not presently widely used. Alkylating agents, predominantly cyclophosphamide [8] and chlorambucil [9], are generally reserved for severe cases because of high toxicity risk (see below) and appear to have the unique property of inducing medication-free disease remission (as opposed to suppression) in a substantial number of cases. A wide range of biologics have been suggested as useful for ocular inflammatory disease, but for a discussion of safety, we will focus on the agents most widely used for ocular inflammation currently: tumor necrosis factor (TNF) inhibitors [10] (predominantly infliximab and adalimumab at the present

time) and emerging agents including interferons [11] and rituximab [12].

Immunosuppression for ocular inflammation is indicated in three general settings: (1) to control inflammation when corticosteroids fail to do so; (2) to prevent corticosteroid-induced toxicity when the dosage of corticosteroid required to control inflammation induces or can be expected to induce clinically important toxicity ("corticosteroid sparing"); and (3) to treat specific high-risk uveitis syndromes expected to respond poorly to corticosteroids alone [13]. However, concern exists about the short- and long-term side effects of immunosuppressive therapy – in particular, the risk of developing severe illnesses such as severe infections or cancer. Despite the well-known, severe, and sometimes cumulative side effects of corticosteroid therapy, there has been a perception by many that the use of immunosuppressive drugs is more risky than the use of corticosteroids. In fact, the motivation for using immunosuppressive drugs is – in most cases – a more favorable safety profile than that with corticosteroids, particularly when long-term therapy is needed. Fortunately, the evidence base addressing concerns about the risks of immunosuppressive drugs has grown in recent years. Data are available from a wide array of extraocular disease cohorts – particularly rheumatologic and transplant cohorts – as well as direct information from ocular inflammation cohorts.

12.1 Short-Term Toxicities of Immunosuppressive Agents

Short-term toxicities with the immunosuppressive drugs in use for ocular inflammation generally are less than with high-dose systemic corticosteroid therapy. However, there are specific potential risks for which surveillance should be conducted, as has been summarized previously by an expert panel [13]. In addition, specific individuals may have difficulty tolerating specific drugs in an idiosyncratic fashion. Also of interest has been the potential risk of opportunistic and commonly occurring infections.

While we review specific agents below, it is worth noting that strong evidence from ocular inflammation patients supports the safety of the general approach. In the Multicenter Uveitis Steroid Treatment (MUST) trial, specific potential risks of immunosuppression were no more commonly encountered in the group randomized to systemic therapy (in which 86 % received immunosuppression) than in the group randomized to fluocinolone acetonide implant therapy, other than perhaps a minor risk of mild infections (see below); the risks were very low in both groups [14].

12.1.1 Antimetabolites

The overwhelming majority of data on the use of antimetabolites has suggested a favorable safety profile. Most side effects that are going to occur present soon after drug initiation are reversible with cessation and only infrequently are severe enough to require drug discontinuation (see Table 12.2). For instance, a large retrospective cohort study of mycophenolate mofetil (MMF) monotherapy for ocular inflammation reported cessation due to side effects at a rate of 0.097 per person-year (PY) [2]. Another study reported an overall discontinuation rate for toxicity of 0.09 per PY over a 6-year follow-up period [15]. Enteric-coated mycophenolate sodium was developed in order to minimize gastrointestinal side effects (the most common treatment-limiting toxicity [2]) while hopefully maintaining similar immunosuppressive benefits and may have even better tolerability [4].

Adverse effects of methotrexate monotherapy have been reported to cause discontinuation at an overall rate of 0.13 per PY; these include gastrointestinal intolerance, hepatotoxicity, cytopenia, and interstitial pneumonia [1]. As with the other antimetabolites, these effects are usually reversible with dose reduction or discontinuation of therapy. A significant irreversible effect of the antimetabolites, particularly methotrexate, is teratogenicity; thus, withdrawal of therapy before planned pregnancy and use of contraception during therapy are mandatory [2].

Similar to mycophenolate mofetil, the most common side effect of azathioprine is gastrointestinal intolerance, which causes discontinuation in a small minority of patients. A large retrospective cohort study of azathioprine monotherapy for ocular inflammation reported azathioprine discontinuation due to gastrointestinal symptoms in 0.06 per PY during approximately 2 years of follow-up [3]. This was followed in frequency by bone marrow suppression (0.03 per PY), elevated liver enzymes (0.03 per PY), and allergic reaction (0.01 per PY), with an overall rate of discontinuation for toxicity of 0.16 per PY (possibly somewhat higher than with mycophenolate mofetil and methotrexate) [3]. Nearly all of these effects were detectable by following established guidelines for drug administration (Table 12.2) and were reversible with dose reduction or discontinuation of therapy [3]. Rarely, a homozygous deficiency of thiopurine methyltransferase (TPMT) can result in severe myelodepression; many clinicians recommend testing for TPMT activity prior to initiating azathioprine therapy, and dose adjustment recommendations have been published [16].

12.1.2 T-Cell Inhibitors

Available data on T-cell inhibitors also indicate a reasonable safety profile. In a large retrospective cohort study of cyclosporine monotherapy for ocular inflammation, side effects resulted in discontinuation of cyclosporine in 0.07 per PY for the entire follow-up period (95 % CI 0.05–0.09) [5]. Renal toxicity and hypertension were the most frequently observed side effects leading to cessation of therapy, occurring at rates of 0.02 per PY (95 % CI 0.01–0.04) and 0.02 per PY (95 % CI 0.009–0.03), respectively [5]. Discontinuation was progressively more frequent with increasing age: compared with patients aged 18–39, discontinuation for toxicity was 3.25 times more common in patients aged 55–64 and was 5.66 times more common in patients above 65 years old (overall $p=0.0005$) [5]. A previous retrospective case series evaluating tacrolimus for ocular inflammation also found a low discontinuation

Table 12.2 Short-term side effects of immunosuppressive medications (grade of recommendation for monitoring: B)

Medication class	Short-term side effects	Frequency of monitoring	Evidence level
Antimetabolites	Gastrointestinal upset[a]	CBC [4[MMF]–8[AZA] weeks]	2++
MTX	Bone marrow suppression[a]	Chemistry [4 [MMF]–12 [AZA] weeks]	2++
MMF	Hepatotoxicity (MTX>AZA>MMF)	Liver enzyme tests (MTX) [6–8 weeks]	2++
AZA	Malaise, myalgia, fatigue, headache		
	Rash, alopecia		
	Teratogenicity		
T-cell inhibitors	Renal toxicity[a]	Blood pressure	2++
CSA	Hypertension[a] (CSA>TAC)	CBC	2+
TAC	Neurologic symptoms[a]	Chemistry	
	Gastrointestinal symptoms (TAC)[a]	Liver enzyme tests	
	Hyperglycemia (TAC)[a]	Magnesium, phosphate	
	Hepatotoxicity	[All every 4 weeks for TAC; chem, Mg, phos every 12 weeks for CSA]	
	Hirsutism, gingival hyperplasia	Lipid panel [periodic]	
	Hypomagnesemia		
Alkylating agents	Bone marrow suppression[a]	CBC	2++
CTX	Cystitis, hematuria (CTX)[a]	Urinalysis (CTX only)	2++
CHB	Ovarian suppression	[Both every 4 weeks]	
	Testicular atrophy, azoospermia		
	Male sterility, alopecia, nausea, vomiting, opportunistic infection		
Biologics			
TNF inhibitors	Infusion/hypersensitivity reactions[a]	CBC	2+
Interferons	Autoantibody formation[a]	Liver enzyme tests	
	Opportunistic infection (rare)	[Both every 12 weeks]	
	Flulike symptoms (nearly universal)[a]	CBC	2+
	Mild leukopenia[a]	Chemistry	
	Psychological disturbances	Liver enzyme tests	
	Fibromyalgia, arthralgia/myalgia	Thyroid function panel	
	Thrombocytopenia	[All every 4 weeks]	
	Fever, nausea, headache		
	Thyroiditis, alopecia, hepatotoxicity		
	Opportunistic infections (rare)		
Rituximab	Infusion/hypersensitivity reactions[a]	CBC	2+
	Leukopenia	Immunoglobulins	
	Granulocytopenia	[Both every 4 weeks]	
	Gammaglobulin decrease		

Side effects and monitoring apply to the entire medication class unless otherwise specified
CBC complete blood count, *MTX* methotrexate, *AZA* azathioprine, *MMF* mycophenolate mofetil, *CSA* cyclosporine, *TAC* tacrolimus, *CTX* cyclophosphamide, *CHB* chlorambucil
[a]Indicates the more common side effects for each class/agent

rate due to toxicity (0.13 per PY), predominantly due to non-cardiovascular and nonrenal side effects, such as neurologic symptoms (e.g., tremor, paresthesias), gastrointestinal symptoms, hyperglycemia, insomnia, and headache [6]. Sirolimus has been associated with cytopenias, hypercholesterolemia, arthralgias, extremity edema, and impaired wound healing [17]. While no immunosuppressive agent is recommended during pregnancy, in a transplant pregnancy cohort, no excess malformations were observed in women receiving cyclosporine during pregnancy [18], which is a potential advantage with respect to antimetabolites.

12.1.3 Alkylating Agents

Regarding alkylating agents, a large retrospective cohort study of cyclophosphamide monotherapy for ocular inflammation reported cyclophosphamide discontinuation at an overall rate of 0.39 per PY (95 % CI 0.31–0.49) [8], substantially higher than reported with antimetabolites or T-cell inhibitors from the same cohort. Toxicities were usually reversible in nature and most commonly included leukopenia (0.20 per PY, 95 % CI 0.14–0.27), thrombocytopenia (0.016 per PY, 95 % CI 0.0032–0.046), anemia (0.036 per PY, 95 % CI 0.015–0.075), and cystitis/blood in the urine (0.073 per PY, 95 % CI 0.040–0.12) [8]. Several other studies have shown the bone marrow suppression of cyclophosphamide to be dose dependent and reversible, with older individuals more susceptible (and hence requiring lower doses to suppress white blood cell levels to the desired therapeutic range). The adverse effects of chlorambucil therapy are similar, with bone marrow suppression to a degree greater than desired being the most common toxicity [13]. Short-term, high-dose chlorambucil therapy, in which the drug is suspended after crossing a given white blood cell count (and thus is a therapeutic end point rather than a toxicity), may have a somewhat different side effect profile [9]. Both cyclophosphamide and chlorambucil can cause alopecia, ovarian suppression, azoospermia, and male sterility [9, 13], and both are embryotoxic.

12.1.4 Biologics

Most of the side effects of TNF inhibitors are mild, consisting of infusion/hypersensitivity reactions such as local erythema at the injection site, atopic dermatitis, flushing, rash, hypertension, fever, or fatigue [19]. These generally do not lead to discontinuation of therapy. Formation of autoantibodies is common but usually not clinically significant [13, 19], although infrequently severe infusion reactions that require discontinuation of therapy do occur with infliximab. Side effects of a fluid infusion can restrict therapy in susceptible individuals, such as those with limited cardiac output, for those agents which are given via intravenous infusion. TNF inhibitors also may have a less unfavorable safety profile in the event of pregnancy than antimetabolites or alkylating agents [20].

Dose-dependent flulike symptoms from interferon-alpha treatment are expected but usually are sufficiently tolerable that discontinuation is not required. In a retrospective study of interferon-alpha treatment in patients with severe uveitis due to Behçet disease, discontinuation due to toxicity occurred in 9.4 % during the total mean follow-up period of nearly 5 years [11]. In addition to flulike symptoms, mild leukopenia (>2,000/μl) was seen in all patients but caused discontinuation in none [11]. Uncommon findings during treatment included fibromyalgia, psychological disturbances, hair loss, thrombocytopenia, headache, mild hepatotoxicity, thyroiditis, fever, and nausea.

Like the TNF inhibitors, rituximab has side effects which are usually mild, are short lived, and do not result in discontinuation of therapy. Infusion/hypersensitivity reactions including hypotension, local erythema, cough, laryngeal edema, and infusion-related rigors occur occasionally [21]. A meta-analysis of patients with lymphoma taking rituximab showed increased risk of severe leukopenia (RR=1.24; 95 % CI 1.12–1.37) and granulocytopenia (RR=1.07; 95 % CI 1.02–1.12), although this did not result in higher infection risk (discussed in next section) [22]. Experience with toxicities of rituximab given for eye disease currently is limited.

12.2 Infection Risk with Immunosuppressive Agents

The extent of increase in the risk of infection, if any, is a frequently cited point of concern when using immunosuppressive medications for ocular inflammation, particularly for the risk of severe opportunistic infection. In the MUST trial, a higher risk of infections requiring a drug prescription was observed in the systemic therapy group (systemic corticosteroids plus immunosuppression in 86 %) than in the implant group (0.60 vs. 0.36 per PY, $p=0.034$). However, these typically were mild infections and none of the patients suffered lasting consequences; it was unclear to what extent the difference reflected an increased likelihood of prescribing drugs for mild infections in patients known to be taking immunosuppressive drugs (since participants and clinicians were unmasked) rather than a true difference in infection incidence [14].

Substantial data exist supporting the safety of monotherapy with either antimetabolites or T-cell inhibitors for ocular inflammation with respect to the risk of opportunistic infections. The Systemic Immunosuppressive Therapy for Eye Diseases (SITE) cohort study reported no observed opportunistic infections in patients treated with mycophenolate mofetil, methotrexate, or azathioprine monotherapy (with or without systemic corticosteroids) [1–3]. This confirmed previous evidence showing no increase in infection risk associated with mycophenolate mofetil monotherapy [15]. The SITE study also showed no increased infection risk associated with T-cell inhibitors, either as a class or for cyclosporine individually [23], consistent with previous studies reporting no association of cyclosporine or tacrolimus monotherapy with increased risk of serious infections [13].

While these results for monotherapy are reassuring, it is important to note that patients sometimes require therapy with more than one agent concurrently. The combination of an antimetabolite with a T-cell inhibitor such as cyclosporine is a common approach because the drugs have different toxicity profiles and have been used together for other diseases such as transplantation [13]. In some transplant cohorts, the combination of mycophenolate mofetil with cyclosporine ($\pm$ corticosteroids) has been associated with a nonsignificant increase in opportunistic infections compared with either agent alone, as well as a nonsignificant trend toward more events with higher mycophenolate mofetil doses (Table 12.3) [24]. The majority of these infections were cytomegalovirus and herpes simplex infections, with less than 2 % being fatal (these observations in transplant cohorts where many participants were severely ill) [24, 25]. The risk of opportunistic infection was substantially lower in an ocular inflammation cohort in which only two patients developed major infections while taking mycophenolate mofetil combination therapy: one with cytomegalovirus retinitis and another with lower limb cellulitis (not clearly an opportunistic infection) [15].

Table 12.3 Immunosuppressive medications for ocular inflammatory disease and infections

Immunosuppressive class	Reported infections with therapy ± (corticosteroids)	Evidence level
Antimetabolites	No clinically important association	2++
T-cell inhibitors	No clinically important association	2++
Combined therapy (antimetabolite and T-cell inhibitor)	Modestly increased risk	2+
Alkylating agents	Increased risk, consider *Pneumocystis* prophylaxis	2++
Biologics		
TNF inhibitors	Modestly increased risk, rule out tuberculosis prior to initiating therapy	1++
Interferons	No clinically important association reported	2++
Rituximab	No clinically important association reported	1++

In contrast to the results with antimetabolites and T-cell inhibitors, cyclophosphamide has been associated with opportunistic infections in ocular inflammation patients, leading to discontinuation in 3.0 % (95 % CI 1.2–7.1 %) of patients in the first year and at an overall rate of 0.026 per PY during 3 years of follow-up (95 % CI 0.0084–0.061) [8]. Infections included *Pneumocystis jirovecii* pneumonia leading to death in 1 (0.5 %) patient, who had been managed according to standard guidelines but who had not taken preemptive *Pneumocystis* prophylaxis with trimethoprim-sulfamethoxazole, as some recommend with alkylating agent or combination immunosuppressive therapy. These findings are consistent with (but less extreme than) the results of a previous randomized controlled clinical trial of 50 patients with Wegener's granulomatosis, which reported infections in 70 % of patients receiving cyclophosphamide, including 30 % who developed *Pneumocystis jirovecii* pneumonia [26]. Substantial granulocytopenia (absolute neutrophil count <1,000 cells/µl) associated with cyclophosphamide is associated with increased risk of bacterial infections, particularly sepsis; most clinicians seek to avoid this complication by holding cyclophosphamide when a white count below 2,500 cells/µl is observed, followed by downward dose adjustment [27], which may explain the much lower risk of infection observed in the ocular inflammation cohort.

The availability of data regarding the risk of opportunistic infections with the biologic agents is growing. The most common sites of infections associated with biologic therapy are respiratory tract infections, skin and soft tissue infections, and urinary tract infections [28]. Presumably because TNF plays an important role in the host defense mechanism against intracellular pathogens, anti-TNF therapy is associated with increased risk of infection with intracellular microorganisms, such as *Mycobacterium tuberculosis*, *Listeria monocytogenes*, and *Legionella pneumophila* [29]. A meta-analysis of TNF inhibitors in 369 patients with Behçet disease reported reactivation of tuberculosis in 4 patients and opportunistic infections in 10 patients. These infections included *Pneumocystis jirovecii*

pneumonia, *Legionella pneumophila* pneumonia, cryptococcal meningitis, varicella zoster infection, CMV colitis, forearm cellulitis, and bacterial endocarditis [19]. A meta-analysis of adults with rheumatoid arthritis participating in clinical trials of infliximab or adalimumab reported a significantly higher risk (OR = 2.0; 95 % CI 1.3–3.1) of serious infections during 22–54 weeks of follow-up, but the absolute risk was low (0.036 % with anti-TNF therapy vs. 0.017 % with placebo) [30]. An absolute risk in this range probably does not represent a clinically important constraint on the use of these agents for ocular inflammation, but clinicians should bear in mind that significant infection occurs occasionally with such therapy.

There are fewer data on the risk of opportunistic infections with interferon treatment, but the available evidence thus far is reassuring. In a retrospective study of interferon-alpha treatment in patients with severe uveitis due to Behçet disease, no opportunistic infections were reported during nearly 5 years of follow-up [11]. This observation is consistent with a previous double-blind clinical trial of gamma-interferon for patients with rheumatoid arthritis, in which no increased risk of opportunistic infections was observed [31].

Likewise, a recent review found no evidence of increased infection risk with rituximab compared to concurrent control treatments in patients with rheumatoid arthritis [32], and a meta-analysis in patients with lymphoma receiving rituximab revealed no increased risk of severe infection (defined as either life-threatening or requiring hospitalization or intravenous antibiotics) with the addition of rituximab to standard chemotherapy regimens (RR = 1.00; 95 % CI 0.87–1.14) [22]. Another meta-analysis reported that the overall pooled odds ratio for serious infection with rituximab treatment was not significantly increased (OR = 1.45; 95 % CI 0.56–3.73) [32]. A randomized, double-blind, placebo-controlled, dose-ranging trial of rituximab showed a slightly higher overall (including both minor and serious) infection rate in placebo-treated patients (1.546 per PY) than in rituximab-treated patients (1.382 per PY) over 24 weeks [21]. The rate of serious infection in the rituximab group was 0.015

per PY higher than in the placebo group, but the absolute rate for both groups still was low (0.052 vs. 0.037 per PY, respectively); there were no reports of tuberculosis or opportunistic infections in either group [21].

12.3 Cancer Risk with Immunosuppressive Agents

Immunosuppression in general has been thought to raise the risk of skin, mucosal, and lymphoproliferative cancers. Proposed mechanisms include interruption of immune surveillance for and destruction of malignant cells, susceptibility to infection with oncogenic infectious agents, damage to DNA (alkylating agents) or to DNA metabolism (antimetabolites), and agent-specific effects on the immune system, which could alter the chances of a transformed cell surviving and proliferating or of an oncogenic infectious agent escaping immune control [33].

A prime example of malignancy related to immunosuppression in general is posttransplant lymphoproliferative disorder (PTLD) in transplant cohorts. PTLD is the second most common malignancy in these patients (after skin cancers) and is linked to Epstein-Barr virus infection in 80–90 % of cases [34]. Pathogenesis probably depends substantially on chronic antigenic stimulation by the graft, as evidenced by the relatively high proportion of transplanted organs with PTLD involvement in the graft, and the substantially higher incidence of this condition in transplant than in autoimmune disease cohorts. Because patients with local ocular inflammation have neither antigenic stimulation nor a graft, they would be expected to have a significantly lower risk of PTLD and likely also would respond favorably to interruption of immunosuppression in most cases [33]. Clinical impression suggests these cases are rare in the ocular inflammation setting.

Regarding the risk of malignancy with each class of immunosuppressive agent, here we discuss cancer incidence with the four major categories of immunosuppressive drugs used in ocular inflammatory disease (see Table 12.4).

Antimetabolites have the best evidence among the immunosuppressive classes to support a lack of clinically important carcinogenicity. Azathioprine has been studied in patients with rheumatoid arthritis, inflammatory bowel disease, and multiple sclerosis and consistently has shown no increased risk of malignancy in these cohorts, other than sporadic reports of PTLD-like cases [33], which in a population study did not occur significantly more often in treated than in nontreated patients (RR = 1.27; 95 % CI 0.03–8.20) [35]. In contrast, azathioprine-treated transplant patients appear to have increased

Table 12.4 Cancer risk with immunosuppressive agents

		Evidence review suggests		Quality of evidence		
	Agent	Clinically important ↑ in cancer risk	May interact to ↑ cancer risk	Evidence level	Strength of association	Dose–response relation
Antimetabolites	Methotrexate	No	No	2++	N/A	N/A
	Mycophenolate mofetil	No	No	2+	N/A	N/A
	Azathioprine	No	Inconclusive	2++	+	+
T-cell inhibitors	Cyclosporine	No	Yes	2++	+	++
	Tacrolimus	No	Yes[a]	2−	++	−
Alkylating agents	Cyclophosphamide	Yes	Yes	2++	++++	++++
	Chlorambucil	Yes	Yes	3	+++	−
Biologics	TNF inhibitors	No	No	2+	+	−
	Interferon	No	No	2−	N/A	N/A
	Rituximab	Unknown	Unknown	2−	N/A	N/A

Modified from Kempen et al. [33]

[a]Conclusion primarily inferred from observations regarding cyclosporine

malignancy risk compared to the general population, particularly with lymphoid malignancies and squamous cell carcinoma of the skin [36]. However, this pattern likely reflects the uniquely high-risk transplant-immunosuppression interaction, which probably does not apply to the setting of ocular inflammation.

Methotrexate also has shown no increased cancer risk in several cohorts with a variety of diseases and has the best evidence in favor of its safety with respect to cancer risk of any of the immunosuppressive drugs [33]. Although PTLD-like cases have been reported with methotrexate, a large observational study following 19,591 rheumatoid arthritis patients over 89,710 PY found no increased risk of lymphoma with methotrexate therapy [37], suggesting that posttransplant lymphoproliferative disorder-like cases must be very rare.

Mycophenolate mofetil (MMF) also appears to have a favorable carcinogenicity profile, although there is less experience with this newer agent. Observational studies of MMF in the post-transplant setting have found a significantly reduced risk of PTLD, improved survival of patients who developed PTLD, and a lower risk of cancer in general when MMF is compared to alternative regimens [33], which has contributed to a preference for immunosuppression using this drug over alternatives in the transplant world.

Most available studies on T-cell inhibitors are from transplant cohorts and show the increased risk of malignancy (especially skin cancer, post-transplant lymphoproliferative disorder, and gastrointestinal cancer), which is typical of transplant cohorts. However, these data are not necessarily applicable to ocular inflammation cohorts, which do not have the chronic antigenic stimulation and other comorbidities associated with transplanted organs [33, 38]. A cohort study of several hundred rheumatoid arthritis patients showed no increased risk of malignancy due to cyclosporine treatment [39]. A 5-year prospective cohort study of psoriatic patients treated with cyclosporine showed a higher risk of leukemia and non-melanomatous skin cancers; however, this was thought to be due to potentiation of the oncogenic effects of psoralen and ultraviolet A treatment by

cyclosporine, rather than due to cyclosporine itself [40]. Thus, in the absence of these accompanying treatments or an organ transplant, such as in uveitis patients, cyclosporine likely would not confer higher cancer risk [33], especially after considering results of the SITE cohort study (see below).

In contrast, alkylating agents consistently have been associated with a higher risk of malignancies. Several studies have shown cyclophosphamide to be associated with substantially increased rates of leukemia, lymphoma, and skin malignancies [the kinds seen with immunosuppression in general (see above)] as well as of bladder cancer likely related to a carcinogenic metabolite, acrolein, that concentrates in urine; and some studies have found an increase in total malignancies [33]. Bladder cancer risk with cyclophosphamide appears to be dose and/or duration dependent and is higher in smokers. Risk can be mitigated by intravenous hydration to prevent acrolein buildup and consequent cystitis, which is thought to increase bladder cancer risk [41]. Simple oral hydration also often is used to accomplish this goal, particularly with daily oral cyclophosphamide therapy. Chlorambucil has been linked to development of cutaneous malignancies – sometimes multiple and recurrent – and also associated with increased incidence of lymphoma and leukemia, the latter possibly occurring more frequently than with cyclophosphamide; however, it is not associated with increased bladder cancer risk [33].

The majority of reports on cancer risk with TNF inhibitors are favorable. Seven large observational studies of tumor necrosis factor (TNF) inhibitors for rheumatoid arthritis, with in aggregate nearly 100,000 PY of follow-up, showed no increased overall risk of malignancy [38, 42–48]. Results in a Crohn's disease cohort also found no increase in cancer risk due to TNF inhibitors [49]. In contrast, a meta-analysis of TNF inhibitors in 5,014 patients with rheumatoid arthritis participating in clinical trials showed a 3.3-fold higher risk of cancer over 22–54 weeks of follow-up, which was theorized to have been the result of an accelerated diagnosis of preexisting cancers given that a significant difference appeared during such a short follow-up period [30].

Data are more limited on interferon-alpha but thus far are reassuring. A retrospective study following patients with uveitis associated with Behçet disease found no increase in malignancy with interferon-alpha treatment over nearly 8 years of follow-up [50], as did a systematic literature review of 338 patients with ocular and systemic manifestations of Behçet disease [51]. At this time, data on rituximab are limited to small clinical studies and case reports and thus are insufficient to draw conclusions, although it should be noted that rituximab is a treatment for B-cell lymphomas.

12.4 Mortality Risk with Immunosuppressive Agents

The risk of death in association with the use of immunosuppressive drugs has been directly evaluated in ocular inflammation patients in a well-powered study (evidence level 2++). The Systemic Immunosuppressive Therapy for Eye Diseases Cohort Study (SITE) retrospectively evaluated overall and cancer-associated mortality due to immunosuppressive therapy in patients with ocular inflammatory disease [23]. Data included demographic, clinical, and treatment characteristics from 7,957 patients with noninfectious ocular inflammation seen at five tertiary ocular inflammation clinics from 1979 to 2005. Corresponding overall and cancer-related mortality were obtained from the US National Death Index in a manner previously described [23].

The SITE study results are summarized in Figs. 12.1 and 12.2, displaying adjusted hazard ratios for each immunosuppressive agent and class of agents studied. Use of antimetabolites as a class was not associated with increased overall mortality (adjusted hazard ratio (aHR) 1.08, 95 % CI 0.86–1.37) or cancer mortality (aHR 0.89, 95 % CI 0.54–1.48). The most common individual antimetabolites (azathioprine, methotrexate, and mycophenolate mofetil) also were not associated with increased overall or cancer mortality. Similarly, use of T-cell inhibitors as a class did not increase risk of overall mortality (aHR 0.81, 95 % CI 0.59–1.11) or cancer-related mortality (aHR 0.78, 95 % CI 0.38–1.59) nor did cyclosporine individually. The latter observation

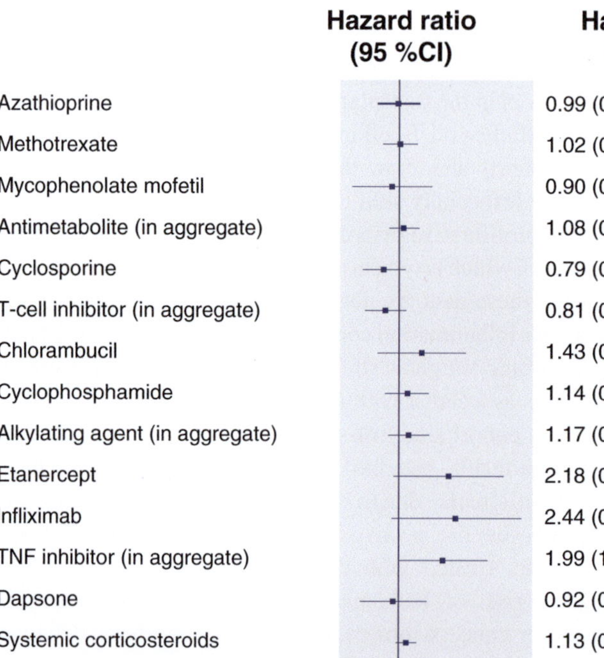

Fig. 12.1 Adjusted relative hazard of all-cause mortality for each immunosuppressive agent and class of agents studied (Ali et al. [20]; reprinted with permission)

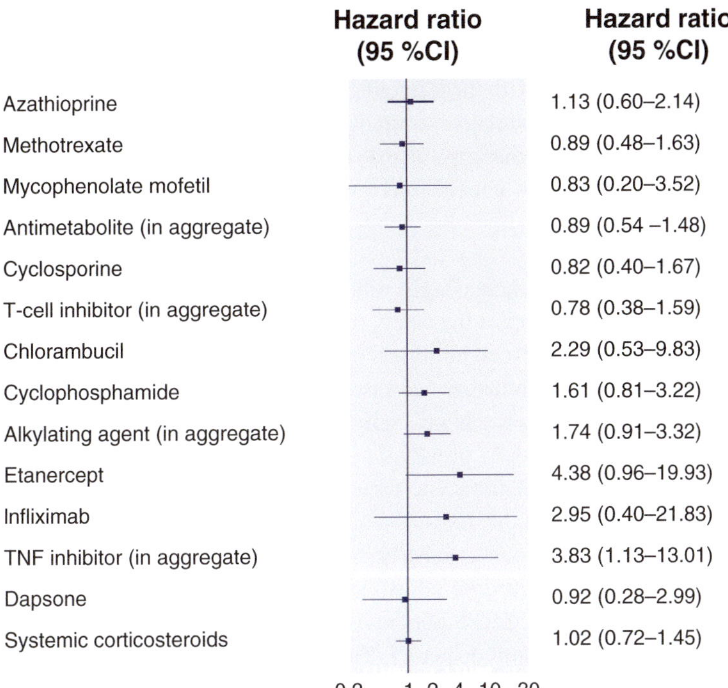

Fig. 12.2 Adjusted relative hazard of mortality attributed to cancer for each immunosuppressive agent and class of agents studied (Ali et al. [20]; reprinted with permission)

was consistent with a retrospective cohort study which showed no increased mortality risk in patients with rheumatoid arthritis treated with cyclosporine [39].

Use of alkylating agents as a class was not associated with significantly increased overall mortality (aHR 1.17, 95 % CI 0.85–1.61), neither was all cancer mortality statistically significantly raised, but statistical power for this outcome was limited (evidence level 2+), and the observed tendency toward increased risk (aHR 1.74, 95 % CI 0.91–3.32) was consistent with the increased risk of cancer observed in other disease cohorts (see above). The results for cyclophosphamide treatment paralleled those for alkylating agents as a class. These findings were consistent with previous reports suggesting that cyclophosphamide treatment may cause a dose-dependent increase in mortality from all cancer types [52, 53], which represents a clinically important constraint on the use of these agents, restricting use to the most serious cases.

The SITE cohort study was not as well powered for evaluating the risk of death associated with TNF inhibitor therapy (evidence level 2-),

which came into use only a few years before the end of follow-up, so results should be regarded as pilot results. However, TNF inhibitors as a class were associated with significant increases in overall mortality (fully adjusted HR 1.99, 95 % CI 1.00–3.98) and cancer mortality (HR 3.83, 95 % CI 1.13–13.01). Individual risk ratios for etanercept and infliximab were similar in magnitude but were nonsignificant in the context of having few observations. The SITE study had very limited information on adalimumab. The SITE results differed from several better-powered observational studies of TNF inhibitors in other populations, which found no increased risk of mortality (see above) [38, 42–44, 46]. A possible explanation of the apparent inconsistency is that ~75 % of SITE patients receiving TNF inhibitor therapy had an associated systemic inflammatory disease vs. ~25 % for the cohort as a whole, and the associated systemic diseases may have increased the risk of death or death from cancer rather than the treatment itself. Further data are needed to provide reassurance that this observation in fact represents an indication for treatment bias rather than a real increase in risk. However, in the meantime, the results from well-powered rheumatologic cohorts seem persuasive of safety vis-à-vis mortality with these agents.

Data regarding the risk of mortality with interferon or rituximab therapy for eye diseases are not sufficient to draw conclusions on the subject.

Conclusion

In summary, an increasingly robust evidence base exists to support the safety of using antimetabolites and T-cell inhibitors in the context of ocular inflammatory diseases, although clinical trial evidence is generally unavailable for reasons which previously have been described [54]. While some patients may not tolerate these medications, usually tolerance problems are encountered early in therapy and are reversible with dose adjustment or cessation of therapy. Most patients tolerate the medications without difficulty. This pattern is in contrast to the well-known and severe toxicity of long-term, high-dose systemic corticosteroid therapy, thus confirming the rationale for the use of these medications as corticosteroid-sparing agents.

Based on the available evidence, alkylating agent therapy does appear to have a higher risk of opportunistic infection and of cancer, which provides a clinically relevant constraint on the use of these agents to the most severe cases of ocular inflammatory diseases, wherein severe vision loss is likely absent control of inflammation. TNF inhibitors appear to have an increased risk of opportunistic infection as well, but the absolute risk thereof is small (at least in a temperate environment), and the majority of data suggest there is no increased risk of cancer. However, concerning preliminary data from the SITE cohort needs to be evaluated further. Interferons have considerable short-term flu-like symptoms which are generally tolerable, but they do not appear to cause a higher risk of severe infection or other major long-term adverse effects; however, data are limited. Rituximab does not often produce short-term toxicity, and the majority of data indicate no increase in infection risk with its use, but data

regarding malignancy and mortality are limited. Further research is needed to elucidate the risk of cancer and mortality in patients taking interferons or rituximab. New immunosuppressive drugs also will need to be evaluated for safety and effectiveness as they become available.

Immunosuppressive therapy, particularly with antimetabolites and T-cell inhibitors and probably also with biologics, offers a safe and reasonably effective alternative to long-term, high-dose corticosteroid therapy and should be used in settings where acceptable dose corticosteroid therapy is inadequate.

References

1. Gangaputra S, Newcomb CW, Liesegang TL, Kacmaz RO, Jabs DA, Levy-Clarke GA, Nussenblatt RB, Rosenbaum JT, Suhler EB, Thorne JE, Foster CS, Kempen JH. Methotrexate for ocular inflammatory diseases. Ophthalmology. 2009;116:2188–98.
2. Daniel E, Thorne JE, Newcomb CW, Pujari SS, Kacmaz RO, Levy-Clarke GA, Nussenblatt RB, Rosenbaum JT, Suhler EB, Foster CS, Jabs DA, Kempen JH. Mycophenolate mofetil for ocular inflammation. Am J Ophthalmol. 2010;149(3):423–32.
3. Pasadhika S, Kempen JH, Newcomb CW, Liesegang TL, Pujari SS, Rosenbaum JT, Thorne JE, Foster CS, Jabs DA, Levy-Clarke GA, Nussenblatt RB, Suhler EB. Azathioprine for ocular inflammatory diseases. Am J Ophthalmol. 2009;148(4):500–9.
4. Deuter CM, Doycheva D, Stuebiger N, Zierhut M. Mycophenolate sodium for immunosuppressive treatment in uveitis. Ocul Immunol Inflamm. 2009;17:415–9.
5. Kacmaz RO, Kempen JH, Newcomb C, Daniel E, Gangaputra S, Nussenblatt RB, Rosenbaum JT, Suhler EB, Thorne JE, Jabs DA, Levy-Clarke GA, Foster CS. Cyclosporine for ocular inflammatory diseases. Ophthalmology. 2010;117(3):576–84.
6. Hogan AC, McAvoy CE, Dick AD, Lee RW. Long-term efficacy and tolerance of tacrolimus for the treatment of uveitis. Ophthalmology. 2007;114:1000–6.
7. Shanmuganathan VA, Casely EM, Raj D, Powell RJ, Joseph A, Amoaku WM, Dua HS. The efficacy of sirolimus in the treatment of patients with refractory uveitis. Br J Ophthalmol. 2005;89:666–9.
8. Pujari SS, Kempen JH, Newcomb CW, Gangaputra S, Daniel E, Suhler EB, Thorne JE, Jabs DA, Levy-Clarke GA, Nussenblatt RB, Rosenbaum JT, Foster CS. Cyclophosphamide for ocular inflammatory diseases. Ophthalmology. 2010;117(2):356–65.

9. Goldstein DA, Fontanilla FA, Kaul S, Sahin O, Tessler HH. Long-term follow-up of patients treated with short-term high-dose chlorambucil for sight-threatening ocular inflammation. Ophthalmology. 2002;109: 370–7.

10. Martel JN, Esterberg E, Nagpal A, Acharya NR. Infliximab and adalimumab for uveitis. Ocul Immunol Inflamm. 2012;20:18–26.

11. Deuter CM, Zierhut M, Mohle A, Vonthein R, Stobiger N, Kotter I. Long-term remission after cessation of interferon-alpha treatment in patients with severe uveitis due to Behcet's disease. Arthritis Rheum. 2010;62:2796–805.

12. Miserocchi E, Pontikaki I, Modorati G, Gattinara M, Meroni PL, Gerloni V. Anti-CD 20 monoclonal antibody (rituximab) treatment for inflammatory ocular diseases. Autoimmun Rev. 2011;11:35–9.

13. Jabs DA, Rosenbaum JT, Foster CS, Holland GN, Jaffe GJ, Louie JS, Nussenblatt RB, Stiehm ER, Tessler H, Van Gelder RN, Whitcup SM, Yocum D. Guidelines for the use of immunosuppressive drugs in patients with ocular inflammatory disorders: recommendations of an expert panel. Am J Ophthalmol. 2000;130(4):492–513.

14. The Multicenter Uveitis Steroid Treatment Trial Research Group, Writing Committee: Kempen JH, Altaweel MM, Holbrook JT, Jabs DA, Louis TA, Sugar EA, Thorne JE. Randomized comparison of systemic anti-inflammatory therapy versus fluocinolone acetonide implant for intermediate, posterior, and panuveitis: the multicenter uveitis steroid treatment trial. Ophthalmology. 2011;118:1916–26.

15. Teoh SC, Hogan AC, Dick AD, Lee RW. Mycophenolate mofetil for the treatment of uveitis. Am J Ophthalmol. 2008;146(5):752–60, 760.e1–3.

16. Relling MV, Gardner EE, Sandborn WJ, Schmiegelow K, Pui CH, Yee SW, Stein CM, Carrillo M, Evans WE, Klein TE, Clinical Pharmacogenetics Implementation Consortium. Clinical Pharmacogenetics Implementation Consortium guidelines for thiopurine methyltransferase genotype and thiopurine dosing. Clin Pharmacol Ther. 2011;89(3):387–91. Epub 26 Jan 2011.

17. Buhaescu I, Izzedine H, Covic A. Sirolimus–challenging current perspectives. Ther Drug Monit. 2006;28(5):577–84.

18. Armenti VT, Radomski JS, Moritz MJ, Gaughan WJ, Philips LZ, McGrory CH, Coscia LA. Report from the national transplantation pregnancy registry (NTPR): outcomes of pregnancy after transplantation. Clin Transpl. 2001;97–105.

19. Fragiadaki K, Giavri E, Sfikakis PP. Anti-TNF agents for Behcet's disease: analysis of published data on 369 patients. Semin Arthritis Rheum. 2011;41(1):61–70.

20. Ali YM, Kuriya B, Orozco C, Cush JJ, Keystone EC. Can tumor necrosis factor inhibitors be safely used in pregnancy? J Rheumatol. 2010;37(1):9–17.

21. Cohen SB, Emery P, Greenwald MW, Dougados M, Furie RA, Genovese MC, Keystone EC, Loveless JE, Burmester GR, Cravets MW, Hessey EW, Shaw T, Totoritis MC, REFLEX Trial Group. Rituximab for rheumatoid arthritis refractory to anti–tumor necrosis factor therapy. Arthritis Rheum. 2006;54(9):2793–806.

22. Lanini S, Molloy AC, Fine PE, Prentice AG, Ippolito G, Kibbler CC. Risk of infection in patients with lymphoma receiving rituximab: systematic review and meta-analysis. BMC Med. 2011;9:36.

23. Kempen JH, Daniel E, Dunn JP, Foster CS, Gangaputra S, Hanish A, Helzlsouer KJ, Jabs DA, Kaçmaz RO, Levy-Clarke GA, Liesegang TL, Newcomb CW, Nussenblatt RB, Pujari SS, Rosenbaum JT, Suhler EB, Thorne JE. Overall and cancer related mortality among patients with ocular inflammation treated with immunosuppressive drugs: retrospective cohort study. BMJ. 2009;339:b2480.

24. European Mycophenolate Mofetil Cooperative Study Group. Placebo-controlled study of mycophenolate mofetil combined with cyclosporine and corticosteroids for prevention of acute rejection. Lancet. 1995;345:1321–5.

25. The Tricontinental Mycophenolate Mofetil Renal Transplantation Group. A blinded, randomized clinical trial of mycophenolate mofetil for the prevention of acute rejection in cadaveric renal transplantation. Transplantation. 1996;61:1029–37.

26. Lacki JK, Schochat T, Sobieska M. Immunological studies in patients with rheumatoid arthritis treated with methotrexate or cyclophosphamide. Z Rheumatol. 1994;53:76–82.

27. Masuda K, Nakajima A, Urayama A, Nakae K, Kogure M, Inaba G. Double-masked trial of cyclosporine versus colchicine and long-term open study of cyclosporine in Behcet's disease. Lancet. 1989;1:1093–6.

28. Furst DE. The risk of infections with biologic therapies for rheumatoid arthritis. Semin Arthritis Rheum. 2010;39(5):327–46.

29. Salliot C, van der Heijde D. Long-term safety of methotrexate monotherapy in patients with rheumatoid arthritis: a systematic literature research. Ann Rheum Dis. 2009;68(7):1100–4.

30. Bongartz T, Sutton AJ, Sweeting MJ, Buchan I, Matteson EL, Montori V. Anti-TNF antibody therapy in rheumatoid arthritis and the risk of serious infections and malignancies: systematic review and meta-analysis of rare harmful effects in randomized controlled trials. JAMA. 2006;295:2275–85.

31. Cannon GW, Pincus SH, Emkey RD, Denes A, Cohen SA, Wolfe F, Saway PA, Jaffer AM, Weaver AL, Cogen L, Schindler JD. Double-blind trial of recombinant gamma-interferon versus placebo in the treatment of rheumatoid arthritis. 1989. Arthritis Rheum. 2008;58(2):S79–88.

32. Kelesidis T, Daikos G, Boumpas D, Tsiodras S. Does rituximab increase the incidence of infectious complications? A narrative review. Int J Infect Dis. 2011;15(1):e2–16.

33. Kempen JH, Gangaputra S, Daniel E, Levy-Clarke GA, Nussenblatt RB, Rosenbaum JT, Suhler EB, Thorne JE, Foster CS, Jabs DA, Helzlsouer KJ. Long-term risk of malignancy among patients treated with

immunosuppressive agents for ocular inflammation: a critical assessment of the evidence. Am J Ophthalmol. 2008;146(6):802–12.

34. Snow AL, Martinez OM. Epstein-Barr virus: evasive maneuvers in the development of PTLD. Am J Transplant. 2007;7:271–7.

35. Lewis JD, Bilker WB, Brensinger C, Deren JJ, Vaughn DJ, Strom BL. Inflammatory bowel disease is not associated with an increased risk of lymphoma. Gastroenterology. 2001;121(5):1080–7.

36. Jensen P, Hansen S, Møller B, Leivestad T, Pfeffer P, Geiran O, Fauchald P, Simonsen S. Skin cancer in kidney and heart transplant recipients and different long-term immunosuppressive therapy regimens. J Am Acad Dermatol. 1999;40(2 Pt 1):177–86.

37. Wolfe F, Michaud K. Biologic treatment of rheumatoid arthritis and the risk of malignancy: analyses from a large US observational study. Arthritis Rheum. 2007;56:2886–95.

38. Birkeland SA, Hamilton-Dutoit S. Is posttransplant lymphoproliferative disorder (PTLD) caused by any specific immunosuppressive drug or by the transplantation per se? Transplantation. 2003;76:984–8.

39. van den Borne BE, Landewé RB, Houkes I, Schild F, van der Heyden PC, Hazes JM, Vandenbroucke JP, Zwinderman AH, Goei The HS, Breedveld FC, Bernelot Moens HJ, Kluin PM, Dijkmans BA. No increased risk of malignancies and mortality in cyclosporin A-treated patients with rheumatoid arthritis. Arthritis Rheum. 1998;41(11):1930–7.

40. Paul CF, Ho VC, McGeown C, Christophers E, Schmidtmann B, Guillaume JC, Lamarque V, Dubertret L. Risk of malignancies in psoriasis patients treated with cyclosporine: a 5 y cohort study. J Invest Dermatol. 2003;120(2):211–6.

41. Talar-Williams C, Hijazi YM, Walther MM, et al. Cyclophosphamide-induced cystitis and bladder cancer in patients with Wegener granulomatosis. Ann Intern Med. 1996;124:477–84.

42. Carmona L, Descalzo MA, Perez-Pampin E, Ruiz-Montesinos D, Erra A, Cobo T, Gómez-Reino JJ, BIOBADASER and EMECAR Groups. All-cause and cause-specific mortality in rheumatoid arthritis are not greater than expected when treated with tumour necrosis factor antagonists. Ann Rheum Dis. 2007;66(7):880–5.

43. Fleischmann RM, Tesser J, Schiff MH, Schechtman J, Burmester GR, Bennett R, Modafferi D, Zhou L, Bell D, Appleton B. Safety of extended treatment with anakinra in patients with rheumatoid arthritis. Ann Rheum Dis. 2006;65:1006–12.

44. Jacobsson LT, Turesson C, Nilsson JA, Petersson IF, Lindqvist E, Saxne T, Geborek P. Treatment with TNF blockers and mortality risk in patients with rheumatoid arthritis. Ann Rheum Dis. 2007;66:670–5.

45. Lebwohl M, Blum R, Berkowitz E, Kim D, Zitnik R, Osteen C, Wallis WJ. No evidence for increased risk of cutaneous squamous cell carcinoma in patients with rheumatoid arthritis receiving etanercept for up to 5 years. Arch Dermatol. 2005;141:861–4.

46. Setoguchi S, Solomon DH, Weinblatt ME, Katz JN, Avorn J, Glynn RJ, Cook EF, Carney G, Schneeweiss S. Tumor necrosis factor alpha antagonist use and cancer in patients with rheumatoid arthritis. Arthritis Rheum. 2006;54:2757–64.

47. Askling J, Fored CM, Brandt L, Baecklund E, Bertilsson L, Feltelius N, Coster L, Geborek P, Jacobsson LT, Lindblad S, Lysholm J, Rantapaa-Dahlqvist S, Saxne T, Klareskog L. Risks of solid cancers in patients with rheumatoid arthritis and after treatment with tumour necrosis factor antagonists. Ann Rheum Dis. 2005;64:1421–6.

48. Askling J, Fored CM, Baecklund E, Brandt L, Backlin C, Ekbom A, Sundstrom C, Bertilsson L, Coster L, Geborek P, Jacobsson LT, Lindblad S, Lysholm J, Rantapaa-Dahlqvist S, Saxne T, Klareskog L, Feltelius N. Haematopoietic malignancies in rheumatoid arthritis: lymphoma risk and characteristics after exposure to tumour necrosis factor antagonists. Ann Rheum Dis. 2005;64:1414–20.

49. Biancone L, Orlando A, Kohn A, Colombo E, Sostegni R, Angelucci E, Rizzello F, Castiglione F, Benazzato L, Papi C, Meucci G, Riegler G, Petruzziello C, Mocciaro F, Geremia A, Calabrese E, Cottone M, Pallone F. Infliximab and newly diagnosed neoplasia in Crohn's disease: a multicentre matched pair study. Gut. 2006;55:228–33.

50. Gueudry J, Wechsler B, Terrada C, Gendron G, Cassoux N, Fardeau C, Lehoang P, Piette JC, Bodaghi B. Long-term efficacy and safety of low-dose interferon alpha2a therapy in severe uveitis associated with Behçet disease. Am J Ophthalmol. 2008;146(6):837–44.

51. Kötter I, Günaydin I, Zierhut M, Stübiger N. The use of interferon alpha in Behçet disease: review of the literature. Semin Arthritis Rheum. 2004;33:320–35.

52. Baker GL, Kahl LE, Zee BC, Stolzer BL, Agarwal AK, Medsger Jr TA. Malignancy following treatment of rheumatoid arthritis with cyclophosphamide. Long-term case–control follow-up study. Am J Med. 1987;83(1):1–9.

53. Baltus JA, Boersma JW, Hartman AP, Vandenbroucke JP. The occurrence of malignancies in patients with rheumatoid arthritis treated with cyclophosphamide: a controlled retrospective follow-up. Ann Rheum Dis. 1983;42(4):368–73.

54. Kempen JH, Daniel E, Gangaputra S, Dreger K, Jabs DA, Kacmaz RO, Pujari SS, Anzaar F, Foster CS, Helzlsouer KJ, Levy-Clarke GA, Nussenblatt RB, Liesegang T, Rosenbaum JT, Suhler EB. Methods for identifying long-term adverse effects of treatment in patients with eye diseases: the Systemic Immunosuppressive Therapy for Eye Diseases (SITE) cohort study. Ophthalmic Epidemiol. 2008;15:47–55.

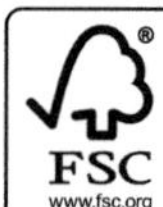

MIX
Papier aus verantwortungsvollen Quellen
Paper from responsible sources
FSC® C105338

If you have any concerns about our products,
you can contact us on
ProductSafety@springernature.com

In case Publisher is established outside the EU,
the EU authorized representative is:
Springer Nature Customer Service Center GmbH
Europaplatz 3, 69115 Heidelberg, Germany

Printed by Libri Plureos GmbH
in Hamburg, Germany